Silenced Angels

Silenced Angels

THE MEDICAL, LEGAL, AND SOCIAL
ASPECTS OF SHAKEN BABY SYNDROME

✧   ✧   ✧

James R. Peinkofer

Foreword by Randell Alexander, MD, PhD

AUBURN HOUSE

Westport, Connecticut
London

Library of Congress Cataloging-in-Publication Data

Peinkofer, J. (Jim)

    Silenced angels : the medical, legal, and social aspects of shaken baby syndrome /
James R. Peinkofer ; foreword by Randell Alexander.

      p. ; cm.

    Includes bibliographical references and index.

    ISBN 0–86569–313–7 (alk. paper)

    1. Battered child syndrome. 2. Battered child syndrome—Social aspects. 3. Battered
child syndrome—Law and legislation. 4. Child abuse—Social aspects. 5. Child
abuse—Law and legislation. I. Title.

    [DNLM: 1. Battered Child Syndrome—Infant. 2. Craniocerebral Trauma—
diagnosis—Infant. 3. Eye Injuries—diagnosis—Infant. 4. Forensic Medicine—
methods. 5. Fractures—diagnosis—Infant. WA 320 P377s 2001]

    RJ375 .P45   2002

    618.92′858223—dc21   2001045105

British Library Cataloguing in Publication Data is available.

Library of Congress Catalog Card Number: 2001045105
ISBN: 0–86569–313–7

First published in 2002

Auburn House, 88 Post Road West, Westport, CT 06881
An imprint of Greenwood Publishing Group, Inc.
www.greenwood.com

Printed in the United States of America

The paper used in this book complies with the
Permanent Paper Standard issued by the National
Information Standards Organization (Z39.48–1984).

10 9 8 7 6 5 4 3 2

Copyright Acknowledgments

The author and publisher gratefully acknowledge permission to use the following material:

- Gael J. Lonergan, MD, for the metaphyseal fracture X-ray and intracranial CT images
  (figures 4.1, 6.1, and 6.5);
- J. Keith Smith, MD, for the intracranial CT images (figures 6.2 and 6.3);
- Mark S. Dias, MD, FAAP, for the intracranial CT image (figure 6.4);
- Alex V. Levin, MD, FRCSC, for the ophthalmologic images (figures 8.1, 8.2, and 8.3);
- Kevin M. Knight and Linda D. Knight for Christian's Shaken Baby Syndrome Poster
  (figure 22.1).

Dedicated to the memory of

GEORGE F. GOODWIN, JR.

a great man, husband, and friend, who would have been a great father,

and

TO SHAKEN BABIES PAST AND PRESENT

your silence is heard

"Ralph felt as if someone had pulled a high-voltage switch inside his brain, one that turned on whole banks of blazing stadium lights. In their raw, momentary glow, he saw a terrible image: hands clad in a violent brownish-purple aura reaching into a crib and snatching up the baby they had just seen. He was shaken back and forth, head snapping and rolling on the thin stalk of neck like the head of a Raggedy Andy doll—and *thrown*."

Stephen King
Insomnia

Contents

✧ ✧ ✧

Figures

✧   ✧   ✧

Foreword

✧　✧　✧

Shaken Baby Syndrome (SBS)—most people have now heard about it, but what is it exactly? Might a child be bounced on a knee and get brain damage? Some have worried that jogging with a child in a backpack might cause SBS. Or tossing him into the air. What about a bumpy cross-country ride in a sport-utility vehicle? Indeed, might any of us have somehow shaken our babies just a little too roughly at some time?

Good news! The word "shaken" in the syndrome does not mean "jiggled." In fact, there is no adequate word in the English language that signifies the violent and repetitive shaking that causes brain injury and bleeding within the head and in the retinas of infants. Well-meaning awareness programs have sometimes made erroneous claims that mild jiggling might cause such injuries. Some parents have become so concerned on hearing these claims that they have shown up at physician's offices and emergency rooms asking for brain imaging of their infants, because they worried they might have unknowingly caused damage through some play activity. When thinking about awareness issues, the ancient medical admonishment should be considered: "First do no wrong."

Severity and timing are the major medical and legal issues that confront us when a child is diagnosed with SBS. The force required to cause the syndrome is severe. Drawing a rough analogy to falls, studies have shown that a child falling out of a third-story window has about a 1 percent risk of death. In contrast, SBS has a 25 percent risk of death. Clearly, the overall sense of violence is much worse with Shaken Baby Syndrome. The American Academy of Pediatrics has pointed out that an observer witnessing the act that results in SBS would believe that the child was going to be seriously injured or killed. SBS is no accident.

Timing is the other important issue. In the worst cases of SBS, resulting in death, the child would probably have lived only one hour, or at most two, before he or she would be dead. However, an even stronger tool is available that uses clinical symptoms to decide the timing. The head injuries of SBS result in immediate symptoms. In the least severe cases, the symptoms are those of a very bad concussion—irritability, decreased appetite, maybe vomiting. In the fatal cases, no meaningful activity is seen, the child is limp or stiff, breathing problems quickly ensue, or the child is unlikely ever to awaken from immediately passing out. Thus any investigator or physician can ask when the child was last acting relatively normal, and know the fatal injuries occurred after that. Often only one adult is present.

With any medical condition, particularly one that entails the legal system, there are bound to be those physicians who have unusual opinions and are willing to express them in the courtroom. There is no medical condition that precisely looks like SBS, complicating proceedings in court: we have heard such diagnoses as DPT shots causing this, West Nile virus, and even mad cow disease. By far, the most common claim is that the child fell off a bed or sofa. In the child abuse business, we refer to these objects as "killer couches" or "killer beds." Everyone else's child seems to fall off this furniture without significant injury, though the child in question has devastating injuries. No doubt, when the doctors ask so soon afterwards, it is difficult to come up with good alibis.

Many doctors do not have much more knowledge about SBS than do well-read laypersons. Occasionally they make erroneous statements or fail to appreciate the situation confronting them. Thus doctors and other professionals and the general public have much to learn about this serious public-health threat to children. This book is an excellent attempt to remedy this lack of knowledge. In reading it for the first time, I was also impressed by some of the historical details of which I was unaware. Having lectured about SBS both in the United States and internationally, I thought I knew nearly all these details. Jim Peinkofer showed me that most of us have a lot more to learn. Perhaps more important than the history of the syndrome or the detailed medical concepts is the human side of this terrible form of abuse, which we learn about in the book's case histories.

Why should you care? Perhaps because child abuse is the second-leading cause of death for children, and SBS is one of the leading causes of child abuse fatalities. Perhaps because a typical case costs at least $100,000 or more in the first year, and someone has to pay those bills. Most likely it is because you care about the safety, health, and potential of children, who should not have, literally, the life shaken out of them.

And be sure to hug your own children tonight.

RANDELL ALEXANDER, MD PHD
Director, Center for Child Abuse
Morehouse School of Medicine
August 2001

Acknowledgments

❖   ❖   ❖

There are a host of people who have assisted in leading me to the place I am today. Your impact and influence on me allowed this book to come to life.

First, thanks to God, from Whom all blessings flow, and Who often leads us down paths we often feel unprepared to travel, yet Who knows there is a lesson in such challenges.

To my wife, Tina; my support, my critical eye, my friend, love of my life. There must have been an angel by my side to lead me back to you. To my son, Jacob, whose birth led me toward child advocacy work; whose personality and wonder at the world leaves me grinning; whose love fills a place in my heart I didn't know existed. To Matthew and Tom Cotton, thanks for your words of support and your questions. Thanks also to Clara Mae Cole.

To my family of origin, Alda and Richard Peinkofer, Robert, Karen, Nicole and Alec Peinkofer, thank you for your love, encouragement, and interest in this project. Your support means everything to me. Thanks also to the Keller and Owen clan for your enthusiasm and love. To the memory of my grandparents, Helen and Robert Keller, Michael and Rose Peinkofer—who helped build my foundation for learning, seeking, and understanding truth.

To Norman Guthkelch, MD, the true originator of how we understand SBS today, my guide on this project, my friend. I literally could not have done this work without you. I am eternally grateful to you.

To the memory of John Caffey, MD who put all the pieces together to create the process of "Whiplash Shaken Infant Syndrome" in 1972. He leaves an important legacy and was a person committed to the welfare of children.

To the memory of C. Henry Kempe, MD who brought "The Battered Child Syndrome" to the forefront of the medical profession in 1962 and whose heritage continues in the name of child advocacy.

To Robert Reece, MD and Randell Alexander, MD, thank you for your initial comments on the manuscript. Your work in allowing others to more deeply understand child abuse injuries and the process of SBS continues to make a significant mark on humanity.

Thank you to the following medical professionals for their input in this project and for clarifying significant medical details for me: Lester Adelson, MD, Ann Botash, MD, Harry Bonnell, MD, Patrick Bray, MD, Goodwin Breinin, MD, Edward Conway, MD, Daniel Davis, MD, Mark Dias, MD, Kent Hymel, MD, Alex Levin, MD, Gael J. Lonergan, MD, J. Keith Smith, MD, Betty Spivack, MD, and Morris Wessel, MD.

Thank you to the following investigative and legal personnel whose commitment to SBS is unfailing: Rob Parrish, JD, Lynn Rooney, JD, Michael Vendola, and Phillip Wheeler. To the memory of Richard Easter.

To Debbie and Sunny Eappen, MDs, thank you for your commitment to SBS prevention. Your loss was immense and captured the attention of the rest of the world. In response, you have turned toward helping others with the creation of the Matty Eappen Foundation, which will ultimately save lives. I am privileged to know you.

To Jacy Showers, EdD, whose work in the field of SBS prevention and commitment to children has been very important.

To Ann-Janine Morey, PhD, thank you for writing *What Happened to Christopher: An American Family's Story of Shaken Baby Syndrome*, the first book ever written about the subject of SBS. It has helped society's understanding of one of life's true tragedies.

Thank you to my academic and life teachers, whose guidance has molded me intellectually, spiritually, and emotionally: Thomas Fronczak, Joseph Gentile, Jonathan Goodwin, Anna May Johnson, Peter Militello, Nancy Newkirk, Raymond Paradis, Susan Saunders, Margaret M. Schram, R. Bruce Simonson, and John Zeller.

Thank you to my professional colleagues: Mary DeGeneffe, MD, Darley Eminem, MD, Bunmi Okanlami, MD, Thomas Soisson, MD, and Robert White, MD, and the nursing staff at St. Joseph Regional Medical Center.

To the following authors, whose writing and experience has provided me with inspiration and motivation that helps me look at the world in a new light: Thomas Moore, Robert Pirsig, Randy Schilts, Stephen Vannoy, and John Walsh.

Thank you to Brian Gensel, JD, for his review of the legal chapters.

Thanks to Lynn Taylor, my editor at Greenwood Publishing, for suggestions and seeing this project through to publication. Special thanks to Bob Kowkabany of Doric Lay Publishers for the significant task of copyediting and page production that added a special touch to this book.

Special thanks to Betty Haines and Vicky Herzog-Urbanski for the years of loving kindness they have provided to infants and children.

To Elizabeth and Mary Beth Phillips, whose tenacity and courage to make positive changes in the lives of our nation's children are inspirational and motivating. Thank you for your work.

To Emily Fisher, mother of Elijah. You have turned the tragedy of loss into something special—the work of child advocacy and child abuse prevention. Thank you for what you are doing.

Thank you to Kevin and Linda Knight for the use of the image of the SBS prevention poster featuring their grandson Christian Knight.

Finally, thank you to the family members on the SBS Internet mailing list and the SBS Alliance. Your stories touched my heart and had a huge effect on my understanding of all the various aspects of SBS. Justice may not have been obtained for many families, but your efforts toward preventing another child from being shaken will speak volumes to those around you.

Introduction

✧   ✧   ✧

"Father Arrested in Baby's Death—Police Say Seven-Week-Old Boy was Shaken." "Babysitter Charged in Infant's Death—Three-Month-Old Showed Signs of Shaken Baby Syndrome." These headlines call to us daily throughout the United States and the rest of the world. Just a decade ago, such cases seemed to occur less often. What happened? Are children being shaken more often, even in light of national efforts for prevention? Or are the media responding more broadly and completely to such cases? Has the family unit or societal pressures changed? Or are we as individuals collectively tuning in and more openly discussing incidents of infant shaking when we hear about them?

Probably all of these factors play a role in the understanding of Shaken Baby Syndrome (SBS). In the May 1999 edition of the journal *Pediatrics*, there was a study on the risk factors for death by injury among infants in the United States related to the specific pathological cause.[1] Brenner and associates analyzed data from the National Center for Health Statistics for the years 1983 to 1991 and found that the leading cause of fatal injury among children less than five years old was death by homicide (23 percent of total deaths). This is an extremely disturbing commentary on our society.

SBS is one of life's worst tragedies. A violent act that takes just a few minutes can cause a lifetime of irreparable damage. Infants who are shaken have high morbidity and mortality rates. The justice system often fails to convict abusers for their crimes. And the families of these infants are left to deal with the aftermath.

People have said that SBS is a tragedy of ignorance. For example, there is ignorance about the way infants should be handled, disciplined, and soothed. Individuals who shake their charges typically are inexperienced in caregiving or are too emotionally unstable to care for dependent babies. Caring for a young child can be overwhelming for anyone, because the demands of children are often considerable. Infants cry frequently, as this is their only mode of communicating basic needs. Older children who are shaken are most likely those struggling with their need to be cared for versus their need for independence.

Shaking incidents occur when an infant is crying, when an infant is part of an abusive environment, or when the caretaker feels that he or she cannot control a child, such as when a toddler refuses a demand. Such caretakers often interpret crying as a sign of overdependency in infants and believe that if they give in to the child's demands, they will spoil the child. To them, physical discipline appears to be the only response to a crying or irritable child. Shaking is the misguided result. Adults too often fail to consider their role in this pattern of behavior. They do not adequately consider the possible causes for crying or that they may use soothing techniques to quiet and calm the child. Infants do respond in positive physiological and emotional ways to soothing voices, loving arms, warm milk, and other sentient moments.

Frequently, the shaking incident that hospitalizes or kills an infant will not be the initial moment of abuse. Infants will become highly anxious and may cry frequently when in the presence of their abuser. This then becomes a vicious cycle. The more anxious the infant, the more he or she will cry, which can lead to further incidents of physical abuse.

SBS can affect any infant, because infants' physical attributes predispose them to such injuries. They have disproportionately large heads, underdeveloped neck muscles, soft brains, copious intracranial space, and loosely attached intracranial nerves. Such attributes, which are beneficial for the rigors of birth, put an infant at greater risk of injury or death if he or she is shaken.

Several factors may put an infant at greater risk for SBS:

- Being the firstborn to young parents who have never before cared for a child.

- Being male. Infant boys have a 60 percent greater risk of being shaken than infant girls.[2] This is partly due to the misguided belief of many caretakers that infant boys should "tough it out" and "not cry so much." Butler also suggests that some parents may believe male infants can withstand rougher handling, even shaking, than female infants.[3]

- Being young. Infants are obviously more at risk for being shaken, because of their weight and size and other previously mentioned physical attributes. But this does not preclude a toddler or older child from being shaken. The diagnosis of SBS reaches its plateau at about the age of two years, and the average victim's age is around six months.[2,3] Young children, at ages four or five years, have been known to be victims of SBS. But typically, violent shaking is a circumstance that affects infants and very young children.

- A disruption in the normal process from being born to going home. Elmer and Gregg found that many abused infants in their study had been born prematurely or had been hospitalized after being born.[4] Another study confirmed their findings and also included any diagnosis of disability where the parents (especially the mother) failed to emotionally accept the infant.[5] Bonding within a family unit does not readily occur when there are complications that require initial separation between parent and child. In fact, the importance of bonding and its relationship to abuse has been identified in many studies over several decades.[6]

- Multiple births. The demands and cries of two or more infants can be emotionally taxing.[7] Becker and colleagues found that a disproportionate number of twins were diagnosed with SBS.[8] The recent Whittle case, in which a woman shook and beat her infant quadruplets, is also a testimony to the risk of multiple infants in the wrong hands.

- A physical impairment or chronic illness. When a child is born with a physical impairment or has a chronic illness that requires frequent clinic visits or hospitalizations, parents or caretakers may find the infant unattractive and unduly burdensome.[9] The inherent pull to nurture may not be present, and the infant may not be emotionally accepted. This creates an environment of high stress and the potential for abuse.

- Being unwanted or unaccepted. Some infants are simply not loved by their parents or caretakers. Such infants are not accepted because they might not meet certain expectations or are the products of unwanted pregnancies, or they may even remind their caretakers of someone else.[10] In such a situation, merely hearing the infant cry can stir an infant's caretaker into a frenzy as he or she mentally relives the past. Steele calls this the "superego identification with [one's] own punitive parent . . . [whereby] the infant is perceived as the [caretaker's] own childhood itself."[11] This is a tenuous relationship at best, and an infant in such a position is at great risk for abuse.

SBS is a tragedy that can be prevented. There are a plenty of ways to soothe a crying infant, just as there are signs of potential danger that parents may be able to perceive when leaving their child with a caretaker. The chapters that follow describe the physiology and history of SBS, and how all of us are affected legally, socially, and emotionally by this tragic form of child abuse. It is the author's hope that this book will save lives and help bring justice upon those who permanently damage the lives of families through a moment of violence.

NOTES

1. Brenner RA, Overpeck MD, Trumble AC, et al. Deaths Attributable to Injuries in Infants, United States, 1983–1991. *Pediatrics* 1999; 103:968–974.

2. Lazoritz S, Baldwin S, Kini N. The Whiplash Shaken Baby Syndrome: Has Caffey's Syndrome Changed or Have We Changed His Syndrome? *Child Abuse and Neglect* 1997; 21:1009–1014.

3. Butler GL. Shaken Baby Syndrome. *J Psychosoc Nurs* 1995; 33:47–50.

4. Elmer E, Gregg GS. Developmental Characteristics of Abused Children. *Pediatrics* 1967; 40:596–602.

5. Klein M, Stern L. Low Birth Weight and the Battered Child Syndrome. *Am J Dis Child* 1971; 122:15–18.

6. Morton N, Browne KD. Theory and Observation of Attachment and Its Relation to Child Maltreatment: A Review. *Child Abuse and Neglect* 1998; 22:1093–1104.

7. Groothuis JR, Altemeier WA, Robarge JP, et al. Increased Child Abuse in Families with Twins. *Pediatrics* 1982; 70:769–773.

8. Becker JC, Liersch R, Tautz C, et al. Shaken Baby Syndrome: Report on Four Pairs of Twins. *Child Abuse and Neglect* 1998; 22:931–937.

9. Dubowitz H, Egan H. The Maltreatment of Infants. In: Straus MB, ed. *Abuse and Victimization across the Life Span*. Baltimore: Johns Hopkins University Press; 1988:32–51.

10. Coody D, Brown M, Montgomery D, et al. Shaken Baby Syndrome: Identification and Prevention for Nurse Practitioners. *J Ped Health Care* 1994; 8:50–56.

11. Steele B. Psychodynamic Factors in Child Abuse. In: Kempe CH, Helfer RE, eds. *The Battered Child*. 3rd ed. Chicago: University of Chicago Press; 1980:49–85.

Part One

MEDICAL ASPECTS OF SHAKEN BABY SYNDROME

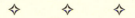

Look for a long time at what pleases you, and for a longer time at what pains you.

—Colette

Whatever you do, do it to the purpose; do it thoroughly, not superficially. Go to the bottom of things. Any thing half done, or half known, is, in my mind, neither done nor known at all. Nay, worse, for it often misleads.

—Lord Chesterfield

CHAPTER ONE

Signs and Symptoms

S HAKEN BABY SYNDROME IS A CONDITION that has only relatively recently been described in the medical literature, and it continues to be missed by health providers. This is alarming, as it means that many abused children are placed back in the care of their abusers. A thorough clinical work-up along with interviews and investigation are essential for a proper diagnosis.

It is usually an infant's parents or caregivers who discover that something is wrong. Many times there is simply a change in behavior, without any sign such as bruising to suggest that trauma has recently occurred—for example, what was a happy-go-lucky baby in the morning may be subdued and withdrawn in the afternoon. If clinicians are initially faced with a child who appears ill but shows no symptoms of any common disease, Reece and Grodin suggest that they should immediately ask themselves whether these could be signs of abuse.[1] If so, they should obtain a head CT scan and check the interior of the infant's eyes for retinal hemorrhaging. Being familiar with the characteristics of SBS and the subtleties of head injury can aid clinicians in making an accurate diagnosis[2] (see chapter 6). Jenny proposes that medical providers should always try to get as much information as possible from emergency medical technicians, and that blood studies should include ruling out coagulopathy (see chapter 12).[3] As soon as possible, a consultation should be obtained with a pediatrician familiar with child abuse cases, and, if possible, with a pediatric radiologist to interpret the radiographs and scans. The diagnosis of SBS is often not made by symptoms, clinical history, or diagnostic images alone, but rather by a combination of all of these. Regular training within medical institutions should be required of all clinicians, as research and observation are continually updated in the field of child abuse injury identification and treatment.

COMMON SYMPTOMS AND SIGNS

Below, listed alphabetically, are some common symptoms that may be noted in a shaken baby. Some symptoms occur more frequently than others.

Apnea

This refers to an interruption in the regular rhythm of respiration. Short periods of apnea may occur in healthy infants, especially during deep sleep. Apnea has sometimes been suggested by perpetrators as their motivation for shaking an infant. They want law enforcement officials to believe that they shook a baby "lightly" in order to break an apneic spell. In fact, it is more likely that the shaking caused the apnea.[4,5] Medical professionals may also see apneic episodes as "near miss" or nonfatal Sudden Infant Death Syndrome (SIDS), in which an infant routinely survives periods of halted breathing.[6] They may go so far as to order an apnea monitor for home use, unaware of the true cause of an infant's problems.

Bradycardia

In this condition, the heart rate slows to fewer than sixty beats per minute. Ludwig and Warman found that 65 percent of the shaken infants they described had bradycardia at initial presentation.[7] Like bradypnea, it can indicate increased intracranial pressure or brain stem injury.

Bradypnea

This refers to abnormal slowness in breathing. It can be a sign of severe injury to the brain stem or of greatly increased intracranial pressure (ICP) though there are other, nontraumatic possibilities. An infant may present in a hospital emergency room with this dramatic pattern of respiration.

Bulging Fontanelle

The fontanelle of a baby's head are the "soft spots," or suture lines. Fontanelle fuse and close by age eighteen to twenty-four months, as the skull develops and hardens. When there is trauma to the brain, infant fontanelle swell and bulge, or become tense; there is an excess of fluid, blood, and swelling within the brain's substance; and there is a natural pushing outward against the fontanelle.

Raimondi and Hirschauer differentiated types of fontanelle into soft, full, or tense.[8] In their study, they found that head-injured infants who had soft fontanelle had a better neurological outcome than those whose fontanelle were tense. They also verified that often a full or tense fontanelle was associated with a unilateral or bilateral subdural hematoma. As intracranial swelling is reduced, the fontanelle becomes soft again, though some infants may experience an overlapping of suture lines.

Coma

This condition is defined as a state of unresponsiveness, and unless it rapidly improves, as after a concussion or a seizure, it is always a sign of serious brain damage. Coma causes deep stupor and poor or no response to external stimuli. Caregivers and clinicians may initially believe that an infant who is comatose after shaking is merely lethargic or in a deep sleep.[9] But the true situation can be assessed in the emergency room by using the Glasgow Coma Scale (GCS). The deeper and more prolonged the coma, combined with an initially low GCS score, the poorer the prognosis (see tables in chapter 6).

Cyanosis

This occurs when an infant is deprived of life-sustaining oxygen. Lips and skin generally turn a bluish purple color, because the hemoglobin in the blood is not oxygenated. This is an emergent condition requiring immediate correction, because the brain cannot be deprived of oxygen for more than a few minutes before irreversible damage occurs.

Eyes Rolling Back or Staring

This is a natural reaction when a severe head injury occurs and there is loss of consciousness. Physicians and emergency medical technicians (EMTs) use flashlights to check pupil reaction and detect nonparallel eye alignment.[10] Abnormalities in either or both of these, particularly if there is a downturned "setting-sun" stare, which is a sign of increased intracranial pressure, indicate serious brain stem injury.

Gastroenteritis

This is not an actual sign of SBS; rather, it is a diagnosis that is often erroneously made when SBS is really the problem. Gastroenteritis means inflammation of the stomach and intestinal tract. A shaken infant may have fed poorly for a few days as a result of injuries due to shaking, and then be brought to a hospital emergency room for treatment on suspicion of gastroenteritis.

Hypothermia

This condition means an abnormally low body temperature (less than 95 degrees F). It is a rare condition and is thought to be due to central nervous system dysfunction.[11] Ludwig and Warman found hypothermia in 45 percent of the infants with SBS they described.[7]

Inconsolable Irritability

An infant can receive a complete clinical work-up for excessive crying and irritability in a hospital emergency room, but nothing may be identified as being physically wrong. Yet it is essential to accept that such an infant is, in fact, experiencing pain or discomfort, as well as emotional stress. Only the abuser is aware of why the infant cries. Unless there is a comprehensive medical evaluation, including an ophthalmologic exam and head CT, and a thorough caretaker interview, which includes an assessment of the family support system in place, the child is at risk for abuse after discharge.

Internal Damage But No External Marks

One pattern typical to SBS is that infant victims frequently have no external signs of abuse. Most physical damage occurs internally. Because of this, infants may be evaluated for occult (hidden) infection. Antibiotics may even be prescribed and the infant discharged home, only to be shaken again. When an abuser has just shaken a child, there may be subtle fingertip bruising in the area where the child has been held. Such marks may be seen on an infant's shoulders, thorax, or back. Children who are shaken may even be held around the neck without leaving a telltale mark of strangulation. Such a manner of shaking can only be confirmed at autopsy by the presence of subcutaneous hemorrhages in the neck.[12]

Lethargy

A shaken infant suffering neurologic trauma often appears sleepy or is hard to arouse. A sense of dullness is evident in the child and is a constant reminder that something is truly wrong.

Seizures and Status Epilepticus

Seizures in a shaken child are a conclusive sign that there has been a serious brain injury. Abusive head trauma can bring on alterations in electrical activity of the brain, leading to seizing. Intracranial complications of SBS, such as hypertension, edema, and hypoxia due to increased ICP may result in seizures. (See the chapter on consequences [chapter 2] for more detail on seizures.)

Status epilepticus can be a characteristic diagnosis in a shaken infant brought to a hospital emergency room. This condition is typified by a rapid succession of seizures without a regaining of consciousness.[13] Medical providers may believe fever or another condition to be the cause of the status epilepticus.

Tensing or Drawing Up of Limbs

An infant's brain, in response to severe trauma, may cause hemiparesis, quadriplegia, or other disabling conditions that affect the limbs. Often arms and legs contract due to any number of neurological responses, including automatic or postural reactions, and reflexes.[14]

Vomiting

Not all shaken infants vomit, but it is a very common response to head injury. There are, of course, many causes of vomiting in infancy besides SBS, but infants with projectile (very forcible) vomiting as their only symptom may be overlooked as having been shaken. Wadford described one case where a three-month-old infant, recently discharged from a hospital with a diagnosis of SBS, had recurrent spells of vomiting.[15] After three follow-up visits to the hospital emergency room, with a plethora of diagnoses, an additional diagnosis was made of pyloric stenosis, which develops progressively as an obstruction of the stomach's pyloric valve, and corrective surgery was performed. Vomiting can also result from fluid and electrolyte imbalance.[13] An infant who suffers from chronic vomiting quickly becomes dehydrated, and an incorrect diagnosis of failure to thrive due to poor nutrition may be made. Consultation with a pediatric gastroenterologist may be necessary to establish a valid diagnosis.

CRYING AND COLIC

When a baby cries, he or she is communicating. This is a concept obvious to most caregivers. Babies do not cry to get back at an adult holding them, or for any other reasons requiring intellectual thought. Crying is instinctual. Most perpetrators of SBS do not realize this, however. Perpetrators forcefully ask babies questions such as "Why won't you stop crying?" or "What's wrong with you?" These adults do not consider a wide variety of techniques to soothe a crying baby and will react tensely and angrily. And the more emotionally tense the adult, the more an infant will cry.

Crying and colic in infants have made their way down through history as often exasperating experiences for parents and other caregivers.[16,17] Colic, often considered to be the reason for an infant's crying, is thought to be a consequence of gastrointestinal irritation or spasm in infants.[18] But infants cry regularly, with the crying peaking between three weeks and three months, and the average infant crying three hours per day.[19,20] Brazelton, in his 1962 groundbreaking study of infant crying, found that infant attachment, partner support, family support, and a positive emotional reaction can be beneficial for mothers dealing with such crying.[16]

Some infants with congenital neurological complications may actually never cry.[21] They may experience a condition that causes macrocephaly or other structural abnormalities. This may even occur in shaken infants, especially if there is damage to the brain stem.

Male caregivers seem to be less prepared to handle an infant who cries. This is partly societal and partly gender-related. Throughout history, women have typically been the primary caregivers to infants and children. The image of men handing over babies to women as soon as they cry has frequently been the subject of stereotype in movies and television. Brewster et al. even went so far as to study the physiological reactions of men to crying infants on videotape and found that men show a greater physiological reactivity than their female counterparts.[22] They concluded that men are more prone to serious child abuse because of their physical responses to crying, which include sweating and an increased heart rate.

Men are, in fact, good caregivers. The abusers of the world are the exception rather than the rule. Often, men just need an understanding of why a baby may be crying and ways to cope positively.

Diagnosis of crying from colic versus abuse can sometimes be difficult for the medical care provider in a hospital emergency room. Consider the following, taken from the powerful documentation of a fatal case of "colic."[23] A nineteen-year-old single mother brought a three-month-old female infant to a hospital emergency room (ER) at two o'clock in the morning, with a complaint of constant crying. The infant was well nourished and well developed, though her mother reported recent spells of vomiting. The baby was not easily consoled during the exam; there were no obvious signs or reason for the crying. Her fontanelle were soft and flat, her pupils responded equally, her heart and lungs were clear and normal sounding, and abdominal, extremity, and neurological exams were all normal. She was given a diagnosis of infantile colic and discharged home with her mother.

Nine hours later, the baby was rushed back to the ER without life signs via emergency medical staff. She never regained consciousness and was pronounced dead soon after arrival. During resuscitation efforts, faint old bruises on her upper arms were noted. When her eyes were examined, she was found to have bilateral retinal hemorrhages and an autopsy revealed subdural hematomas. Her cause of death quickly became identified as Shaken Baby Syndrome.

The authors who reported this case call for medical personnel to build into their evaluation, diagnosis, and treatment of crying infants an assessment of parents' and caregivers' emotional states and available support systems. Symptoms as described by caregivers may not lead a medical provider to consider SBS as a diagnosis. Yet the potential for abuse is very real, and thorough exams of both the child and his or her parents can be lifesaving. Crying is a sign of physical or emotional discomfort in infants and children. Adult clues to their own discomfort can be more difficult to read.

NOTES

1. Reece RM, Grodin MA. Recognition of Nonaccidental Injury. *Ped Clin N Amer* 1985; 32:41–60.

2. Dykes LJ. The Whiplash Shaken Infant Syndrome: What Has Been Learned? *Child Abuse & Neglect* 1986; 10:211–221.

3. Jenny C. Abusive Head Trauma: An Analysis of Missed Cases. Second National Conference on SBS. September 1998.

4. Johnson DL, Beal D, Baule R. Role of Apnea in Nonaccidental Head Injury. *Ped Neurosurg* 1995; 23:305–310.

5. Noorda C, Carlile J, Lazerson J. An Apneic Infant with Blood in His Eyes. *Hosp Prac* October 15, 1987; 169–170.

6. Berger D. Child Abuse Simulating "Near Miss" Sudden Infant Death Syndrome. *J Ped* 1979; 95:554–556.

7. Ludwig S, Warman M. Shaken Baby Syndrome: A Review of 20 Cases. *Ann Emerg Med* 1984; 13:104–107.

8. Raimondi AJ, Hirschauer J. Head Injury in the Infant and Toddler. *Child's Brain* 1984; 11:12–35.

9. American Academy of Pediatrics. Shaken Baby Syndrome: Inflicted Cerebral Trauma, *Pediatrics* 1993; 92:872–875.

10. Menkes JH. Introduction. In: Menkes, JH, ed. *Textbook of Child Neurology*. 4th ed. Philadelphia: Lea & Febiger; 1990:1–27.

11. Wahl NG, Woodall BN. Hypothermia in Shaken Infant Syndrome. *Ped Emerg Care* 1995; 11:233–234.

12. Bird CR, McMahan JR, Gilles FH, et al. Strangulation in Child Abuse: CT Diagnosis. *Radiol* 1987; 163:373–375.

13. Thomas CL, ed. *Taber's Cyclopedic Medical Dictionary.* 14th ed. Philadelphia: FA Davis Co.; 1981:1361.

14. Long TM, Cintas HL. *Handbook of Pediatric Physical Therapy.* Baltimore: Williams & Wilkins; 1995:80.

15. Wadford PJ. General Anesthetic Considerations for the Infant with Shaken Impact Syndrome and Pyloromyotomy: A Case Report. *J Amer Assoc Nurse Anesth* 1995; 63:450–454.

16. Brazelton TB. Crying in Infancy. *Pediatrics* 1962; 29:579–588.

17. Carey WB. Colic: Exasperating but Fascinating and Gratifying. *Pediatrics* 1989; 84:568–569.

18. Wessel MA, Cobb JC, Jackson EB, et al. Paroxysmal Fussing in Infancy, Sometimes Called "Colic." *Pediatrics* 1954; 14:421–434.

19. Harley LM. Fussing and Crying in Young Infants. *Clin Ped* 1969; 8:138–141.

20. Illingworth RS. Three Months' Colic. *Arch Dis Child* 1954; 29:165–174.

21. Coker SB. Babies Who Don't Cry. *Clin Ped* 1992; 31:357–359.

22. Brewster AL, Nelson JP, McCanne TR, et al. Gender Differences in Physiological Reactivity to Infant Cries and Smiles in Military Families. *Child Abuse & Neglect* 1998; 22:775–788.

23. Singer JL, Rosenberg NM. A Fatal Case of Colic. *Ped Emerg Care* 1992; 8:171–173.

CHAPTER TWO

Consequences

I T IS A SAD AND ALARMING FACT that between 60 and 70 percent of infants identified as having been shaken are faced with dire consequences, including death. The rest of the children may seem to recover well from being shaken, but they still have residual effects. Truly, the lives of not just the victims, but of their entire families change as a result of a brief act of violence. Millions of dollars are expended each year in the rehabilitation of shaken infants and toddlers. The expenses include costs for equipment and services, costs for daily care, and even more importantly, emotional costs.

MAIN CONSEQUENCES

Listed below alphabetically are some of the main consequences that a shaken infant may face. Some occur more frequently than others.

Attention Problems

Because the brain has some resiliency in response to traumatic injury, there are children who experience minimal aftereffects following an incident of shaking. One such effect might be an attention disorder with or without hyperactivity. With an attention disorder, children may appear to ignore what a parent or caregiver is saying to them. They may also be easily distractible and need careful monitoring and clear instructions on adult expectations.

Certain stimulant medications, such as methylphenidate (Ritalin), can help a child experiencing attention problems to focus by counterbalancing the stimulation chemicals of the brain that are overproduced. Parents or caregivers should consult their physician to discuss behavioral or medical options to assist with their child's needs. Before a diagnosis of attention deficit is formally made, the child should receive psychological testing and evaluation. School personnel should be aware if a child is diagnosed with an attention disorder, so that special programs or consideration can be arranged.

Balance Problems

Balance is controlled by three areas of the body's nervous system: the basal ganglia, the cerebellum, and the inner ear (fluid in the eustachian tubes must maintain a consistent level for balance to effectively occur). Damage to any of these areas may result in poor balance.

Physical and occupational therapy can help correct deficits in a child's balance, which may cause him or her to have difficulty standing or to walk in an uncontrolled way. Coordination and strengthening therapies can help the child achieve smoother mobility. If the problem primarily stems from the inner ear, a masking agent, such as a device that produces "white noise," may assist in maintaining balance and coordination.

Blindness

Many types of visual deficits may develop as a result of SBS. Retinal hemorrhaging may resolve without any lasting ill effects, but it may leave permanent scarring with partial or complete blindness.

Cortical trauma may result from any type of injury to the cortex of the brain, including contusion, edema, or hemorrhage, and usually results in severe loss of vision. Though the eye and optic nerve may be functional, the cortex of the brain is unable to effectively process visual information. Annable described several types of visual deficits that may result from cortical injury, such as gaze disorder (strabismus), visual field defects, or total blindness.[1] Any injury to the occipital region of the brain may also threaten vision, because this is the area that controls that function. Visual deficits may also occur in conjunction with other disabilities, such as cerebral palsy, wherein a child is more likely to experience optic atrophy, lazy eye (amblyopia), or eye jerks (nystagmus).[2]

Children with visual disability or blindness caused by SBS will benefit from regular visits to an ophthalmologist experienced in the area of ocular injuries resulting from child abuse. Parents or caregivers will then be able to feel more comfortable with the care their child is receiving from a provider with access to specialized resources.

Cerebral Palsy

This condition identifies a group of disorders that affect a child's motor skills—his or her ability to perform and control normal movements. Poor balance, weakness, stiffness, and lack of coordination are all aspects of cerebral palsy (CP).

A child may be affected on different sides or parts of the body. Hemiplegia is CP that affects an arm and leg on one side of the body, diplegia affects both legs, and quadriplegia affects all four limbs. These are all considered "pyramidal" (spastic) CP, as the pyramidal tract of the brain is often affected.[3] Muscle control may be spastic (rigid movement), hypotonic (floppy movement), or ataxic (poor balance and coordination).

Extrapyramidal CP occurs when there is damage to the basal ganglia section of the brain. Such a child has no muscle control (athetoid), with the limbs moving in an abrupt and involuntary fashion. One study found that 92 percent of children diagnosed with extrapyramidal CP held a concurrent diagnosis of mental retardation.[3]

CP in infants and toddlers is diagnosed after certain developmental milestones fail to be met and muscle tone and movement are abnormal. There is no exact measurement that can predict the eventual severity of the effects of CP, though by age two a child can be diagnosed as hemiplegic, diplegic, or quadriplegic.[2]

Parents or caregivers are encouraged to allow an afflicted infant or toddler to socialize with other children, especially others with disabilities, because this will emotionally support the child's instinctual need for independence from within a largely dependent body.

Deafness or Hearing Loss

Children who are shaken may suffer damage to the eighth cranial nerve, which controls hearing, as well as to the bones of the inner ear and the cochlea, responsible for converting sounds from mechanical impulses to chemical and electrical impulses sent to the brain. A child's hearing may be tested in an audiology follow-up. Deficits in hearing range from mild impairment to profound deafness. If the child has some residual hearing, hearing aids can amplify sounds and voices. Cochlear implantation has also helped many children with hearing loss. Regular visits to an audiologist and speech therapist will help children who were deafened by shaking learn to adjust to this disability. Sign language is an excellent adjunct for the infant or toddler learning communication, giving him or her a way to let feelings and needs be known to a parent or caregiver.

Death

Death in SBS most commonly occurs as a result of cerebral edema and/or hemorrhage with a resulting uncontrolled increase of intracranial pressure. Children under the age of six months have a greater risk for dying as a result of being shaken.[4] Overall, infants and toddlers have a 25 to 30 percent chance of dying after a shaking incident. This consequence of SBS can be the most devastating for families. When a child is born, parents or caregivers have dreams for the child's future. When the child is suddenly and tragically taken away, there is a deep void. Many parents struggling with the daily routines of caring for children severely disabled as a result of SBS emphasize their thankfulness that at least their children are still alive. Parents who lose a child to death have only memories.

There are also children who suffer a "late death." These are children who have suffered massive brain injury and die years later, such as a child with only brain stem functioning that finally ceases; a child who succumbs to increased intracranial pressure when a shunt can longer support her neurological changes; or a child who dies from pneumonia after living with devastating neurological damage for twelve years from being shaken at age five months.[5] The outcome for a shaken infant is something that can never be predicted. There are children who are expected to live, those who are expected to die, those who make recoveries that are called "miracles," and others whose young bodies cannot take the trauma of living with their injuries. *Hope* is a concept that is dovetailed with *love*. Providing a hopeful, loving environment is the best any parent or caregiver can do, no matter how many days, months, or years.

One question that often haunts families dealing with a shaken child's death is how much the child suffered during the moment of shaking. Some parents and caregivers are comforted with the belief that their children did not suffer. Others wonder if their children experienced pain and fear. Studies show that most children who are severely head-injured do not experience lucid moments prior to losing consciousness, except in older children with epidural hemorrhage, who can experience brief lucid moments after unconsciousness. Infants also do not have the mental capacity to understand the process of aggression prior to becoming unconscious. Infants do, though, respond physiologically to *ongoing* stressors, as cortisol is released in the brain.[6] Cortisol is a hormone that coats the brain as an instinctive response to stress.

Emotional Problems

An SBS victim may experience subsequent emotional problems. This is a subtle complication, because an underlying shaking incident may never be discovered or diagnosed. There are children who are shaken, become unconscious, may experience lethargy or vomiting, and recover. Years later, the child may experience emotional problems, such as explosive anger, self-injurious behavior, or depression, but parents or caregivers are not aware of the basis for such complications. Later in life, a child who has been shaken may develop an attachment disorder. Psychiatric evaluation and treatment may be needed as a shaken child grows.

The harmful emotional effects of abuse can be lessened. Parents and caregivers should watch for changes in their children's behavior. Loving family members can offer structure and guidance to a child whose basic trust issues were dramatically altered. Therapists and other mental health professionals can help with understanding emotional problems and guide with treatment options.

Gastrointestinal Problems

Many children who are shaken are left with poor oral motor function and hence are unable to chew or swallow.[2] Children may aspirate (inhale) food or liquid instead of swallowing, or they may experience gastroesophageal reflux, wherein food is regularly brought back up from the stomach into the esophagus. This can cause severe irritation in the tract from the caustic effects of stomach acid and may lead to excessive weight loss.

When a child has such problems with eating and processing foods, a gastrostomy tube (G-tube) or G-button may need to be placed directly into the stomach. One type of G-tube is the percutaneous gastrostomy (PEG) tube. A needle is inserted into the stomach, and the PEG is passed over the needle, all done under anesthesia.[2]

Children also may have problems processing food in their intestines and bowels, and may even experience constipation. Changes in diet, medications, and laxatives prescribed under a physician's care may help alleviate such problems. Registered dieticians are also invaluable resources.

Hydrocephalus

One complication of traumatic brain injury is an excessive buildup of fluid in and around the ventricles of the cranial space. Cerebrospinal fluid (CSF) is constantly being produced and absorbed in the brain. If there is a problem with reabsorption, CSF backs up and causes enlargement of the brain, and subsequently the head. This condition is known as hydrocephalus.

Hydrocephalus is treated through the use of a shunt, a small tube inserted into one of the ventricles of the brain. The opposite end of the shunt is placed in either the abdominal cavity or the jugular vein for drainage and reabsorption. Shunts may become clogged and require replacement or repair. They may also become infected; 80 percent of the cases in which infection develops occur within six months of the shunt placement surgery.[7] Persistent headaches, nausea, and vomiting are signs of problematic shunt functioning.[8]

Another treatment for the buildup of CSF involves a rerouting within the ventricular system by endoscopic third ventriculostomy.[9] Such a procedure is much more invasive, but the long-term success rate is high, especially in children over two years of age. Infants usually receive a shunt placement initially, with endoscopic treatment suggested later.[7]

Hypersensitivity

Infants and children who have been shaken can be hypersensitive in various ways. Hypersensitivity to touch means that an infant cannot distinguish between types and degrees of touch and may withdraw in a self-regulatory fashion.[2] Slow, patient, loving hands will eventually help the infant accept a caregiver's touch. Hypersensitivity to sound can keep an entire family tiptoeing. Infants with this condition frequently wail with discomfort when distressed by noise. Hypersensitivity to temperature may occur if there is a dysfunction in the body's self-regulatory and circulatory processes. Hands and feet frequently become cold or hot. Caregivers need to be extra conscious of this when dressing a hypersensitive child.

Learning Disabilities

Children with learning disabilities may appear, act, and think as normal children until they are faced with regular mental-processing challenges in the classroom. This can be another subtle complication from a shaking incident that is never discovered. Children with learning disabilities cannot process complex information adequately or smoothly. Writing, reading, mathematical computations, and other types of learning can become significant hurdles. Great care and patience are required when working with a child with a learning disability. Such a child will probably require an individualized educational plan (IEP), whereby many disciplines are brought together to develop the right tools to effectively educate the child. There are several types of learning disabilities: visual (problems distinguishing shapes or colors); language (problems with word or sentence formation); reading (misreading or problems with pronunciation); attention (poor at following instructions); and computational (problems with math). Learning disabilities can be diagnosed by psychological testing.

Mental Retardation

Mental retardation from shaking is far different from Down's Syndrome, a congenital birth defect that worldwide affects thousands of children each year. If there has been significant brain trauma from being shaken, a child may not have the ability to learn as other children. Mental retardation means that a child has below-average intelligence, with an intelligence quotient (IQ) below 70, the average IQ being 100. The child's IQ may actually drop as he or she becomes older.[10]

Mentally retarded children may later learn to care for themselves, live on their own, hold jobs, and go shopping. But in a small percentage of cases the brain damage is too severe for them to do so. Children can be mentally retarded in conjunction with other SBS injuries, such as blindness, deafness, or cerebral palsy. Evaluation and planning by a team of professionals, including a pediatrician, speech therapist, clinical psychologist, special education teacher, and social worker, are vital for the successful functioning of a mentally retarded child and his or her family. An IEP at the child's place of learning will maximize intellectual and social potential. Parents or caregivers should focus on gross motor skills, such as those involved in running, swimming, or ball playing, as fine motor skills can be difficult and frustrating for the child.[3]

Microcephaly

In this condition, the head is abnormally small, with a circumference that is two standard deviations below the mean for same gender and age.[2,11] Shaking can cause an infant's brain to slow down its rate of growth, and the protective skull will slow down in tandem. The prognosis is poor for microcephalic children, most of whom will be severely disabled and may have other physical complications.

Paralysis

Some children who survive a shaking episode may be totally paralyzed and be confined to a wheelchair for the remainder of their lives. Such children may have sustained injuries to the spinal cord or brain, which coordinates movement. They will be dependent on their caregivers for everything and will not progress through the normal developmental milestones. These children may be more prone to tantrums, as they are unable to move freely and may become frustrated as toddlers desiring to be more independent. Physical and occupational therapies may allow for maximal use of limbs in paralyzed children, but often neuromuscular messages are not transmitted or are slow to transmit. Such a dramatic injury may also affect the child's vocal cords and capabilities for chewing and swallowing, and a feeding tube may be required. If there is a speech deficit and there are no developmental delays or mental retardation, a child can ultimately learn to use a speech board. A ventilator is often required, because the basic instinct of respiration can be altered in shaking injuries. Paralysis affects the entire family financially, emotionally, and socially. Care at a regional rehabilitation center can help a family slowly adapt to the changes brought on by a child's paralysis and learn vital information associated with caregiving.

Persistent Vegetative State

Though rare in occurrence, this condition is emotionally the most difficult for an infant's family, and in a surviving child, it is by far the worst possible consequence of SBS. When an infant's brain suffers severe damage, it may experience excessive fluid buildup, ventricular atrophy, chronic hemorrhage, or other dynamic changes. In response to such trauma, the brain may shut down, leaving only the brain stem to function. Such a child has no awareness of the outside world. Activities such as eating and drinking, moving spontaneously in bed, reacting to sights and sounds, and sometimes even breathing are all very limited or impossible. The child is in a persistent vegetative state, and the body can only be kept alive artificially with breathing tubes, feeding tubes, and so on. The child's body will continue to grow, but there is little hope for rehabilitation, and death can be expected within months to years.[10]

Respiratory Difficulties

A child's brain may be damaged in an area that controls the function of the throat. If the gag reflex is lost, for example, the child cannot clear his or her lungs. Children may also aspirate, or breathe in, their saliva or food and could ultimately develop pneumonia. A tracheostomy may be done to bypass the mouth and throat and allow for a separate airway. This involves surgically cutting a hole and placing a temporary or permanent tube in a child's trachea. Permanent tracheostomy tubes are more for children who have severe problems with aspiration.[2] Families will need to learn the details of caring for a tracheostomy tube, which includes regular suctioning, cleaning, and dressing. Chronically debilitated children may ultimately need a ventilator, an apparatus that breathes for the child. This is a life-sustaining measure, but it makes the child more susceptible to lung infections.

Seizures

Also known as convulsions, seizures can occur with any brain injury. Seizures are caused by a sudden flurry of neuron activity, which blocks normal brain functioning. They are common with cerebral palsy.

Epilepsy is a condition in which a child has recurrent convulsant or nonconvulsant seizures, caused by partial or generalized electrical discharges in the brain. Epilepsy in shaken infants is caused by damage to the brain. It is usually a lifelong impairment and manifests in various forms.

Electroencephalograms (EEGs) measure brain activity during seizures and when seizures are absent. Most children with epilepsy and cerebral palsy have abnormal EEG patterns.[3]

A child may experience generalized or partial seizures. Generalized seizures (formerly known as grand mal) are the most demonstrative and involve the entire cerebral cortex of the brain. Seizures will be tonic-clonic, the tonic element producing body stiffening and loss of consciousness, and the clonic element alternating between relaxation and tensing of the body's muscles. Incontinence and deep sleep often follow such seizures.[3]

Partial, or focal, seizures (formerly known as petit mal) are limited to a small area of the cortex and produce involuntary, sudden movements in one area of the body. They occur in such a way that is nonintrusive to the child. There are several types of partial seizures. With simple-partial seizures, a child experiences unusual sensations, such as sudden jerky movements of one body part, distortions in hearing or seeing, stomach discomfort, or a sudden sense of fear, but consciousness is not impaired. With complex-partial seizures, however, a child experiences impaired consciousness and will appear dazed. Purposeless behaviors called "automatisms" may be observed, such as random movements, staring, or lip-smacking. Generalized absence seizures are characterized by lapses in consciousness for several seconds. During this time, a child will appear to be staring into space with eyes rolled upward. These may evolve into other seizure types, such as complex-partial or tonic-clonic.

Brain injury in SBS may also be followed by infantile spasms. Unlike normal startle reactions, an infant's head will suddenly drop forward while its trunk and legs "jackknife" upward. These spasms will occur frequently throughout the day and disappear around the age of twenty-four months. Infantile spasms can lead to a more disabling condition called Lennox-Gastaut Syndrome, which is characterized by frequent seizures.

Status epilepticus is a condition characterized by a steady set of seizures, where consciousness is not regained between convulsions. Any seizure that lasts more than five minutes should be viewed as a medical emergency. Shaken infants brought to hospital emergency rooms are often given an initial diagnosis of status epilepticus.

Seizures in infants who have been recently shaken are associated with blood in the subdural and subarachnoid spaces of the brain and intracranial pressure. As the intracranial injuries resolve, there should be a resolution of the seizures as well, though some infants may still experience twitching or jerking in the face, hand, or leg. A fever in a brain-injured child can also bring about a seizure (febrile seizure).[9]

Seizures can be very troubling for parents or caregivers, but knowing what to do during a seizure can change a situation of panic into one of structured calm.[2] Being prepared for seizures is the main thing that parents or caregivers can do for their child. The following is a positive system to use when seizures occur: calm; turn; allow; time; support; and document. First of all, the adults should remain *calm* in order to give maximum support to the child. Next, they should carefully *turn* the child onto his or her side, in order to avoid a choking hazard. Then, they must *allow* the child to go through the seizure without restraint. Light touches and calming words can help both caregivers and child (if conscious) remain calm. It is important to *time* seizures, noting both when they happen and how long they last. A child's neurologist will need such information. When the seizure is finished, the child needs loving *support*. Emotional security is an important element in seizure management. Finally, caregivers should *document* the type of seizure and whether there were any complications. Caregivers who have possible questions about the seriousness of a seizure should immediately contact a pediatrician.

Most seizures can be controlled with an antiseizure medication, such as Phenobarbitol, Dilantin, Tegretol, Klonopin, or Depakote. Ketogenic diets, which dramatically reduce carbohydrates and proteins and maximize fat intake, have been known to help control seizures. Careful monitoring needs to be done using a registered dietician. To get to a state of ketosis, a child must go on a fast. When a person fasts, there is an accumulation of ketone bodies, known as ketosis, which increases the body's acidity level (acidosis) and can control seizures. It is often used when antiseizure medication does not effectively control seizures or is not a preferred treatment by parents or caregivers. The ketosis balance within the body must be maintained, and caregivers need to be thoroughly educated. Often such a diet begins when a child is hospitalized with a medical condition related to an injury as a result of a shaking incident. The child can be carefully monitored in a controlled setting. Some parents and caregivers of shaken children are true advocates of this diet and state that it cuts down not only the number of seizures the children experience, but the amount of medication that must be taken as well. It is best to read carefully on this subject and discuss it with a medical provider before such a diet is begun.[12]

ACTH injections are an invasive treatment for seizures, but seem to be effective when other treatments fail.[13] Finally, Vigabatrin, though not approved by the FDA, can help as an adjunct in treatment of some types of seizures, such as infantile spasms.[14]

Speech Problems

Even shaken infants who have sustained traumatic brain injury before beginning to talk may be left with the potential for later development of speech deficits. Often the problem will manifest when children go to school or when their speech is tested when they are older. Speech disturbances appear in many forms. Children may have difficulty processing information and expressing themselves effectively, a condition known as aphasia. Problems with articulation may be due to a disability in facial and mouth control. A child caught up in a pattern of abuse may have had an injury to the frenulum, the thin membrane attached from the underside of the tongue to the floor of the mouth. Such a child may be "tongue-tied" as a result and articulation can be challenging. Children with cerebral palsy or who are mentally retarded may suffer from stuttering (dysfluency). Often, the more excited a child becomes, the more he or she will stutter. Children should never be reprimanded for stuttering but may need to be reminded to talk more slowly.

CONSULTATION AND FOLLOW-UP

A multitude of medical and social personnel may be involved in the care of a child with SBS. An effective team of individuals will work collaboratively to ensure the best possible outcome for a shaken child and his or her family. Some members of the multidisciplinary group will be consulted for only a short time; others will follow the child for months or years. It is vital that families of shaken children are comfortable enough to ask pertinent questions or share their feelings with any member of a multidisciplinary team. This provides not only a caring atmosphere, but a professional one as well. Below is an alphabetical list of the disciplines comprising such a collaborative team.

Audiology

For a child with suspected hearing loss, an audiologist will administer a hearing test and, based on the results of this, will make formalized recommendations for treatment. A brain stem auditory evoked response (BAER) is a type of hearing test that is done during an EEG.[15] An audible click is produced, and a neural response from the brain should be seen in the form of sound waves. Hearing tests can show mild, moderate, or severe hearing loss.

Chaplaincy

Hospital ministry can provide great comfort for families in need of emotional and spiritual care. Chaplains are available for all types of needs: to pray, to listen, to handhold, to guide, and to serve communion. Most hospitals have a quiet meditation room or chapel where families may gather for prayer or worship services. Chaplains are an important part of the hospital interdisciplinary team to assist families and others through emotionally difficult times. Prayer groups and guidance can also support hospital personnel and clinicians affected in their own way by SBS.

Gastroenterology

Because brain injury may cause subsequent problems in a child's gastrointestinal process, a gastroenterologist may be consulted. He or she will help determine whether feeding tubes or surgery is necessary, especially if there was abdominal trauma related with the shaking incident. Chronic gastrointestinal problems are followed up on an outpatient basis with a gastroenterologist.

Neurology

Because the brain is such a complex organ, injury to any of its parts may cause significant problems, such as seizures, which are a result of faulty neurotransmission. Neurologists are specialists who can help manage seizures and other neurological deficits experienced by hospitalized and outpatient children by tracking a child's EEG, prescribing medication, aiding in the interpretation of CT and MRI scans, and so on. Outpatient management depends on the severity of neurological difficulties the child is experiencing. Visits may occur on a regular basis or only a few times a year.

Neurosurgery

A neurosurgeon can determine the best process for correcting the presence of intracranial bleeding. Shunts, burr holes, and craniotomies are ways to evacuate collections of blood within the cranium. Neurosurgeons perform the surgery and follow up with the child after hospitalization to ensure successful management of intracranial trauma.

Nursing

Though not specialists that are formally consulted, nurses are with a shaken child and his or her family from the outset of their appearance in a hospital emergency room. Nurses provide the backbone of the medical care a child receives and often assist with the emotional needs of the family.

Often the first medical contact with the child and family at a hospital, nurses are in a unique information-gathering position. Their documentation of the initial injury history can make the difference in how a case proceeds.[16] In an outpatient or hospital setting, nurses are in an important position "for the early identification of families at risk for SBS, the early recognition of victims of SBS, and the management of patients suspected of SBS."[17]

Nurses can also make a difference in how a family remembers their experience of the child's hospitalization. They can create special touches for injured children by placing soft toys in their hospital bed, by comforting with a touch, and by soothing with calming words. These are the types of emotional "medicine" unique to the profession of nursing.

Nutrition

When a child is unable to eat because of brain trauma or other abusive injuries, a nutritionist will work with a gastroenterologist to supply the child with the appropriate types of nutrition. Sometimes children will be unable to chew, even if they knew how prior to the shaking incident. In such cases, alternative means will be found to provide nutrition, such as liquid or soft food diets. Nutritionists help ensure that the child receives the calories necessary for growth and rehabilitation.

Ophthalmology

Since most shaken children have intraocular trauma, they will be seen by ophthalmologists. Many different types of ocular injury may occur to a shaken child, so it is often best for a shaken child to be seen by a pediatric ophthalmologist. These specialists often have expertise in child-abuse-related injuries and can provide state-of-the-art care. Surgery may be needed to correct damaged vision, as caused by detached retinas. Otherwise, frequent outpatient appointments will assist in managing eye injuries caused by shaking.

Orthopedics

Unless there have been concurrent fractures in a child who has been shaken, orthopedists may not be consulted until later in the child's development. As a child grows, there may be complications in his or her limb movement. For example, a child with cerebral palsy may experience hip dislocation. Surgery may be able to correct this, in order to avoid osteoarthritis later. Orthopedists can guide parents and caregivers in the appropriate support of legs, feet, arms, and hands through the use of braces. Strengthening exercises may also be suggested.

Pediatrics

Pediatricians of shaken children are involved in their care from their arrival in the hospital emergency room. A child's pediatrician is notified of the incident and formally admits the child to the hospital in person or over the phone, if the admission is in the middle of the night. Residents and/or ER physicians provide initial care, and the pediatrician then performs the day-to-day management of the child, writes orders for other specialists to become involved, and arranges for any special procedures to be done. In an intensive care unit, the child may have a medical director who also writes orders and is key in managing his or her care needs. Children who survive shaking tragedies will follow up with their pediatricians closely after they are discharged.

Psychiatry or Psychology

Hospital emergency rooms often have mental health workers on their care teams. Involvement of a psychiatrist or psychologist in the initial process is important, because this specialist will support the family of a shaken child. Ongoing therapy for family members is beneficial for working through their emotions while getting their lives back together. The mental health worker may also have a chance to interview or converse with the perpetrator of the shaking crime. Thorough documentation may then play a significant role in efforts to prosecute such cases.

Pulmonary and Respiratory Therapy

Pulmonologists offer guidance with the management of heart and lung functioning. Children who are shaken may be unable to breathe on their own and may need to be intubated or put on a ventilator. These specialists will make these decisions, perform the procedures, and provide follow-up care.

In the hospital setting, respiratory therapists check blood gases, set appropriate oxygen flow, and interpret vital oxygen counts. Respiratory therapists can also help arrange home oxygen for children being discharged.

Social Work

Social workers have a multifaceted role in the management of a shaken child. A social worker will be a member of the team that initially evaluates the injured child and interviews family members. Child Protection Services will become involved, and social work may or may not be the discipline to coordinate their involvement.

Social workers also provide brief counseling and support for families affected by SBS. Such a discipline will also be the key in arranging home-care services, transportation, follow-up with community agencies, short-term extended care facility placement (if necessary), and assistance with financial services.

Social workers have a much different role today than in years past. They work along with other disciplines to maximize family integration and to advocate for the child. Such efforts may often be mutually exclusive. Social workers have been stereotypically viewed as working against families in crises over abuse cases. The safety of the child is paramount, however.

NOTES

1. Annable WL. Ocular Manifestations of Child Abuse. In: Reece RM, ed. *Child Abuse: Medical Diagnosis and Management.* Philadelphia: Lea & Febiger; 1994:138–149.

2. Miller F, Bachrach SJ. *Cerebral Palsy: A Complete Guide for Caregiving.* Baltimore: Johns Hopkins University Press; 1995.

3. Batshaw ML, Perret YM. *Children with Handicaps: A Medical Primer.* 2nd ed. Baltimore: Paul H. Brookes Pub.; 1987.

4. Duhaime AC, Alario AJ, Lewander WJ, et al. Head Injury in Very Young Children: Mechanisms, Injury Types and Ophthalmologic Findings in 100 Hospitalized Patients Younger Than 2 Years of Age. *Pediatrics* 1992; 90:179–185.

5. Parrish R. Personal communication, May 1998.

6. Begley S. How to Build a Baby's Brain. *Newsweek.* Special Edition, Spring/Summer 1997; 28–31.

7. Dias MS, Li V. Pediatric Neurosurgical Disease. *Ped N Amer* 1998; 45: 1539–1578.

8. Guertin SR. Cerebrospinal Fluid Shunts: Evaluation, Complications, and Crisis Management. *Ped Clin N Amer* 1987; 34:203–217.

9. Lawton KH, Meyers M, Donahue EM. Current Practices and Advances in Pediatric Neurosurgery. *Nurs Clin N Amer* 1997; 32:73–96.

10. Bonnier C, Nassogne MC, Evrard P. Outcome and Prognosis of Whiplash Shaken Infant Syndrome: Late Consequences after a Symptom-free Interval. *Dev Med Child Neurol* 1995; 37:943–956.

11. Menkes JH, Till K, Gabriel RS. Malformations of the Central Nervous System. In: Menkes JH, ed. *Textbook of Child Neurology.* 4th ed. Philadelphia: Lea & Febiger; 1990: 209–283.

12. Berryman MS. The Ketogenic Diet Revisted. *J Am Diet Assoc* 1997; 97(suppl): S192–194.

13. Holden KR, Clarke SL, Griesemer DA. Long-term Outcomes of Conventional Therapy for Infantile Spasms. *Seizure* 1997; 6:201–205.

14. Zamponi N, Cardinali C. Open Comparative Long-term Study of Vigabatrin vs. Carbamazepine in Newly Diagnosed Partial Seizures in Children. *Arch Neurol* 1999; 56: 605–607.

15. Batshaw ML, Perret YM. Hearing. In Batshaw ML, Perret YM. *Children with Handicaps: A Medical Primer.* Baltimore: Paul H. Brookes Pub.; 1987.

16. Jackson L, Miller CL. Recognizing the Symptoms of Shaken Baby Syndrome. *Nursing and Allied Healthweek* (San Antonio) July 1996; 1:8–9.

17. Wyszynski ME. Shaken Baby Syndrome: Identification, Intervention, and Prevention. *Clin Excel Nurse Prac* 1999; 3:262–267.

CHAPTER THREE

Cutaneous Manifestations

T HE WORD *CUTANEOUS* REFERS to the skin and the underlying layers of muscle. Blunt impact will tear, shear, and crush skin. What happens to the skin
depends on the force and nature of the impact. External manifestations
can include abrasions (scrapes), contusions (bruises), and lacerations (cuts or
tears). Internal bleeding may occur as a result of blunt impact. Listed below,
alphabetically, are the various types of inflicted blunt-force injury that may occur
concomitantly with other SBS injuries.

INFLICTED BLUNT-FORCE INJURIES

Abrasions

An abrasion results when skin is scraped away and left chafed. This often
occurs when an infant is thrown down or dropped after being shaken. Abrasions
are caused by friction from sliding across a surface, as from a bedsheet or a rug.

Bruising

Bruises, also known as contusions or ecchymoses, depending on the severity
of the injury, are injuries to the blood vessels beneath the skin. The underlying
blood vessels are crushed or torn, leaving the top surface of the skin intact.
Pinching or deep pressing can cause skin bruising, but most commonly bruises
are caused by a blow. The tissue between the skin and the underlying bone are

crushed together. Bruises on the abdomen and other soft areas of the body are rare, because there is no supporting bone.

Bruising typically assumes the shape of the object of injury, such as small, round circles of grab marks, a recognizable handprint, or the loop marks of a cord.[1–3] The development of a bruise depends upon the severity of the injury, the skin pigmentation of the infant, and the supply of blood vessels to the injured area.

Timing or aging bruises can be difficult, though an approximation of when an injury occurred can be made. Chemical change in the hemoglobin of red blood cells causes a bruise to change coloration over time. A bruise initially appears as a reddish or red-purple area for the first twenty-four hours. It will then change to a brownish purple or blue-purple and remain that way for one to three days. On days four through seven, the bruise becomes brownish green. A bruise that is one to two weeks old is yellow-brown, becoming light brown soon afterward. The bruise will disappear anywhere from two to four weeks after the initial injury, depending upon the amount of blood present to be reabsorbed and the adequacy of the blood supply to the damaged area to make the needed repairs.[4]

Estimating the age of bruising on a child is not an exact science. Bruises inflicted at the same time on a child will even heal at different rates, showing differing colors.[5] Yet multiple bruising in a central, clustered area indicates repetitive abuse.[6] The main message is that bruises on an infant are suggestive of abuse, as are bruises on a toddler not limited to bony structures, such as shins, foreheads, knees, or elbows.[7–9]

Shaken infants are usually relatively free from external bruising, which is one reason that a diagnosis of SBS can be overlooked. The marks of fingertips or thumbs around an infant's chest and back may be the only signs of being held and shaken violently.

Burns

Children who are shaken are often caught up in a vicious circle of repetitive abuse. In such cases, bruises, lacerations, and even burns can be common. Burns usually can be identified by an educated, experienced observer. Cigarette burns are naturally circular and ragged in appearance, and burns from heaters will take on the markings of a grate. These are known as contact burns.[10]

Other types of burns include immersion (usually in very hot bath water) and scalds from splashes with hot liquid. Intentional burns from water or other liquids can be distinguished from accidental burns, as there is a line of demarcation from where a child has been forced to remain in place. Accidental immersion or scalds will show splash marks from the child actively trying to escape injury.

Frenulum Tearing

The frenula are folds of skin in the mouth that attach in three separate areas. The frenulum of the tongue is attached to its underneath down to the soft floor of the mouth cavity. The frenula of the lips attach from underneath each lip to the bridge of the teeth on both the upper and lower jaws. Frenula are strong membranes, but they may be torn when a pacifier is jammed into the mouth or the mouth is struck.[11] A newly torn or healed frenulum is a sure sign of abuse.

Lacerations

Lacerations are areas of skin that are broken or torn. Bite marks (easily identifiable) and cuts by an inanimate object are examples of lacerations. Over a period of days after an incident of abuse, the lines of lacerations are seen more clearly, as accompanying bruises evolve as well.[6]

Petechial Injury

Petechiae appear as red, pinpoint, hemorrhagic spots on the skin where an injury has occurred. Blood has actually broken from the vessels and has been forced up through the skin by pressure from squeezing. In cases of strangulation, for example, petechiae appear on the neck and face of the victim. Petechiae can occur within various internal organs as well and are representative of abuse.

DIFFERENTIAL DIAGNOSES

To the eye of the novice, cutaneous manifestations from some diseases or disorders may be mistaken as signs of abuse.[12-16] Examples of these include bullous impetigo identified as cigarette burns; Mongolian spots confused with extensive bruising on the buttocks; dermatitis considered a scald burn; or a bleeding disease or disorder identified as bruising from abuse. Such misdiagnoses can occur with intracranial, intraocular, and skeletal findings as well. To avoid such misdiagnoses, thorough histories of injuries need to be taken, clinical findings discussed between disciplines, and differential diagnoses ruled out. When a misdiagnosis occurs, all individuals connected with a case are adversely affected, though this does not compare with the seriousness of a case in which actual abuse is overlooked or not diagnosed. The outcome in such a situation can be deadly.

NOTES

1. Jaudes PK. Psychosocial Emergencies. In: Strange GR, Ahrens W, Lelyveld S, Schafermeyer R, eds. *Pediatric Emergency Medicine.* New York: McGraw-Hill; 1996:657–662.

2. Richardson AC. Cutaneous Manifestations of Abuse. In: Reece RM, ed. *Child Abuse: Medical Diagnosis and Management.* Philadelphia: Lea & Febiger; 1994:167–184.

3. Ellerstein NS. The Cutaneous Manifestations of Child Abuse and Neglect. *Am J Dis Child* 1979; 133:906–909.

4. Reece RM, Grodin MA. Recognition of Nonaccidental Injury. *Ped Clin North Am* 1985:32:41–60.

5. Stephenson T, Bialas Y. Estimation of the Age of Bruising. *Arch Dis Child* 1996; 74: 53–55.

6. Wissow LS. The Medical History and the Physical Examination. In: Wissow LS, ed. *Child Advocacy for the Clinician.* Baltimore: Williams & Wilkins; 1989:49–66.

7. Kerns DL. Child Abuse. In: Mayer TA, ed. *Emergency Management of Pediatric Trauma.* Philadelphia: WB Saunders Co.; 1985:421–434.

8. Pascoe JM, Hildebrandt HM, Tarrier A, Murphy M. Patterns of Skin Injury in Nonaccidental and Accidental Injury. *Pediatrics* 1979; 64:245–247.

9. Sugar NF, Taylor JA, Feldman KW, Puget Sound Research Network. Bruises in Infants and Toddlers: Those Who Cruise Rarely Bruise. *Arch Pediatr Adolesc Med* 1999; 153:399–403.

10. Hyden PW, Gallagher TA. Child Abuse Intervention in the Emergency Room. *Ped Clin N Amer* 1992; 39:1053–1081.

11. Monteleone JA, Brodeur AE. Identifying, Interpreting, and Reporting Injuries. In: Monteleone JA, Brodeur AE, eds. *Child Maltreatment: A Clinical Guide and Reference*. St. Louis: GW Medical Publishing; 1994:1–26.

12. Oates RK. Overturning the Diagnosis of Child Abuse. *Arch Dis Child* 1984; 59:665–666.

13. Bays J. Conditions Mistaken for Child Abuse. In: Reece RM, ed. *Child Abuse: Medical Diagnosis and Management*. Philadelphia: Lea & Febiger; 1994:358–385.

14. Kaplan JM. Pseudoabuse—The Misdiagnosis of Child Abuse. *J Foren Sci* 1986; 31:1420–1428.

15. Wheeler DM, Hobbs CJ. Mistakes in Diagnosing Non-Accidental Injury: 10 Years' Experience. *BMJ* 1988; 296:1233–1236.

16. Kirschner RH, Stein RJ. The Mistaken Diagnosis of Child Abuse: A Form of Medical Abuse? *Amer J Dis Child* 1985; 139:873–875.

CHAPTER FOUR

Fractures in Shaken Baby Syndrome

I N INFANTS UNDER TWELVE MONTHS OLD, fractures are highly suggestive of abuse.[1] Even infants who crawl or are able to walk do not produce enough force in their own movements to cause a fracture. Unless there is some underlying medical condition associated with increased risk, a fracture in an infant should be a clinical red flag to a medical provider.

In much of what is written about fractures in children, the term *long bones* is used, to refer to all the limb bones of the legs and arms, except the small bones of the hands and feet. Each long bone comprises three sections: the shaft (diaphysis), the ends (epiphyses), and cartilage (metaphysis) that lies between. When an infant is shaken, one or more of these connections can sever or become damaged.

Two possible mechanisms of shaking can produce injuries to young bones. An infant may be held by the thorax or shoulders and shaken, causing the limbs to flail and producing fractures or lesions in the long bones. Or an infant may be grasped by the forearms and shaken, whereby the stresses and strains on these "handles" will cause such injury.

Healing time of trauma to the long bones depends on the severity and duration of the injury. The process usually takes four to twelve weeks.[2] It is important that any broken bones or bone lesions be immobilized to help union and prevent deformity. When fractures are due to child abuse, X-ray examination often reveals evidence of multiple fractures in various stages of healing. Dating fractures often depends on the significance of four clinical aspects, as described in table 4.1.[3,4]

TABLE **4.1** *The Four Clinical Aspects of Fractures*

Days after Injury	Clinical Findings
3–7	Soft tissue inflammation and swelling may be seen on an infant or the infant's radiograph
7–14	The periosteum (outer lining) of the bone may produce new bone
10–14	Recent fracture lines appear as clearly defined and sharp, but fractures in the process of healing are poorly defined
14–21	Callus (new bone) formation will begin to appear over the ends of injured bones, which may ultimately remodel their shape

DIFFERENTIAL DIAGNOSES

Infants may be suffering from an underlying bone disease, and this possibility must always be considered during a medical evaluation of fractures before a diagnosis of SBS is made. Osteogenesis imperfecta (OI) is a congenital disorder characterized by defects in the connective tissues and bone matrix. It has been frequently associated with child abuse injuries, because an infant affected by this condition may bruise easily and experience multiple fractures from minimal trauma. Healing occurs at a normal rate. A trained physician, however, can easily rule out this disease after a series of tests.[5,6] OI has four different inherited types, all of which are characterized by blue sclerae (whites of the eyes) and osteoporosis, except for Type IV, where sclerae are normal appearing. OI is an extremely rare disorder.[7] Clinicians should remember that no other condition exactly replicates the collection of injuries found in SBS.[8] For example, retinal hemorrhaging is not a feature of OI, and hence if this is noted in an infant, then abuse must be considered and is highly suspect.

Birth trauma fractures are usually noted immediately after birth or during the weeks following. If the question of child abuse arises, there should be a record of any such previous injuries, there being no incentive to conceal them. Fractures can also be dated by observing any healing callus and periosteum reaction that have already begun.

A disease best known from years past is rickets, in which a vitamin deficiency causes bones to become brittle. Other conditions that can produce lesions and fractures in the bones of infants and children include syphilis, scurvy, infantile cortical hyperostosis (also known as Caffey Disease), osteomyelitis, leukemia, and copper deficiency. Clinicians should do thorough lab work and take accurate histories from caregivers in order to rule out any medical conditions that may be the cause of fractures in children.

TYPES OF FRACTURES

After the "battered child" concept was first introduced in the early 1960s, hospitals began to standardize their practices on when to suspect abuse and when to X-ray.[9] These methods have been understood more completely in recent years, and there are now clinical standards by which medical professionals abide.

A variety of injuries to young, growing bones are seen daily by physicians throughout the world. Listed below, alphabetically, are examples of the types of fractures and lesions that may occur from shaking.

Avulsion Fractures

These occur when a bone is pulled or torn away from its connecting tissue. One common site of avulsion fractures is within an infant's spine, where the intense whiplash movement of shaking causes the vertebrae's connecting segments to be pulled away from their supports. Avulsion fractures can also occur in other bones due to pulling, twisting, or shaking.

Bucket-Handle Fractures

Caffey was the first to describe this fracture in his original article on injuries of the long bones coupled with subdural hematomas in infants.[10] In any bone, a mineralized portion can look like a bucket handle on a radiograph. This appears on the edge of the bone between the metaphysis and epiphysis. Such a classic metaphyseal lesion is indicative of abuse.

Radiologists originally thought that corner fractures were another kind of fracture occurring in the same area of the bone as bucket-handle fractures, but Kleinman found that these fractures were one and the same, depending on the angle at which the radiograph was taken.[11]

Clavicular Fractures

The clavicle can break during an episode of shaking if an infant is held by the shoulders and the perpetrator's thumbs press on these bones. The force of shaking combined with the pressure of thumbs can result in clavicular fracture at its midshaft. Midshaft fractures are common in children who have fallen, however, so they need to be associated with other injuries to be labeled as signs of abuse.[12] Fractures from the midshaft to the distal (end) portion of the clavicle will produce a calcification formation similar to that of metaphyseal injuries. These are representative of shaking injuries.

Corner Fractures

As described above, this injury is actually a metaphyseal lesion and can also be seen as a bucket-handle fracture, depending on the angle of radiograph view. Radiologists may continue to describe these metaphyseal lesions as corner fractures. This type of fracture appearing on a radiograph is often the basis for a child-abuse diagnosis.

Diaphyseal Lesions

When an injury to a diaphysis, the shaft of a long bone, occurs in an infant, there is bleeding from under the thin covering of the bone, known as the periosteum. The bleeding creates an expansion of the periosteum, which in turn causes new bone growth. This is known as a diaphyseal lesion. The resulting image on a radiograph is a diffuse, craggy-appearing mass.

Diaphyseal lesions occur four times more frequently than metaphyseal lesions.[13] These injuries can occur from a direct blow to the area or a jerking of the bone.[7] Treatment is effective if the bone is immobilized for optimal healing to occur.

Dislocations

A dislocation refers to the abnormal position, or displacement, of a bone from its joint. In child abuse and shaking injuries, it is known as traumatic dislocation. Often what appears to be a dislocation is actually a separation of the epiphyseal growth plate. This is more definitive of an injury caused by abuse.

Epiphyseal Lesions

The normal process of ossification in growing infant bones involves the formation of bone from tissue and other substance. Epiphyseal growth describes the process of a secondary bone-forming center inside and at each end of the long bones. This is appropriately known as the epiphyseal growth plate. If the epiphyseal plate is injured and the bones are not immobilized, resultant deformity can be severe. Usually, the younger the child, the more potential for a halting of the growth process.[7]

"Greenstick" Fractures

This type of fracture is specific to young children, occurring when a long bone breaks on one side, but only bends on the other. Aptly named, a greenstick fracture appears just as a young twig or sapling that is bent and snaps on one side. These fractures may be innocently acquired, as when toddlers fall during play.[1]

Humerus Fractures

A fracture or ring of calcification around the metaphysis of the humerus, in an infant with a questionable mechanism of injury, should immediately raise suspicion for abuse. The humerus is the segment of the upper arm that is one of the long bones frequently subject to injury, through direct impact, shaking, or pulling of the upper arm. Transverse, or right-angled, fractures can occur from direct impact, when a child is hit with an object or slams into an immobile object.

Shaking injuries may affect the humerus in a variety of ways. The best known is when the child is grasped by the thorax and shaken, with the long bones flailing violently. It is in such cases that the periosteum or metaphysis of the bone can be displaced.[11] The multiple attachments from the underlying chest and shoulder muscles influence the degree of displacement of proximal (those closest to the body) humerus fractures. An infant may have been held by the upper arms or forearms, creating the torsional effects that cause serious humeral injury.

When an infant's arm is pulled or twisted, spiral fractures may occur in the humeral shaft. Often no fracture or displacement is noted on an initial radiograph, because there has not been enough time for calcification to take place.

An infant who cries and has a "dropped" or underused arm needs a thorough exam, as well as initial and follow-up X-rays to see if periosteal lesions are present. Once treated and immobilized, a humeral fracture can be expected to unite completely in six to eight weeks.

Impact Fractures

These occur from direct trauma when an infant is slammed onto a hard surface after an incidence of shaking, one end of a fractured bone being driven into another. Realignment or surgery may be necessary to correct this type of fracture.

Metaphyseal Lesions

The metaphysis is the section of bone between the diaphysis (shaft) and the epiphysis (end portion). Trauma in the region of the metaphysis of a long bone is called a lesion because there may be a thickening of the outer region or a squaring of its edges, rather than an actual fracture line (see figure 4.1).[11] Such lesions appearing on radiographs are often referred to as bucket-handle or corner fractures.

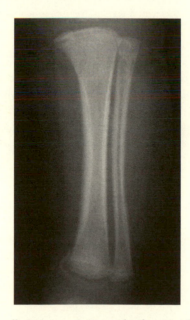

FIGURE **4.1**   *Bucket-Handle Fracture. An example of proximal and distal left tibial metaphyseal fractures. There is also a metaphyseal fracture of the distal left fibula.*

In 1960, Altman and Smith first proposed the concept of infant shaking as a cause for the appearance of metaphyseal lesions.[14] They also called for further investigation, using a skeletal survey, because metaphyseal lesions were indicative of trauma. These injuries usually do not become displaced and heal quite rapidly, but the affected part of the limb should be immobilized to prevent further damage. One concern is that the adjacent epiphyseal growth plate may close, and then the bone will not grow equally with the same bone in the other arm or leg. The course of the growth may be tracked by repeated X-rays.

Multiple Fractures

When there are two or more breaks in one bone, multiple fractures are present. With shaking injuries, this can commonly occur in the ribs, skull, and long bones. Some fractures may be older than others, or they may have occurred concurrently.

Periosteal, or Subperiosteal, Lesions

The periosteum is a tissue covering of young, growing bones. It contains minute blood vessels and cells, serving as the bone's supporting structure. When a bone is injured, the cells, called osteoblasts, generate new bone formation, and the periosteum will push out in a balloonlike manner, seeking to contain bleeding and growing calcification. Such an injury is also known as subperiosteal lesion, because there is bleeding from beneath the periosteum covering of a bone.

Approximately seven to fourteen days following injury, the process of ossification begins. Yet four to twelve weeks are necessary for total healing of subperiosteal lesions. On a radiograph, subperiosteal lesions appear as thick and craggy, usually around the diaphysis (shaft) of a bone. Healing takes place when the bone is rendered immobile by casting. If left untreated, significant alterations in bone growth can occur, leaving a child permanently disabled.

Periosteal new bone can also be seen in normal infants between the ages of six weeks and six months. Carty describes this new growth as distinguishable from the growth seen in abused bones, as normal bone formation is restricted to the shaft of the bone and is smooth in appearance, whereas bone formation after abuse extends into the metaphysis and can be ragged.[15]

Rib Fractures

Infant ribs, as with other growing bones, are supple and tend to compress with elasticity. Hence, rib fractures are rarely seen in minor injuries in children. In the absence of a history of a motor vehicle accident or bone-affecting disease, rib fractures in infants are usually indicative of abuse. Rib fractures also have been reported *not* to be a direct result of cardiopulmonary resuscitation (CPR).[16,17]

During a shaking episode, an infant is usually held around the thorax and shaken. When a perpetrator shakes, his or her hands can squeeze the child's rib cage severely. Ribs, during shaking, commonly fracture at the posterior area, where they are connected to the spinal column, which is structurally their weakest area. They may also fracture at the lateral (side) areas of the ribs.

There are twelve pairs of ribs in the human body. Generally, rib numbers four through nine are the most commonly injured in abused infants and children. Rib fractures in the first position, though unusual, are caused only by severe trauma, because they are very well protected by the shoulder, lower neck musculature, and clavicle, and require a much greater force to fracture. First-rib fractures have been found to be more related to shaking than to other forms of abuse.[18]

Rib fractures that are recent in origin—up to seven days old—may not be seen on a radiograph of the chest. There is usually only 50 percent X-ray sensitivity to rib fractures noted on initial exams. Repeating chest X-rays ten to twelve days after an initial study can identify rib fractures in the process of healing, as calcification will be present, making the fracture much easier to see.[19] A thickness of the outer layer of the ribs may also be seen and will appear as nodules or bumps where bone has been reabsorbed.

Kleinman states that when a rib fracture is found, it is critical that a nuclear bone scan is performed and read by competent clinicians to ensure that there are no other fractures.[12] Multiple rib fractures in various stages of healing are proof of repetitive abuse. There also may be fracturing within two sections of the same rib. Such an injury can cause a "flail chest," where the broken bones are free-floating.[12]

It is estimated that rib fractures are present in 20 to 25 percent of fatal cases of shaking. These percentages are lower in nonfatal cases.[20]

Skull Fractures

Skull fractures are one of the more common fractures that occur in child abuse. Skull fractures are difficult to produce in an infant, because the cranium not only is pliable, but has three lines of sutures ("soft spots" or fontanelle), and significant trauma must occur to cause a simple linear fracture. Sutures are nature's way of protecting the infant during the birth process, widening or compressing to protect the brain from direct trauma. As an infant grows, these sutures eventually fuse to become a hard covering, over a period of about two years. Birth-injury skull fractures, though rare, may occur from hours of compression by the vaginal walls during labor or, more likely, from the use of forceps or vacuum extractors in the birth process.

An infant's skull can fracture in several ways. The most common, and not always indicative of abuse, is the simple linear skull fracture. It is so named because it proceeds in one continuous line without branches. It can appear straight, zigzagged, or angled.[21] Simple linear fractures will be contained within the skull region where they occur and will not cross suture lines. Such fractures heal within three to six months, and the fracture line may be resolved completely.

Complex or multiple fractures are a problematic finding and are usually indicative of abuse if no substantial history is given for their cause. They are usually indicative of repetitive blows to an infant head caused by an impact injury after an incident of shaking. Hobbs defined such fractures as "two or more distinct fractures of any type or a single fracture with multiple components."[22] Branched linear fractures are included in this category. Complex fractures are often known to cross suture lines, or they may radiate outward in several lines from an initial area of impact (known as a stellate configuration).[21] They can also be bilateral, with breaks occurring on both sides of an infant's head. Often in complex fractures, the underlying dura of the brain is disrupted and there is intracranial bleeding. Silverman described the leptomeningeal cyst, which may arise if cerebrospinal fluid leaks into the arachnoid membrane that has been pushed slightly into the open fracture.[21]

A depression fracture, where skull fragments are displaced inwardly, may result from a blow to the head or when the head strikes an object. Forceps applied with too much pressure can cause such fractures at birth.[21] Some depression fractures are known as ping-pong fractures, because they resemble the indentation of a ping-pong ball on a radiograph.

Swischuk reported that vascular grooves (markings of intracranial veins) may sometimes be mistaken for a skull fracture.[23] He stated that in young infants, vascular grooves could be pronounced on a radiograph, especially in the frontal region. Upon reexamination from various views, a skull fracture can be ruled out because the grooves in this area "assume a configuration, which defies differentiation from fracture." Fractures remain more consistent from view to view.

Growth fractures occur as the line of a break actually widens with time. This is highly indicative of abuse, because growth fractures do not occur from minor falls.[6] Falls in infants and children have been studied copiously over the last two decades. Data from these studies show that major injuries, including skull fractures, do not occur from a fall two to three feet from a bed or couch, especially onto a carpeted floor.[24–26] Falls down stairs have also been examined in a large group of children, and even then skull fractures were rarely produced.[27,28]

Spinal Fractures or Lesions

Spinal cord injury occurs at a low rate in child abuse, less than 3 percent. Infants' anatomical features help protect them from serious spinal injury during battery and shaking. An infant's head and weak neck muscles allow the head to freely "give" during shaking. Perpetrators' fingers actually may support the spine of an infant when shaking occurs, which can diminish the risk of spinal injury as well. The vertebrae within the spinous process (the prominent points of the posterior ends of each vertebra) are wedge-shaped and freely move, and the ligaments within the spinal area are supple. These features prevent the spine from merely snapping during shaking. The trauma of the event is displaced evenly throughout the entire length of the spine.[29]

In his groundbreaking book *Diagnostic Imaging of Child Abuse*, Kleinman detailed several injuries that may occur to the spine in abused children. He examined how, during violent episodes of shaking, the spinous process can be avulsed, or pulled away, from its connecting segments.[12] The hyperflexion (or excessive bending) motion of the spine during shaking causes the avulsion to occur. Metaphyseal lesions and subsequent calcification of the injuries will occur within seven to twelve days following injury to the spinous process.

Other injuries may occur in the high cervical area of the spine, formally referred to as the C1–C5 cervical plexus area. Piatt and Steinberg described how one perpetrator shook a fifteen-month-old by the head, leaving her with flaccid quadriplegia.[30] In such cases, the spinal cord is pulled enough to elongate it, known as distraction.[29]

Bleeding can also occur within the epidural and subdural spaces of the spinal column, though such bleeding is not always indicative of trauma. In the late 1960s, Towbin first questioned spinal bleeding that was found during autopsies of infants who had suffered "crib death."[31] He speculated that the "mechanical forces" of hyperflexion caused the majority of spinal injuries found in dead infants that were studied in autopsy. A year later, Harris and Adelson discounted this by claiming that infants in their study died from spinal epidural venous congestion and not physical trauma.[32] Shaking was not considered.

Prior to being transferred to a hospital, an infant who has been shaken should be immobilized with appropriate-sized cervical collars and pediatric immobilization devices. Careful scrutiny of the entire spine is important when a child is brought to the hospital for injuries caused by abuse, especially shaking, because it is an area of the body that often goes unchecked.[33] In an infant who has died from an incidence of shaking, spinal injuries may be revealed during autopsy. Studies have suggested that the entire spine be carefully scrutinized during SBS-related autopsies and that removal of the C1–C5 en bloc allows for a more thorough investigation for hemorrhage.[34]

On CT scans, and less often on MRI images, spinal injury may not be seen because of the elasticity of the spinal column and soft cartilage. This condition is known as spinal cord injury without radiologic abnormalities (SCIWORA).[35] MRI scans often reveal injury to the spinal cord because of the buildup of edema and hemorrhage. Children should always have AP and lateral views of the spine during skeletal surveys if abuse is suspected, because hemorrhaging can occur in the upper cervical region of the spine.

Spiral (Torsion) Fractures

This type of fracture appears diagonally as a coil or spiral on a radiograph. The mechanism of this injury is a forceful pulling or turning, with a twisting motion.[36] Spiral fractures can occur in accidental injuries in ambulating children. Carefully obtaining a history of the injury is imperative, because great force is needed to cause such a fracture.

✧   ✧   ✧

Any fracture in a shaken infant is likely to lead to the discovery of other fractures. This is the nature of abusive patterns. Complete evaluation, treatment, and follow-up by medical personnel will lead to successful recovery in most cases.[37] Diagnostic imaging has come a long way over the years in being able to find and treat fractures. The specialty of pediatric radiology has also brought forth a new set of skills in the evaluation of cases of abuse.

NOTES

1. Tower CC. The Physical Abuse of Children. In: Tower CC, *Understanding Child Abuse and Neglect.* Boston: Allyn & Bacon; 1989:54–77.

2. Gwinn JL, Lewin KW, Peterson HG. Roentgenographic Manifestations of Unsuspected Trauma in Infancy: A Problem of Medical, Social and Legal Importance. *JAMA* 1961; 176:926–929.

3. O'Connor JF, Cohen J. Dating Fractures. In: Kleinman P, ed. *Diagnostic Imaging of Child Abuse.* Baltimore: Williams & Wilkins; 1989:103–113.

4. Chapman S. The Radiological Dating of Injuries. *Arch Dis Child* 1992; 67:1063–1065.

5 Ablin DS, Greenspan A, Reinhart M, Grix A. Differentiation of Child Abuse from Osteogenesis Imperfecta. *Am J Roentgenol* 1990; 154:1035–1046.

6. Nimkin K, Kleinman PK. Imaging of Child Abuse. *Ped Radiol* 1997; 44:615–635.

7. Sinal SH, Stewart CD. Physical Abuse of Children: A Review for Orthopedic Surgeons. *J South Orthop Assoc* 1998; 74:264–276.

8. Alexander, RA. Junk Science in the Courtroom. Third National Conference on SBS, September 2000.

9. Baker DH, Berdon WE. Special Trauma Problems in Children. *Rad Clin N Amer* 1966; 4:289–305.

10. Caffey J. Multiple Fractures in Long Bones of Infants Suffering from Chronic Subdural Hematoma. *Am J Roentgenol* 1946; 56:163–173.

11. Kleinman PK, Marks SC, Blackbourne BD. The Metaphyseal Lesion in Abused Infant. *Am J Roentgenol* 1985; 146:895–905.

12. Kleinman P. Bony Thoracic Trauma. In: Kleinman P, ed. *Diagnostic Imaging of Child Abuse.* Baltimore: Williams & Wilkins; 1989:67–89.

13. Ozonoff MB. Skeletal Trauma. In: Ozonoff MB, ed. *Pediatric Orthopedic Radiology.* 2nd ed. Philadelphia: WB Saunders Co.; 1992:604–689.

14. Altman DH, Smith RL. Unrecognized Trauma in Infants and Children. *J Bone Joint Surg* 1960; 42-A:407–413.

15. Carty HM. Fractures Caused by Child Abuse. *J Bone Joint Surg* 1993; 75-B:849–857.

16. Feldman KW, Brewer DK. Child Abuse, Cardiopulmonary Resuscitation, and Rib Fractures. *Pediatrics* 1984; 73:339–342.

17. Merten DF, Cooperman DR, Thompson GH. Skeletal Manifestations of Child Abuse. In: Reece RM, ed. *Child Abuse: Medical Diagnosis and Management.* Philadelphia: Lea & Febiger; 1994:23–53.

18. Strouse PJ, Owings CL. Fractures of the First Rib in Child Abuse. *Radiol* 1995; 197: 763–765.

19. Merten DF, Carpenter BLM. Radiologic Imaging of Inflicted Injury in the Child Abuse Syndrome. *Ped Clin N Amer* 1990; 37:815–837.

20. Bonnell H. Personal communication, July 1998.

21. Silverman FN. The Skull. In: Silverman FN, ed. *Caffey's Pediatric X-ray Diagnosis: An Integrated Imaging Approach.* Vol. 1. 8th ed. Chicago: Year Book Medical Pub.; 1985:3–88.

22. Hobbs CJ. Skull Fracture and the Diagnosis of Abuse. *Arch Dis Child* 1984; 59:246–252.

23. Swischuk LE. The Normal Pediatric Skull: Variations and Artifacts In: Gwinn JL, ed. *The Radiologic Clinics of North America Symposium of Pediatric Radiology.* Philadelphia: WB Saunders Co.; 1972:277–290.

24. Helfer RE, Slovis TL, Black M. Injuries Resulting When Small Children Fall Out of Bed. *Pediatrics* 1977; 60:533–535.

25. Lyons TJ, Oates RK. Falling Out of Bed: A Relatively Benign Occurrence. *Pediatrics* 1993; 92:125–127.

26. Reiber GD. How Far Must Children Fall to Sustain Fatal Head Injury?: Report of Cases and Review of the Literature. *Am J Forens Med Path* 1993; 14:201–207.

27. Joffe M, Ludwig S. Stairway Injuries in Children. *Pediatrics* 1988; 82:457–461.

28. Williams RA. Injuries in Infants and Small Children Resulting from Witnessed and Corroborated Free Falls. *J Trauma* 1991; 28:1350–1352.

29. Case M. Spinal Injury in SBS. Second National Conference on SBS, September 1998.

30. Piatt JH, Steinberg M. Isolated Spinal Cord Injury as a Presentation of Child Abuse. *Pediatrics* 1995; 96:780–782.

31. Towbin A. Spinal Injury Related to the Syndrome of Sudden Death ("Crib Death") in Infants. *Am J Clin Path* 1968; 49:562–567.

32. Harris LS, Adelson L. "Spinal Injury" and Sudden Infant Death: A Second Look. *Am J Clin Path* 1969; 52:289–295.

33. Cullen JC. Spinal Lesions in Battered Babies. *J Bone & Joint Surg* 1975; 57-B:364–66.

34. Gleckman AM, Kessler SC, Smith TW. Periadventitial Extracranial Vertebral Artery Hemorrhage in a Case of Shaken Baby Syndrome. *J Forensic Sci* 2000; 45:1151–1153.

35. Pang D, Wilberger JE. Spinal Cord Injury Without Radiographic Abnormalities in Children. *J Neurosurg* 1982; 57:114–129.

36. Philip PA, Traisman ES, Philip M. Musculoskeletal Injuries in Child Abuse. *Phys Med & Rehab* 1995; 9:251–268.

37. Kleinman P, Nimkin K, Spevak MR, et al. Follow-up Skeletal Surveys in Suspected Child Abuse. *Am J Roentgenol* 1996; 167:893–896.

CHAPTER FIVE

History of Abuse
and the Role of
Shaken Baby Syndrome

Perpetrators of abusive acts against children typically got away with their crimes until the late 1950s and early 1960s, because child abuse was an issue not readily identified or widely discussed among medical professionals. It was not until the late 1960s and early 1970s that governmental legislation, medical recognition, and social concern regarding child abuse truly became a standard. Prior to this, hundreds of thousands of children over many centuries suffered at the hands of their supposed caregivers. When physicians initially tried to put a name to physical abuse and openly discuss the topic in medical journals, there was a hesitancy to label it as such, for fear of ostracism by the medical community and public liability. Yet the few who did risk their professional reputation provided important hindsight for today's reader.

THE EARLY YEARS

In 1860, Ambrose Tardieu, professor of forensic medicine at the University of Paris, who apparently acted as a consultant to examining magistrates in surrounding cities, described thirty-two cases of child abuse, of which eighteen were fatal.[1] His paper, translated as "Medicolegal Study of the Cruelty and Mistreatment Inflicted on Children," exposed the extent of their injuries and the variety of ways in which they were inflicted. Though he did not specifically mention shaking, Tardieu noted that some of the victims had been "pulled all over the place" and mentioned lesions on the arms and chest due to rough handling. Tardieu seemed to have made the best of incomplete autopsy findings, or none at all. He noted that one finding was an "effusion of blood" over the surface of the brain, a condition known as acute subdural hematoma (SDH), and in another case he drew attention to a "collection of serous fluid," a description that is suggestive of a chronic SDH. Though German pathologist Rudolph Virchow had described examples of chronic SDH three years earlier, he had regarded them as inflammatory "pachymeningitis hemorrhagica" and thought the presence of blood was a secondary phenomenon. Following Tardieu's investigations, several of the perpetrators were convicted, and three were actually executed. But no one followed up on his pioneer work.

West, a London physician, identified child physical abuse in 1888 without actually labeling it as such.[2] He was stumped by the skeletal injuries in a set of siblings from one family and ultimately decided the cause of the injuries was from rickets—an appropriate diagnosis of that time. Though he did not accurately identify the injuries as physical trauma, he put the wheels of recognition into motion for other physicians.

An early case of a shaken infant was documented in 1928 in Rochester, New York.[3] "D.M." was the eight-month-old female subject of an article written by John Aikman, a doctor at Genessee Hospital. The girl's birth history (eight pounds, full-term), medical history, and family history (mother and father living and well) were normal, and she was "well-nourished and developed" (thirteen pounds and on malted milk) upon presentation. "D.M." was admitted "with a history of coma for one day," appeared ill, cried when handled, had a "slight contusion about the right eye and several spots of ecchymoses on the neck, face and limbs," and flaccid paralysis of the left arm. She had no evidence of fractures, no bulging fontanelle, and equal and reactive pupils. The girl was given an intramuscular injection of whole blood to counter the effects of her bruises. The following day, she took a turn for the worse. She showed a deviated gaze, "with her head turned to the right," and had bulging fontanelle, left arm rigidity, and left leg paralysis. A lumbar puncture showed "many red blood cells" and a lymphocyte count of 64 percent. On day two, "D.M." had an eye examination by another doctor, Frank Barber, who diagnosed retinal hemorrhaging. On day three, the girl's spinal fluid was said to be of little value "due to an accidental hemorrhage," which was attributed to an initial traumatic lumbar puncture. Aikman did not detail what medical or surgical interventions he used with this girl, but several weeks later, her left leg had improved, gradual improvement had begun in her left arm, and she had gained two-and-a-half pounds. She was discharged home after thirty-six days in the hospital. Aikman was perplexed that an apparently healthy child would suddenly develop a "cerebral hemorrhage." He outlined and ruled out various differential diagnoses, and then ended his description of this case abruptly with an identification of the cause of the girl's hemorrhage—her father. He had been arrested and convicted for extreme cruelty after he killed another of his children with "a blow of his fist." Aikman reported that any "injury was repeatedly denied" in "D.M.," but that this was a justifiable cause for her intracranial and intraocular bleeding. He concluded the article by encouraging other medical providers to consider injury as an option in such cases. This is a special look at an early case of an infant showing the classic signs of being shaken and being caught up in a pattern of violence.

In 1946, John Caffey, a pediatric radiologist, broke new ground by detailing the curious combination of subdural hematoma with fractures of the long bones in infants and children he was seeing in his practice, in an article in the *American Journal of Roentgenology*.[4] It was significant for drawing the attention of radiologists and other medical professionals to an unusual combination of injuries in infants and toddlers, detailing six cases of multiple fractures in young bones. All the infants had subdural hematomas, and in two of the cases retinal hemorrhaging was also found. Several of the cases also had severe bruising, which was not explained by the children's parents. He hinted at the possibility of "intentional illtreatment." Caffey also detailed and coined the terms "bucket-handle lesions" and "corner fractures." Though Caffey did not identify the subdural hematomas and fractures as signs of abuse, he wanted to do so, but feared that making such a claim would be too great a risk professionally and that colleagues would turn their backs on him.[5] To suggest that parents and other caregivers would intentionally inflict injury on babies and young children was incomprehensible at the time, because the topic of violence in the home was never discussed.[6] Caffey was a man ahead of his time, and he finally received the recognition he wished for in 1972, when he fully described another condition and coined the term for it: Whiplash Shaken Infant Syndrome.

THE 1950s

In 1950, Edward Lis and George Frauenberger examined a ten-week-old infant with bilateral subdural hematoma and multiple rib and scapula fractures.[7] Their conversation with the infant's parents about the cause of the injuries elicited no mention of trauma, however, and the final diagnosis was given as "unknown etiology." The child recovered with "no residual effects." These doctors had recognized that there had been physical injuries, but failed to explore the social issues that were the obvious cause of these. The case went uninvestigated, as was typical of the time.

Also in 1950, Marcus Smith reported on a case of a four-month-old female who was found, after four hospitalizations, to have subdural hematoma with multiple fractures.[8] The girl's initial troubles began when she was discharged home eleven days after her cesarean birth. At home, she was on a diet of Similac formula and orange juice, as was common at the time. She was brought to the hospital at age ten weeks with swelling of her right lower leg and was diagnosed with scurvy. She was given large doses of vitamins C and D and sent home. Two weeks later, she was brought back with large areas of swelling over her skull and was hospitalized for oral and IV vitamin C administration. One month later still, when visiting relatives in a different state, she was hospitalized with a swollen left arm. X-rays showed multiple fractures of the left arm, skull, and right tibia. Follow-up X-rays at a different hospital showed rib fractures as well. All fractures had considerable callus formation, identifying them as being old. A subdural tap of her brain was performed, and bloody subdural fluid was removed. After two weeks of subdural tapping, a craniotomy was performed, and the girl progressed well. Smith stated that no trauma was identified, but questioned the fact that the girl "had made a long trip by train and had been handled by sitters and relatives." This was surely another case of unrecognized abuse, obvious by today's standards.

The year 1953 brought a different slant on infant trauma. Frederic Silverman became the first physician in medical literature to take a stand by questioning the cause of skeletal injuries in infancy.[9] His article was also the first to describe an actual shaking event by a parent. Silverman reviewed three cases of unrecognized skeletal trauma in infants. Case 2, the most troubling, detailed the short life of a seven-month-old female named "W.P." She would now be recognized as at risk for abuse since her birth in October 1949, because she was a twin with a birth weight of three pounds, four ounces, who remained hospitalized for two weeks. By age five months, the girl had gained appropriate weight but was found to have significant tenderness in her lower extremities. On several occasions, she appeared to be in pain, crying out, frowning, and seeming "nervous and jittery." She was hospitalized at age seven months in May 1950 due to a thirty-hour-old burn from a hot iron. The girl's mother claimed that an older sibling had caused the accident by pushing the girl's bassinet against an ironing board, causing the iron to fall into it and burn the baby. Upon examination, it was found that "W.P." could not sit up on her own, was dirty, and had an ulcer on her genitalia. Though she was seven months old, "she handled herself much like a 3-month-old baby." X-rays showed a seven- to ten-day-old left humeral fracture and multiple healing fractures of both femurs and both tibias. A subdural hematoma was suspected but never proven.

When interviewed after these findings, the girl's mother explained her injuries as follows:

> In November 1949, after an automobile ride, the patient was found to be pale and very limp. The mother's attempts at resuscitation in this and in many subsequent similar episodes [were] limited to violently shaking the baby, usually holding her by the arms. This was done for the first time in November 1949, and the baby survived both the primary difficulty and the treatment. . . . In January 1950, the child had several episodes in which the arms and legs became caught in the slats of the crib; no trauma was admitted in freeing the baby. . . . In February 1950, the mother fell downstairs with the baby in her arms. She attempted to shield the baby but did not know whether in her excitement she squeezed the baby hard or not. In the six weeks prior to admission, the baby's bassinet collapsed three times. . . . A nineteen-month-[old] sibling was said to play vigorously with the baby, pulling at the arms and legs and occasionally sitting on the baby. The most critical episode, however, was thought to have occurred approximately one month prior to admission when the nineteen-month-old sibling fed the baby some cotton. The baby choked and the mother picked her up by the legs, inverted her and shook and slapped her violently several times before the baby coughed up the cotton. Demonstrating the fashion in which

she held the child inverted by the legs, the mother gave an excellent demonstration of a crack-the-whip technique.

Silverman reported that "W.P." was followed up in the outpatient clinic and appeared to be doing well. X-rays in June 1950 showed healing metaphyseal lesions and resorption of callus formation. X-rays were also performed on her twin brother and were negative for recent or old fractures. Sadly, somehow the relationship between the mother of "W.P." and the clinic deteriorated, and follow-up ended. Social Services made unsuccessful attempts at locating the child; it was found that she had died of "bronchopneumonia" in September 1950. The girl's parents did not permit autopsy. In conclusion of his report, Silverman focused on the "sudden fall/sudden catch" mechanism as a primary cause of unrecognized traumatic injury in children. He cautioned other medical providers not to be overly confrontational with parents so as not to put a child in danger or "precipitate a crisis in a difficult family situation."

This report was followed by a brief commentary by Edward Neuhauser, MD, who proposed three mechanisms for skeletal fractures and lesions in young children: obstetrical injuries, as from breech extraction; careless parenting, as when an "intoxicated father" tosses the child back and forth with a family friend; and self-inflicted injuries, such as "rib fractures in the presence of respiratory difficulty, pneumonia, or tracheal obstruction," known as "fatigue fractures." This unfortunate annotation not only incorrectly described physical injury in children, but also helped sustain the belief that parental child abuse could never actually occur.

Roy Astley wrote an article, also in 1953, about multiple skeletal lesions in six infants.[10] He determined that such injuries were caused by an underlying structural abnormality, without any overt trauma. All the infants he described came from "healthy families." Two were born prematurely. All had metaphyseal defects in various bones of their bodies. One girl had a "routine wrist radiograph" performed at age seven months. At fourteen months, she was found to have abnormal rearward curvature of the spine, called thoraco-lumbar kyphosis; metaphyseal fractures of the right radius, both ulnas, and right femur; and two rib fractures. At twenty-six months, she still had kyphosis, as well as metaphyseal fractures of the right tibia, humerus, and scapula; cortical thickening at both ends of the left humerus; and a clavicle fracture. At three years old, she had four new rib fractures and residual deformities from previous injuries. Finally, at four years of age, the girl had two black eyes "that had occurred spontaneously." Astley went on to write that "she was said to have tended to bruise easily and for trivial reasons since her early months," yet no bleeding disorder was identified. The parents of all the children he described obviously deceived Astley, who searched for medical reasons for the injuries rather than recognizing them as signs of abuse.

Paul Woolley and William Evans were the first team representing pediatrics and radiology to discuss traumatic skeletal lesions. Their 1955 article in the *Journal of the American Medical Association* discounted the "skeletal fragility" claim proposed by Astley and instead focused on parental abuse.[11] They described the nature of the households where abuse cases occurred, a first in the medical literature. The authors stated that abuse cases come from both stable households (with cases of "unavoidable" episodes of injury) and households where one or both parents were "aggressive, immature, or emotionally ill." Their clinical summary of the infants and their caregivers provides an important historical legacy.

In 1956, Englishman Leslie George Housden published *The Prevention of Cruelty to Children*.[12] Throughout this book, he presented cases of children of various ages who were abused by their caretakers. In one case, he described a mother who brought her two-year-old boy to a doctor with bilateral arm fractures. Initially, the mother claimed the child fell. When later questioned by the police, she confessed, "I lost my temper and got hold of his two arms and pulled him and shook him all the way from the dining room to the kitchen. I shaked [*sic*] him so hard I heard something crack in his shoulder." We are not told the outcome of this early report of shaking, nor if the boy suffered any neurological damage from the incident.

In 1957, W. J. Weston, writing from Australia, described three infants—ages two weeks, four weeks, and ten months—who had humeral, radial, ulnar, and femoral fractures.[13] Weston suggested that the youngest cases were probably obstetrical injuries, though the four-week-old had an "easy labor" without complications. Nonetheless, this infant had femoral and ulnar metaphyseal fractures. The ten-month-old was the subject of rough handling, because one of the parents' relatives "used to play with this child with great vigour and threw him up into the air on many occasions." The boy's parents told the doctor he fell several times on his shoulder. Later, the boy returned to the hospital with a new humeral fracture. This is one of the first articles to allude to a shaking injury. It is interesting to note that the parents used the excuses, still so common today, of other people mishandling the victim or of rough play.

A second article to appear in 1957 came from a radiology-pediatric team from San Francisco.[14] Henry Jones and Joseph Davis compiled forty-two cases of "trauma lesions" in infants (five of their own and thirty-seven previously published) to show the similarities in the skeletal injuries. This article was the first to openly point to the "number of factors which unfavorably affect the infant–adult relationship." The authors used tables to show the variety and locations of fractures. Rib fractures were the most frequent and were misdiagnosed by the authors, who wrote, "It has been suggested that the lesions may be inflicted by an older sibling bouncing up and down on the prone infant, an apparently not uncommon form of childish amusement." The multiplicity of fractures was also described, the mean number being five fractures per case. In the follow-up of these cases, 83 percent were found to be "living with skeletal lesions healed," 10 percent "died," and 7 percent had "conditions not stated." Jones and Davis also called for further investigation of skeletal injuries in infants brought to hospitals with subdural hematomas, saying, "Early diagnosis can make it possible to prevent further traumatic episodes."

Samuel Fisher broke ground in 1958 with a paper that "calls attention to the need of suspecting willful mistreatment of children by a parent."[15] He knew that the four cases he identified in the article were abuse-related and described them in detail. There was one particularly unfortunate case of a one-year-old girl who ultimately died at the hands of her father, having slipped through the cracks of protection. She was initially seen for several fractures and lesions of the bones of her ribs, arms, and legs, and it was noted that her parents had long delayed seeking care for her. Two weeks after her discharge from the hospital, Fisher reported the case to the authorities based on his conversation with the parents' neighbors. When investigated, the girl's father "was very rude and uncommunicative and they were unable to prove mistreatment." Five months later, the infant's pediatrician was called to her house, to find her dead. Autopsy showed an appalling catalog of injuries: further abnormalities of the metaphyses and periosteum of the long bones, multiple rib fractures, facial bruising and lacerations, lacerations of fingers and toes, kidney hemorrhage, deformed bones, and subdural hematoma. Further investigation revealed that the girl's multiple fractures had begun at age five months and had been treated at a different medical facility. This was an early identification of an infant who was shaken, beaten, and caught up in an abusive environment. The girl's parents ultimately pleaded guilty to murder (the mother had covered up for the father) and were sentenced to a penitentiary. Fisher presented two cases of what he believed were "accidental" fractures to distinguish them from abusive injuries, yet with today's knowledge, both cases can be viewed as obviously nonaccidental. The author called for early identification of "trauma by adults . . . so life may be saved."

THE 1960s

Donald Altman and Richard Smith welcomed the new decade with another landmark in the arena of child abuse.[16] In their 1960 article, they outlined previous articles on infant trauma and added five cases of their own—four abuse and one obstetric. They were the first to note that the mechanism of shaking would produce injuries to the metaphysis and periosteum of the bone: "Although a shaking or twisting type of injury will produce metaphyseal infractions, more severe injuries, such as striking or throwing a child, may well result in frank long or transverse fractures." They did not, however, consider any intracranial or intraocular damage that could occur from shaking. They then described radiographic changes and called for close inspection of fractures to determine if they were of varying ages. Finally, they made a statement about prevention, saying that physicians should be persistent about recognizing the causes of trauma in order to prevent subsequent injury or "more serious complications in these children." It was also recommended that physicians should work in close cooperation with "enlightened authorities" to remove children from environments where the abuse originated.

The next year (1961) brought a new perspective on child abuse: the call for a medical, social, and legal partnership. Three doctors (John Gwinn, Kenneth Lewin, and Herbert Peterson) collaborated on an article dealing with infant trauma identified on X-rays.[17] They described the appearance of bones over time during the process of healing, emphasizing that different stages of healing in different locales were conclusive in determining repetitive abuse. They also outlined the physical changes in the ends of the bones (metaphyseal/epiphyseal lesions and corner fractures) that occur from "joggling." They concluded their article by calling for physicians, legal authorities, and social-service agencies to work together to rescue children caught up in abusive environments, where repeated injury was the rule rather than the exception.

On July 7, 1962, the *Journal of the American Medical Association* (*JAMA*) published a landmark article. The prior autumn, in October 1961, a team of physicians led by C. Henry Kempe presented a symposium on child abuse at the American Academy of Pediatrics near Chicago titled "The Battered Child Syndrome"; physical child abuse was finally out in the open and given a name.[18] The team's subsequent article in *JAMA* exposed the back-hallway conversations of doctors, the failure-to-prosecute legal cases, and the "just-happened" stories given by parents. For example, an article published by a different group of authors that same year, describing the host of injuries that hospitalize children, failed to mentioned abuse as a cause, though fractures and multiple injuries occurred in a large percentage of the cases; these were attributed to falls.[19] Kempe and his colleagues outlined what constitutes child abuse and provided several case histories of children who had suffered at the hands of their caregivers. They stated that Battered Child Syndrome occurred mostly to children under age three and included "fractures of any bone, subdural hematoma, failure to thrive, soft tissue swelling or skin bruising, in any child who dies suddenly, or where the degree and type of injury is at variance with the history given regarding the occurrence of the trauma." They gave examples of radiographs depicting the types of fracture seen in abuse and examined the many alternative diagnoses that could wrongly be made, such as scurvy producing brittle bones. This article was also the first to completely detail the psychological profile of the abuser and how doctors could intervene to protect the abused child.

Kempe and associates pulled together a host of former journal articles alluding to abuse under one heading and gave it a name. Their article was published in one of the most popular medical journals and brought abuse out into the light as a tragedy that needed exposure—the tragedy formerly known as "unrecognized trauma."

From that time on, articles on child abuse appeared with regularity. New names were given to this issue, such as "willful trauma to young children," "Battered-Baby Syndrome," and "the Maltreatment Syndrome in children."[20–22]

In 1963, an article was produced on child abuse by an interdisciplinary team representing pediatrics, radiology, and social work. This team collaborated to identify child abuse on multiple levels, including the family dynamics of abuse.[23] It critically examined the histories given in many cases of abuse and concluded that such explanations given "were insufficient to account for [the] skeletal injuries."

A year later, A. C. Fairburn and A. C. Hunt wrote about the "new" concept of the battered baby but gave most of the credit to John Caffey, calling this his

"Third Syndrome."[24] They illustrated seven infant cases and tried to combine the disciplines of medicine, law, and psychiatry to make a more accurate diagnosis of abuse or neglect. In case number 4, they described a three-week-old girl who died after being abused by her mother. She showed the classic injuries of today's standard of SBS. The only admission the mother made was that the bruising on her infant was caused by "nervously holding her." The mother also held suicidal and homicidal thoughts prior to the abuse—an entity now known as postpartum depression.

Though child abuse was now openly given a place within the field of medicine, physicians still failed to consistently report cases of abuse to legal authorities. Katherine Bain, then deputy chief of the Children's Bureau of the Department of Health, Education, and Welfare in Washington, D.C., called for physicians to be proactive in suspected cases of abuse by assuming responsibility for reporting such findings.[25] She discussed a "model state law" that was being developed that would lay down the principles of reporting, and lauded Children's Hospital of Los Angeles for the way it worked with abused children. There, physicians, social workers, law enforcement, and juvenile court personnel worked together cooperatively to bring protection to an abused child. By contrast, Bain noted that in Boston, only 9 percent of referrals to the Massachusetts Society for the Prevention of Cruelty to Children came from hospitals. This poor statistic was exceeded years later in New York City, where for a period of *two years* there were no reports of child abuse made to the city's Child Protective Agency.[26]

It was not until 1966 that the American Academy of Pediatrics offered its guidelines for reporting, which included mandated physician reporting; prompt investigation of cases; removal of or close supervision of the child victim; central registry documentation of abusive parents or caretakers; and protection of hospitals and physicians from legal suits.[27]

Toward the end of this groundbreaking decade, there appeared a brief letter in *Lancet* from M. J. Gilkes and Trevor Mann, two ophthalmologists seeking to understand the combination of intracranial and ocular manifestations in the "battered baby."[28] They postulated that retinal hemorrhaging occurred from extreme rise in intraocular pressure, though in response, other authors suggested a viral etiology.[29] Gilkes and Mann discussed the case of a child who had been swung vigorously by the feet and then "sustained cranial trauma by impact" (the first reported case of Shaken Impact Syndrome). They also reported having had a conversation in London with an American ophthalmologist, Goodwin Breinin, who suggested that retinal hemorrhaging was similar to the retinopathy often seen in crushing injuries to the chest and "may arise by gripping the child by the chest and shaking violently." This was the first accurate description of how retinal hemorrhaging is produced in what is today called Shaken Baby Syndrome. Still an active ophthalmologist at the New York University Medical Center, Breinin does not recall the chance encounter with Gilkes and Mann while on his 1966–1967 sabbatical in England.[30] In his early interest in pediatric ophthalmology, he studied and treated the ophthalmologic effects of head trauma and peripheral trauma involving the bones of the body. He did not see the retinal hemorrhaging as a unique finding at the time, even though this encounter with Gilkes and Mann resulted in a significant contribution to the understanding of Shaken Baby Syndrome, as it is known today.

As the 1960s closed, an important book titled *Neurology in Pediatrics* was published.[31] Patrick Bray, the book's author and a pediatrician turned neurologist, included a chapter called "Postnatal Injury (Direct)." On page 197 he made reference to shaking as the cause of subdural hematomas:

> Some have suggested that bridging veins are torn or sheared when a small child is shaken by an angry parent or custodian. The fact that babies with subdural hematomas more often come from economically deprived families suggests not that they are suffering from malnutrition and hence are more prone to bleeding with injuries, but that the complete psychologic and social disturbances in their environment more commonly lead to violence.

Now retired, Bray states that he does not remember the source of the reference on shaking, but violence in the home as a factor for infant head injury was a topic that he and his colleagues discussed regularly.[32] His book sold well, as it was the only one of its kind at the time.

THE 1970s

The new decade brought forth more advances in recognizing, reporting, and documenting cases of physical child abuse. Shaking as a means of abuse was at the crest of being fully explained.

In 1970, New York City reported 2,800 cases of abuse, with new guidelines given for physicians and hospitals to follow—a far cry from the city's earlier paucity of reports.[33] These guidelines suggested that potentially abusive parents be identified in all hospitals and clinics by using a predictive questionnaire or other technique. Childcare drop-off centers for crisis relief for parents were recommended, though training of staff was not addressed. Lay counselors and aides from the community were also suggested as useful support for needy parents at both the individual and group level. Mothers Anonymous, later Parents Anonymous, was a model program newly formed in California. Finally, communities were called upon to develop teams of specialists, experts in child abuse diagnosis and treatment, to be located in child protection centers or hospitals and provide central direction and coordination for all persons involved in abuse cases.

It was a decade during which child abuse programs were being developed, discussed, and researched. The thrust of prevention efforts focused on treating the abusive family as a unit and providing rehabilitative services. Henry Kempe, Ray Helfer, and Vincent Fontana, who, among others, had pioneered child abuse identification in the 1960s, now implemented prevention programs in their own cities and across the nation.[34-36] For example, Kempe devised the home visitation program, wherein nurses or caseworkers would visit at-risk homes to ensure proper care of children and guide parents in the daily demands of child care. Laws were also honed to protect children as well as medical and social service professionals. Ever since the problem of physical child abuse was first identified, physicians, especially, had a hesitancy to report suspected cases. Mandatory laws passed in the 1970s made it possible for such professionals working with children and their families to make "good faith" reports without recrimination of civil actions against them. In the late 1960s, California developed the first model program for mandated child abuse reporting.[26]

In 1971, an article was written that would set the course for subsequent study of Shaken Baby Syndrome.[37] A. Norman Guthkelch, a British pediatric neurosurgeon, proposed that subdural hematomas in infants were often caused by shaking at the hands of their caretakers. His article, titled "Infantile Subdural Hematoma and Its Relationship to Whiplash Injuries," combined case studies, forerunner articles, and keen insight on the part of the author to provide groundbreaking information. His evidence for the causative nature of shaking injuries was threefold. First, he mentioned the case of an American neurosurgical colleague who had himself sustained a subdural hematoma, without any sort of direct blow to the head, when on a ride at a fairground that stopped and restarted very suddenly. Then he quoted a report from a social worker of a mother who shook her children "in a blind rage." Finally, he distinguished, in his own series of cases of chronic subdural hematomas proven to be due to child abuse, between two groups: one with obvious external marks of violence and fractures of the limbs, the other with few, if any, external marks of injury. He thought the children in the second group had sustained whiplash injuries as a result of being shaken by their caretakers.

Guthkelch remembers: "After speaking with Ingraham and Matson in the United States [who had pioneered the identification and treatment of subdural hematomas and been puzzled by the frequency with which they recurred], a light went off in me. Of course!—these cases of shaking are Ingraham and Matson's 'unexplainable' recurrent subdural hematomas in infants who have no marks of injury."[38] Guthkelch knew that infants had a greater propensity for subdural hematomas than adults, and he found that some of them may have been shaken. He described a case in which a six-month-old boy arrived at the Hull Royal Infirmary in England with bilateral retinal hemorrhages and bulging fontanelle. This gave rise to the suspicion that the boy might also have a subdural hematoma, which, in fact, was later confirmed. These signs and symptoms today are the hallmarks of SBS. Guthkelch also presented a social slant within this article, something his counterparts had not done. He stated that it was often the case, years ago, that many British parents would think nothing of giving their child "a good shaking" for the purpose of discipline. He warned in this 1971 article that the repercussions of shaking infants and children could be far more dangerous than direct blows to their young brains, describing an experiment that Ayub Ommaya had originally suggested to him, in which liquid paraffin wax and desiccated coconut were mixed in a flask. Shaking the flask caused the contents to continue swirling for many seconds, whereas delivering a hard blow caused only limited motion.

Today, retired and living in the United States, Guthkelch comments: "I've always wanted to do a study on the forces required to tear a bridging [cerebral] vein from its connection with the sagittal sinus, as I don't believe that it needs the impact force to cause subdural hematoma. I think shaking alone could rupture the connection. During neurosurgery, these veins can easily tear, even when the dura mater is gently lifted from the brain."[38] Guthkelch also discussed Ommaya's work in 1968, in which primates were used in the study of whiplash injuries.[39] Anesthetized primates were placed in a small vehicle with rollers on a track. Their skulls were opened, and a clear "window" was placed over the opening. With their necks secured, the primates were accelerated and decelerated in the vehicle. Using high-speed film, it was shown how the primates' brains were jolted about, causing significant damage. Their heads did not impact any object or their own bodies. Yet there were resultant subdural hematomas.

Guthkelch wrote a letter in 1995 to the *British Medical Journal* (*BMJ*) in response to an article by Carty and Ratcliffe, who named John Caffey as the first to describe whiplash injury as the cause of intracranial trauma in infants.[40] Guthkelch stated "the first mention of shaking of infants as a cause of subdural hematoma appeared in the *BMJ* in a paper that I wrote almost a year before Caffey's paper was published. . . . Unlike Caffey, I never believed that such shaking was playful; rather, I suggested that it was thought of as a socially more acceptable form of correction than a beating."[41] Guthkelch should be credited with being the first to describe the condition of SBS. His pioneer contribution is also important because he asked other heath-care providers to watch for signs of subdural hematomas in infants and children and to consider shaking in the differential diagnosis.

Australia picked up interest in Guthkelch's proposal and published an article echoing the claim that medical providers should always be suspicious of abuse in cases of infants with subdural hematomas.[42]

In 1972, John Caffey formalized the description of the condition then known as Whiplash Shaken Infant Syndrome, detailing several cases of shaken infants and their injuries.[43] Though he was not the first to describe the causation of the syndrome, he was the first to assign it a name and expound on the combination of injuries infants suffer as a result of being shaken. Guthkelch had mentioned retinal hemorrhaging as an identifier of subdural hematoma in his 1971 article; Caffey now proposed that these should be regarded as part and parcel of SBS. He went further by identifying various shaking mechanisms that he thought would produce such a condition. He gave the accurate example of gripping an infant by the thorax or around the arms and shaking, as well as the inaccurate descriptions of "overvigorous burping," "tossing the baby in the air," playing "crack the whip," playing "skin the cat," playing "riding the horse," rough play by older siblings ("spinning him dizzy"), using toys and devices that caused jolting or whiplash motions, giving rides in vehicles of recreation that jolted the infant, having repeated convulsions and rhythmic habits such as head rolling or banging. Except for Ommaya's study of whiplash in primates, there were no studies or witnessed accounts written of these traumatic events at the time of Caffey's article. Not knowing how the injuries of SBS were caused, he suggested this extensive list by which physicians could take note.

He reviewed twenty-seven cases of shaking, which he gleaned from his practice and from other sources, the bulk of which (fifteen) were related to the 1956 case of an infant nurse who had assaulted children in her care over a period of eight years. He also called upon physicians to keep a watchful eye out for infants and children with head and eye trauma, as "whiplash-shaking appears to be practiced widely in all levels of society for many different reasons . . . [and] warrants a massive nation-wide educational campaign to alert everyone responsible for the welfare of infants on its potential and actual pathogenicity." Unfortunately, this did not come until almost twenty years later.[44]

In the same year (1972), O'Neill and associates gave a presentation on the patterns of injury in the Battered Child Syndrome to the American Association for the Surgery of Trauma. They described how shaking infants "while suspended by the arm or leg" produced periosteal, metaphyseal, and epiphyseal lesions.[45] They also reported that in the abused children they saw, 80 percent had repeat injuries, and greater than 90 percent of the parents and caretakers gave an inaccurate or evasive description of the history of the injuries. These physicians encouraged other providers to use their clinical judgment well when considering the diagnosis of abuse: "The responsibility of a physician is simply to make a diagnosis and report, and not to do otherwise."

In 1974, Caffey's second article on Whiplash Shaken Infant Syndrome was even more descriptive, and he used the case of the infant nurse and her victims as a foundation for the rest of the article.[46] The deaths of two of the murdered girls, Cynthia Hubbard and Abbe Kapsinow (known in the article as Baby H, age thirteen days, and Baby K, age eleven days), were detailed, including their autopsies, which Caffey obtained from pathologist Michael Kashgarian at Yale University. Both infants had bilateral subdural hematomas with subarachnoid hemorrhaging. The autopsies also found that Baby H's eyes had retinal hemorrhaging and optic nerve edema; Baby K's eyes were not examined, though her clinical examination at the hospital showed "ocular fundi invisible—bleeding?" The rest of the article examined more closely the history of both subdural hematoma and retinal hemorrhaging. Caffey also discussed his meeting with Ommaya, the original investigator of whiplash injuries using primates, as a result of his first article on the syndrome. They accurately described how the manual shaking of infants could produce damaging rotational effects to the brain. Caffey suggested that some cases of Sudden Infant Death Syndrome (SIDS) "may have suffered, not admitted, manual shaking which caused no physical signs of external trauma." He broke his syndrome down into two different types: *Infantile Whiplash Shaking Syndrome*, which produced intracranial bleeding, intraocular bleeding, and lesions of the long bones in the absence of external trauma; and *Latent Whiplash Shaken Infant Syndrome*, wherein a "habitual, prolonged, casual shaking . . . may produce an insidious progressive clinical picture." Here, "mild" shakings over time may produce cerebral motor deficits or vision or hearing impairments when a child becomes older. Caffey's accomplishments in this area of child abuse were considerable, and he left behind an important medical and social legacy on his death in 1978.

Following these important articles, several authors made comments about SBS and offered follow-up clinical support. Collins reviewed Caffey's original article and reinforced the need for a nationwide educational campaign about the dangers of shaking children.[47] Oliver presented three cases of microcephaly in children whom he believe were shaken, causing stunted cranial growth.[48] And Hussey commented on the unusual manifestations that were being seen in physical child abuse, including SBS, and how "prompt change in the child's custody is a radical but necessary first step."[49] He also was one of the first to mention in the medical literature that babysitters were potential perpetrators of abusive injuries to children.

The advent of computed tomography (CT) in the mid-1970s shed new light on identifying the traumatic processes within infant, child, and adult brains. Radiologists and physicians could now see bleeding, fractures, and contusions two-dimensionally. Until then, medical professionals had relied on subdural taps on young brains in hopes of finding the underlying cause of tense or bulging fontanelle. CT now allowed for a more accurate diagnosis of head trauma in children.

Ellison and associates were among the first to report on abusive head injuries using CT, presenting several cases of cerebral contusions.[50] One father of a ten-week-old male admitted to shaking the baby, whose "head had struck a hard surface." The boy had multiple bruising, was lethargic, and had multiple fractures in various stages of healing. He was ultimately discharged home, another example of the medicolegal climate of the 1970s.

Zimmerman and colleagues in 1978 discussed the benefits of using CT to identify the presence of acute interhemispheric subdural hematoma, a now well-regarded feature of Shaken Baby Syndrome.[51] Their article was important, as it highlighted shaking as a mechanism for the radiologist to consider in diagnosing injuries.

The International Year of the Child closed the decade in 1979, and Taylor and Newberger offered their suggestions for the next decade in an article in the *New England Journal of Medicine*.[52] They reviewed current problems that they saw with child abuse issues in the United States and the rest of the world, and they called for world action by reallocating governmental funds (such as defense funds) to child-abuse prevention, treatment, identification, and education. They concluded, "Although all will agree that children represent the future of the world, it is clear that throughout most of the world the welfare of children lags behind as a priority."

1980s AND BEYOND

Key persons sharpened their identification and prevention skills in this new decade, and newcomers added to the wealth of information about abuse already established. Shaken Baby Syndrome became a regularly discussed entity of abuse in the medical literature. Studies on the mechanics of shaking brought important, yet controversial, findings. Prevention of SBS was first proposed. People discovered the medical, legal, and social complexities that were created as a result of shaking an infant. And insights were given about the long-term physical effects a shaken child could experience. The development and standard usage of magnetic resonance imaging (MRI) and other new diagnostic tools, such as bone scintigraphy, assisted medical professionals in understanding the complexities of the human brain and skeleton. These tools became invaluable in the diagnosis of SBS.

The pioneers of SBS investigation and research are highlighted below. Their firsthand accounts of infant abuse led the way to the greater understanding of SBS that exists today.

1980: Bennett and French

The authors detailed normal CT findings in a fifteen-month-old girl who had been shaken and was brought to the hospital with bradycardia (abnormally slow heart rate), irregular respiration, widening skull sutures, and bilateral retinal hemorrhaging.[53] This article provided a rare glimpse of a witnessed shaking event: The girl's father had been seen by the nursing staff at the hospital "violently shaking the child by her arms because she had not finished her lunch." He admitted that this was not the first episode of shaking. They called for "careful diagnostic consideration in all infants with unexplained convulsions and/or coma."

1983: Benstead

Shaking of infants was now highlighted as a criminal act and worthy of prosecution and conviction.[54] Benstead gave three case reports that detailed the victims, the perpetrators, and the outcomes. He called for complete investigation and diagnosis of infants who had subdural hematomas without evidence of external trauma. He openly called shaking an act of "criminal (albeit concealed) violence." He also encouraged complete interviewing in any case of infant death, even with grieving parents who may claim "cot death."

1984: Ludwig and Warman

One of the most frequently cited articles about Shaken Baby Syndrome was written by this team from Children's Hospital of Philadelphia and Children's Hospital National Medical Center of Washington, D.C.[55] This was also the first article to alter the condition's name to the more layperson-friendly term Shaken Baby Syndrome. The authors examined twenty cases of abuse of children "solely by being shaken"; shaken children who also had multiple trauma were excluded from the study. On arrival at the hospital, 80 percent of these children had either unilateral or bilateral retinal hemorrhaging, 55 percent had gastrointestinal problems, 60 percent had respiratory difficulties, 55 percent had bulging fontanelle, and 80 percent had central nervous system problems. Over 80 percent of the infants in the study had either bloody cerebrospinal fluid or a positive subdural tap. This article also detailed the characteristics of both the victim and the perpetrator. The average age of the infants was six months (70 percent were boys and 30 percent girls). There was a death rate of 15 percent and a morbidity rate (lasting problems such as blindness or a motor deficit) of 50 percent; only 35 percent recovered with no apparent deficit. Parents of these children gave a variety of excuses for such injuries, including prior accidental injuries, resuscitation attempts, and rough play. Ludwig and Warman called for medical providers to be careful not to assume a viral cause for the symptoms of infants who showed no external trauma, and noted that the use of a head CT scan would be a "key diagnostic study in identifying SBS." The editors of the journal *Emergency Medicine* highlighted the Ludwig-Warman article in the autumn of 1984 and called for the development of more effective methods of early diagnosis and prevention of SBS.[56]

1985: Billmire and Myers

In this first teaming of physician and social worker to focus specifically on abusive head trauma, the authors performed a chart and CT review of eighty-four infants under one year of age.[57] They found that solitary skull fractures or concussions without intracranial bleeding accounted for the majority of accidental injuries suffered by the subjects of the study. Half of the infants with skull fracture *and* concussion were abused. Any intracranial bleeding or intracranial injury that occurred was indicative of an abused infant (90 to 100 percent of infants with intracranial sequelae). Retinal hemorrhaging was found in 90 percent of the infants who had been shaken, but none of the accidental cases.

1985: Frank, Zimmerman, and Leeds

This team reported on four cases of infants who had been shaken or squeezed.[58] None of the children had skull fractures, and only one had subdural hematoma, but all had cerebral edema, changes in the ventricular system, and retinal hemorrhaging. This article made the point that in hostile home environments, physical child abuse includes other siblings. Ultimately, all four of these infants were removed from their homes. The authors also warned of misdiagnosis or "unsuccessful appeals in the courts," which would allow the child back into an abusive household.

1986: Dykes

This author was the first to compile a review of medical literature on Whiplash Shaken Infant Syndrome and provided information on the incidence of the hallmark injuries found in SBS.[59] Her research demonstrated that anywhere from 38 to 100 percent of shaken infants were found to have had subdural hematomas when hospitalized for their injuries, and between 67 and 100 percent had retinal hemorrhaging. The mortality ranged from 7 to 33 percent; 33 to 57 percent of the survivors had significant morbidity; and only 33 to 36 percent ultimately regained normal neurological functioning. Dykes reported that skeletal fractures had "received little attention in the recent literature and there are no data as to its incidence in this syndrome." She called for physicians to incorporate regular ocular checks in infants and children when they come for office visits to rule out any trauma. As Caffey had done twelve years earlier, Dykes also urged the commencement of a nationwide campaign on the dangers of shaking infants.

1986: Alexander, Schor, and Smith

Magnetic resonance imaging (MRI) came into regular use in the early 1980s, and this team of physicians was the first to describe its capabilities in diagnosing intracranial injuries in child abuse.[60] They also compared it with CT, finding that MRI was more useful for diagnosing subdural hematomas and had greater sensitivity, clarity, and flexibility in detecting brain pathology, whereas CT scans had the advantages of being less expensive, speedier, and better at bone imaging, and was equally good at detecting subarachnoid hemorrhaging. They encouraged MRI usage, if available, saying that the device was clearly their "method of choice for the detection of intracranial injuries, particularly those associated with shaking-induced trauma."

1987: Duhaime, Gennarelli, Thibault, et al.

This study rocked the foundation on which SBS was formed and has henceforth cleaved in two the way medical personnel and others view abusive head injury attributed to shaking.[61] Forty-eight infants and children (mean age eight months, 65 percent male) were studied. Eighty-one percent had retinal hemorrhaging plus subarachnoid and/or subdural hematomas. In 58 percent of those studied, an impact injury occurred either by fall, strike or fall plus shaking, or strike alone, as described by the caretakers. In 62 percent of the cases, there was actual evidence of blunt trauma, such as skull fracture or soft-tissue contusion. Those with mortal injuries (27 percent) all showed subarachnoid hemorrhage, subdural hematoma, diffuse cerebral edema, and cranial contusion at autopsy.

The team then went further than others had to test the theory that infants are "particularly susceptible to injury from shaking because of a relatively large head and weak neck." They constructed models of one-month-old infants implanted with an accelerometer to measure both shaking and impact. The heads of the models were filled with cotton and water, the necks were measured accurately and secured with resin, and the bodies were stuffed and weighted. Three types of necks were used—hinged, flexible rubber, and stiff rubber—all tested with and without a thermoplastic "skull." Each model was subject to violent shaking alone and with impact against a metal bar or padded surface. Both male and female "shakers" participated in the experiment to study the difference in amount of force generated according to gender. Data collected from sixty-nine shaking episodes and sixty impact episodes showed that "accelerations due to impact are significantly greater than those obtained by shaking . . . on average, impact accelerations exceed shake accelerations by a factor of nearly 50 times." The mean acceleration rate for shaking was 9.29 gravitational (G) forces, and for impact, 428.18 G forces. They concluded that in order for SBS to occur, children had to be "thrown into or against a crib or other surface, striking the back of the head and thus undergoing a large, brief deceleration," causing intracranial injury. Excluding the illustrative model that Guthkelch had used at Ommaya's suggestion, the only study to date that had tested whiplash injuries had been done by Ommaya nearly twenty years previously, using primates.[39] One important outcome of this study was to scientifically refute the possibility of brain injury occur-ring from the sorts of play activities originally suggested by Caffey.

1987: Hanigan, Peterson, and Njus

A variation on the SBS theme, Tin Ear Syndrome (TES), was proposed by this team in the journal *Pediatrics*.[62] A grayish discoloration of the ear that follows a blow from a hand or fist is one reason for the name "tin ear." The authors noted three cases of children between ages two and three years who had cerebral edema, retinal hemorrhaging, tin ear (subperichondrial hematoma), and ipsilateral (same side as impact) subdural hematoma. All three children died of their injuries. The authors postulated that children suffering from TES had sustained "a blunt injury to the ear, resulting in significant rotational acceleration of the head, stretching and tearing of the cortical veins . . . uncontrollable intracranial hypertension, and tentorial herniation." They even described a mathematical model to show the rotation of the head and brain in TES, saying that "the forces required to produce the tin ear syndrome would have to be sufficiently directed to the region of the ear and of such magnitude as to preclude inadvertent injury."

1987: Vowles, Scholtz, and Cameron

Diffuse axonal injury (DAI) in infants was the subject of a ground-breaking article by these three authors.[63] Such an injury occurs from the stretching of axonal nerves in infants' growing brains when infants are shaken. A stretching mechanism produces what are commonly called retraction balls in swollen axons. Swelling occurs over a period of many days. The authors found that DAI fre-quently occurs with cerebral contusional tearing and subdural hematoma, though bleeding may be minimal due to the shearing of the nerves and not to the blood vessels. DAI can be identified on MRI scans but only finally confirmed dur-ing microscopic investigation at autopsy.

1987: Kleinman

A pediatric radiologist, Paul Kleinman detailed hundreds of examples of what signs of child abuse look like in radiographs, CTs, MRIs, and other vehicles of diagnostic imaging in the first book on the topic, *Diagnostic Imaging of Child Abuse*.[64] This very important contribution broadened an issue with which many professionals had limited experience. Large sections were devoted to abusive head trauma as well as SBS, a topic of great interest to Kleinman. This text helped fill the need of medical and legal professionals for a single reference on the "radio-logic alterations occurring with abuse." The second edition was printed in 1998.

1989: Bruce and Zimmerman

These authors took the 1987 Duhaime group study one step further, stating that infants who were "considered to be the result of shaking injury now appear more likely to be the result of shaking impact injury."[65] In fact, they concluded that shaking alone could not produce abusive traumatic brain injury, which they termed Shaken Impact Syndrome. The authors supported Duhaime's study with the mechanical dolls and the conclusion that injuries resulted from "throwing or striking the infant after shaking." They stated that follow-up CT and MRIs are vital in the management of the shaken impacted infant, offering guidance for management of intracranial pressure. They also proposed that shaking impact injury could occur in any child at all levels of society.

1989: Hadley, Sonntag, Rekate, and Murphy

These authors suggested renaming SBS the Infant Whiplash-Shake Injury Syndrome.[66] They studied thirty-six infants who had sustained nonaccidental head injury; of these, thirteen infants had been shaken without evidence of impact—shaking in its pure form. Of these thirteen, 100 percent had retinal hemorrhaging and subdural hematoma. Because of this, the authors disputed the 1987 Duhaime et al. study that claimed that impact was a necessary component of SBS. There was a higher-than-average fatality rate (62 percent), and a high rate of cervical spinal hematoma was also noted at autopsy. Hadley and colleagues stressed that pathologists should take care to look for injuries in all parts of the cranium and spine.

1990: Alexander, Crabbe, Sato, et al.

This medical team from Iowa, which included a pathologist, welcomed the new decade with two articles on Shaken Baby Syndrome.[67,68] Their first article dealt with the nature of serial abuse and stated that 71 percent of shaken infants had suffered prior abuse or neglect (33 percent had been previously shaken). Siblings were also shown to be at risk for abuse. They recommended that other professionals be thorough in investigating possible cases of SBS in order to "reduce the risk to children and in addressing appropriate criminal sanction."

The second article dealt with trauma from shaking alone versus shaking with impact. They studied twenty-four infants with severe brain injury as a result of shaking and concluded that shaking alone is sufficient to cause the life-threatening injuries typically seen in SBS. Most infants who sustain impact will have a resultant bruise or mark on the scalp or will sustain a skull fracture. In their series, 50 percent of the infants were found to have an impact injury in addition to shaking.

1990: Spaide, Swengel, and Scharre

In one of the most complete descriptions for its time, these authors illustrated, using two cases, the medical, biomechanical, social, and legal aspects of SBS.[69] They described the symptoms of which to be aware in an infant with subdural hematoma, subarachnoid hemorrhage, and skull fracture. They also described the characteristic retinal hemorrhages and discussed the physical consequences of shaking infants. They reviewed the mechanisms of shaking injury, proposed differential diagnoses, commented on SIDS compared with SBS, and urged family physicians to watch carefully for signs of SBS, which could be done if the provider "maintains a high index of suspicion, weighs the clinical findings against the history reported by the parents [or caretakers], examines the eyes early and keeps the findings of the entire patient in mind."

1991: American Academy of Pediatrics

In one of the first unified statements on child abuse, a committee on diagnostic imaging of child abuse published its guidelines in the journal *Pediatrics*.[70] The group proposed that imaging studies be obtained when there is an indication of physical abuse and reviewed several types of diagnostic study. The first was skeletal imaging. Recommendations were made on the process of the imaging studies as well as the type. Skeletal surveys for all cases of suspected abuse should be mandatory in children less than two years of age. Intracranial injury should be evaluated initially by CT, but MRI is the favored imaging system due to its sensitivity. Finally, the team recommended guidelines for diagnostic imaging professionals to use when working with families of injured children, such as adequately preparing families for the process of imaging, including an explanation of restraints, and directing specific questions about indications for imaging studies back to the referring physician.

1992: Showers

The call for a nationwide prevention program on SBS had first come from Caffey and then from Dykes. Their hopes came true with the "Don't Shake the Baby" program based in Ohio.[71] Showers's program included posters, advertisements, and information packets to make new parents and the general public aware of the dangers of shaking infants. In her description of the program, Showers used previous studies to show that 25 to 50 percent of teens and adults were not aware of the dangers of shaking, saying that "the need for education has never been more clear." This program has been successful and continues to be used in hospitals and clinics and by social service agencies.

1993: American Academy of Pediatrics

This was an important year for SBS prevention and education, as the American Academy of Pediatrics provided a statement on its findings on this "serious form of child maltreatment."[72] The statement, created by a committee of medical professionals who specialized in physical child abuse, reviewed the historical, etiological (causative), and clinical facts that are key findings in SBS. They offered guidelines for diagnosing injuries by either clinical or radiological findings. They also reported on the medicolegal management of post-trauma patients and their families, and they called for careful follow-up, which "requires integration of specific clinical management and community intervention in an interdisciplinary fashion."

1993: Brown and Minns

A review article written by these pediatric neurologists acknowledged the difficulty physicians have when asked their opinion in court on accidental versus nonaccidental injuries.[73] They covered a range of injuries found in cases of physical child abuse, detailing bruising, skull fractures, brain injuries, and retinal hemorrhages. They focused on the specific findings of SBS and the associated medicolegal aspects. They also commented on the clinical management and long-term effects of such injuries.

1994: Fischer and Allasio

This physician and social worker pair reviewed cases of infants shaken during a span of six years.[74] Of twenty-five cases, they were able to get complete information on ten. All the subjects of the study initially suffered intracranial and intraocular bleeding. Seventy percent were left with significant impairment, ranging from spastic quadriplegia to blindness. On follow-up, of the remaining 30 percent with "normal" conditions at the time of discharge, only one had no physical limitations. The authors also found that 29 percent of the initial group were "sent back to the homes in which they were abused," and 67 percent of these children were abused again. The authors admitted that their study was small, but it clearly showed the dramatic effects of SBS on children and their future.

1995: Starling, Holden, and Jenny

This group from Denver, Colorado, performed a study specifically targeting the perpetrators of SBS cases.[75] This was an important marker in understanding the social and legal aspects of this type of abusive head trauma. The authors found that men (fathers and boyfriends of the mother) are at 2.2 times greater risk (over 68 percent more likely) to commit crimes of shaking. Female babysitters made up 17 percent of the perpetrators in their study, and biological mothers were responsible for 13 percent of the shaking incidents. Male infants accounted for 60 percent of the 127 shaking victims that were studied, which follows a national trend. One finding, which was counter to the experience of others, was that the infants who died were older than those who survived, a mean of eight months versus six months. Finally, the authors looked at the matter of timing. Ninety-seven percent of the perpetrators were with the infants when symptoms following shaking began: "this suggests that symptoms occur soon after the abuse, and do not evolve over a period of hours to days."

1995: Bonnier, Nassogne, and Evrard

In one of the first efforts to identify the long-term effects of shaking on an infant, this medical team from Brussels provided a thorough account of thirteen cases of SBS over a period of four to fourteen years.[76] Only one infant in this series (8 percent) died. Other aftereffects included mental retardation (93 percent); learning disabilities (93 percent); psychomotor retardation (75 percent); psychiatric problems (50 percent); microcephaly (33 percent); tetra/hemiplegia (25 percent); blindness or visual impairment (33 percent); and epilepsy (33 percent). Many of the shaken children at follow-up may have had normal neurological examinations but tended toward low IQs, hence the diagnosis of mental retardation. Only one child in this study (a five-year-old) "seemed to be clinically normal and problem-free." The authors found that hemiparesis was the first condition to be detected after a "sign-free interval," around the age of eighteen months. It is during this time that children are developing social and coordination skills, hence it is then that "deficits in the emergence of language, constructional ability and spatiotemporal exploration" arise. Another trend in the long-term effects of shaking was that behavioral difficulties became "detectable three to six years after the shaking and were always associated with neurological signs in this series." The authors concluded that a sign-free interval does not necessarily constitute a good prognosis after a diagnosis of SBS.

1996: Duhaime, Christian, Moss, and Seidl

This group also studied the long-term effects of shaking on infants.[77] They identified eighty-four cases of Shaking-Impact Syndrome over a ten-year period at Children's Hospital in Philadelphia. They were able to locate and study fourteen of these children five to fifteen years after being injured. The authors presented information on the histories given at the time of injuries, the physical examination and radiological findings, and the outcomes of the children. Twelve of the fourteen children (87 percent) initially had retinal hemorrhaging. One child (7 percent) died from respiratory complications at age eight; eight children (57 percent) were left moderately to severely disabled; and five children (36 percent) were identified as having a good outcome. Yet, of those children labeled as having a good outcome, "3 have repeated grades or require tutors, and 2 have behavioral problems." This study was significant, as it correlated the infants' initial medical diagnoses with their outcomes. Some infants were unresponsive after shaking and remained vegetative or severely impaired; others, who required initial intubation, were severely or moderately impaired on follow-up. Infants who had CT findings of "diffuse hypodensity," a generalized loss of gray-white matter differentiation in the brain, fared much worse than infants with "focal hypodensity or contusion," where there was a specified area of injury.

1996: Gilliland and Folberg

In a counter to the 1987 Duhaime study on impact injuries in shaken infants, these authors contended that, in a prospective postmortem study, nine of eighty pediatric head-injury deaths were victims of exclusive shaking—without impact.[78] Duhaime and others had proposed that it was not possible to shake an infant to death without having a final impact blow, but Gilliland and Folberg stated that, though they constituted a minority of the total cases, exclusively shaken infants could be distinguished by having no skull fractures or soft-tissue contusions of the scalp. They also found an increased frequency of retinal hemorrhaging in shaken infants in comparison with impact-only injury.

1997: Lazoritz, Baldwin, and Kini

These authors reviewed the current trend of findings in SBS and compared their series of seventy-one shaken infants with the original twenty-seven described by Caffey in 1972.[79] They found that well over 50 percent of the perpetrators of shaking were male, compared with the 78 percent female noted by

Caffey. They also found that admissions of shaking or trauma were more frequently made today than reported in Caffey's original paper, where he said, "usually there is no history of trauma of any kind." And finally, they found that rib and skull fractures were more common in shaken infants than in Caffey's reports, which described only metaphyseal and periosteal lesions of the long bones and vertebral compression fractures. Lazoritz and his colleagues pointed out that the concept of Shaken Baby Syndrome has been broadened to include impact injuries, the description of "all forms of abusive head trauma," the change in child-care trends (including care by the mother's boyfriend or the father "who may or may not be living in the home"), and noted the wide increase of awareness of this syndrome. The authors called for the syndrome to be labeled as Shaken Infant Syndrome and to include both shaking-alone and shaking-plus-impact injuries.

1998: Duhaime, Christian, Rorke, and Zimmerman

In the aftermath of the famed Boston au pair case of 1997, these authors collaborated to write a comprehensive article on SBS, which they believed should be called Shaking-Impact Syndrome.[80] The article provided a thorough review of the syndrome to assist physicians in their ability "to recognize its characteristic features," including biomechanics, epidemiology, physical and radiologic findings, management and outcome, timing of injuries, autopsy findings, and differential diagnoses.

1998: Alexander and Smith

In the journal *Infants and Young Children*, this pair from Iowa produced one of the most comprehensive and well-written articles on SBS in medical literature.[81] It included the history of the syndrome, its epidemiology, diagnostic imaging, biomechanics, medicolegal issues, and prevention. Two informal descriptions of SBS in this article were used to show the gravity of shaking an infant. With the difference in size between an infant and an adult, the authors remarked that the equivalent would be a man being shaken by a two thousand-pound gorilla. They also defined the biomechanical mechanism during an incidence of shaking as an infant being violently thrust back and forth, with the perpetrator extending his or her arms at a rate of three times per second. Finally, to make the concept of SBS clearer, the pair pointed out that the 20 to 25 percent death rate in SBS is much higher than was seen in a study of infants who fell two, three, or four stories—only 1 percent.[82]

1998: Lancon, Haines, and Parent

Another thorough description of the syndrome appeared the same year in the little-known journal *New Anatomist*.[83] These authors described SBS as a part of the broader problem of child abuse and neglect, of which there is an annual rate of 1.1 million cases in the United States. They also considered other social aspects of the syndrome, such as the age and sex of the victim, a review of the "common perpetrator," and the need for preventive efforts throughout the country. They described the anatomical features of shaking injuries, including a complete depiction of head, eye, and skeletal injuries.

1998: Conway

This author successfully reviewed the process of SBS in all its aspects.[84] He provided tables, graphs, and images for parents and professionals alike to understand in detail what happens to infants when they are shaken. Conway emphasized the importance of intracranial pressure stabilization in shaken infants, as such pressure is most damaging to the brain and can ultimately cause death. He also emphasized the need for thorough investigation of SIDS cases and described how to distinguish SIDS from SBS. This article would be highly useful for anyone seeking a comprehensive understanding of the nature of this syndrome.

1998: Dias, Backstrom, Falk, and Li

This group from the Children's Hospital of Buffalo emphasized the importance of performing serial radiography on the shaken infant.[85] Prior studies and reports from the medical literature had claimed that the presence of intracranial abnormalities after a shaking incident would show on CT scans six to forty-eight hours postinjury. This team was the first to examine the timing of intracranial changes on serial radiographic studies in infants after they had been shaken. They found that acute subdural hematoma was the most common intracranial abnormality noted in victims of SBS "and is nearly always present on the first scan obtained an average of 2.4 [hours] after the injury is reported." They found that chronic subdural hematoma may evolve within twenty hours, but typically within three to twelve days of the injury. Past studies had suggested a timeframe of one to four weeks for chronic cases to show on CT or MRI scans. This study from Dias et al. made available new information for medical professionals to use in the treatment of shaken infants and for investigators and prosecutors to use in the investigation of timing of injuries.

1999: Jenny, Hymel, Ritzen, et al.

Five experts in the fields of diagnostic imaging and pediatrics authored this important article dealing with missed cases of abusive head trauma (AHT).[86] The study began after a fourteen-month-old child was diagnosed with an abusive head injury—eight months after the initial assault, and after evaluation through seven medical visits and two cranial imaging studies had failed to diagnose the abuse. The authors reviewed 173 charts of head trauma. In fifty-four (31.2 percent) of these cases, AHT was not recognized. Unfortunately, 38 percent were reinjured after the missed diagnosis, and 40 percent experienced medical complications. Five children in the study had died and the authors concluded that at least four of the deaths could have been prevented with proper diagnosis. Children had such clinical signs as vomiting, seizures, irritability, lethargy, bruising, and respiratory difficulties. Improper diagnoses included gastroenteritis, accidental head injury, rule-out sepsis, otitis media (ear infection), seizure disorder, reflux, apnea, upper respiratory infection, hydrocephalus, meningitis, and unknown origin bruising.

There were also errors in radiological readings. Jenny and colleagues found that more cases were missed among white infants younger than six months from intact families. They concluded that even more would have been missed if the infants had normal respiration, no seizures, and no facial or scalp injury. They made the following suggestions to assist in the diagnosis of AHT:

1. Medical personnel should be alert to bruises and other cutaneous manifestations on the faces and heads of infants.

2. Head trauma should be considered as a possibility when evaluating infants with symptoms such as vomiting and irritability. (Physicians should measure the head, palpate fontanelle, and so on.)

3. During lumbar punctures, look for xanthochromia, as this can represent older blood from previous trauma.

4. Pediatric radiologists should be consulted in cases of suspected child abuse.

5. A retinal examination should be standard practice when faced with an infant with "nonspecific symptoms of illness."

2000: Reece and Sege; DiScala, Sege, Guohua, and Reece

These two sets of authors published retrospective reviews of accidental versus intentional injuries of children in the January issue of *Archives of Pediatric and Adolescent Medicine*.[87,88] The first article reviewed the findings of 287 medical records over a five-year period of children with head injuries admitted to one hospital. Age, injury types and mechanisms, mortality, length of stay in the hospital, and disposition after discharge for each case were categorized and compared. Statistically significant findings in abused children included intracranial bleeding; retinal hemorrhaging; cutaneous, skeletal, and visceral injuries; and death. Abused children were found to have been hospitalized three times as long as accidental cases. Over 30 percent of the abuse cases were returned home (the perpetrators were not identified). Reece and Sege concluded that if a child is brought to the hospital with severe signs and symptoms, and if the parent or caretaker gives no history or says there was only a short fall, child abuse should be strongly suspected. The authors also felt that if there was no major accidental trauma, retinal hemorrhaging seemed to be diagnostic of abuse.

The second article looked at all cases of child abuse and accidental injury from the National Pediatric Trauma Registry over a ten-year period. Over sixteen thousand cases were reviewed and compared. Like Reece and Sege, this team found that certain aspects of child abuse were unique. They observed, for example, that the clinical finding of retinal hemorrhage, "in absence of documented history of major trauma, such as motor vehicle crashes, should be considered diagnostic of child abuse." The severity of injuries from abuse was greater than from accidents, as was the death rate—"a sober reminder that abusive acts are intended to cause harm." The authors called for prompt evaluation of children suspected as being abused, improved education for medical professionals on all aspects of physical abuse, and improved documentation of child abuse findings.

CONCLUSION

This historical review shows that our perception of the nature of physical child abuse, as well as Shaken Baby Syndrome, has changed considerably over the years, as noted by the progress of significant contributions over the years by imminent researchers, clinicians, and authors. There has also been a dramatic reversal in society in our understanding of and reaction to child abuse. Gone are the days of hushed whispers of questionable acts. Now there is mandated reporting and vigilance for questionable findings. This does not mean that all medical and social service providers will follow the rule of "what is best for the child," or that diagnostic mistakes will not be made, yet ours is a different society from fifty years ago. Generally, the identification and follow-up protection of abused children is better. In many areas, though, problems remain. Child protective services act on cases readily, but not always thoroughly; medical providers recognize abuse injury more deftly, but not always consistently; prosecutors target perpetrators of child injury more openly, but are not always supported in the end judicially.

Society is at a place where child abuse can be significantly reduced, by the coordination of activities on an interdisciplinary level. Prevention programs can and do work. Tougher laws can make people stop and think of consequences. Education offers alternatives. These are the avenues, but each citizen must be ready to travel.

NOTES

1. Tardieu A. Etude medico-legal sur les services et mauvais traitements exerces sur des enfants. *Annales de la Hygiene Publique et Medicine Legale* 1860; 13:361–398.

2. West S. Acute Periosteal Swelling in Several Young Infants of the Same Family, Probably Rickety in Nature. *BMJ* 1888; 1:856–857.

3. Aikman J. Cerebral Hemorrhage in Infant, Aged Eight Months: Recovery. *Arch Peds* 1928; 45:56–58.

4. Caffey J. Multiple Fractures in Long Bones of Infants Suffering from Chronic Subdural Hematoma. *Am J Roentgenol* 1946; 56:163–173.

5. Elmer E. Personal communication, September 1998.

6. Griscom NT. John Caffey and his Contributions to Radiology. *Radiology* 1995; 194: 513–518.

7. Lis EF, Frauenberger GS. Multiple Fractures Associated with Subdural Hematoma in Infancy. *Pediatrics* 1950; 6:890–892.

8. Smith MJ. Subdural Hematoma with Multiple Fractures: Case Report. *Am J Roentgenol* 1950; 63:342–344.

9. Silverman FN. The Roentgen Manifestations of Unrecognized Skeletal Trauma in Infants. *Am J Roentgenol* 1953; 69:413–426.

10. Astley R. Multiple Metaphyseal Fractures in Small Children (Metaphyseal Fragility of Bone). *Brit J Radiol* 1953; 26:577–583.

11. Woolley PV, Evans WA. Significance of Skeletal Lesions in Infants Resembling Those of Traumatic Origin. *JAMA* 1955; 158:539–543.

12. Housden LG. *The Prevention of Cruelty to Children.* New York: Philosophical Library Incidence; 1956.

13. Weston WJ. Metaphysial Fractures in Infancy. *J Bone & Joint Surg* 1957; 39-B: 694–700.

14. Jones HH, Davis JH. Multiple Traumatic Lesions of the Infant Skeleton. *Stanford Med Bull* 1957; 15:259–273.

15. Fisher SH. Skeletal Manifestations of Parent-Induced Trauma in Infants and Children. *Southern Med J* 1958; 51:956–960.

16. Altman DH, Smith RL. Unrecognized Trauma in Infants and Children. *J Bone Joint Surg* 1960; 42-A:407–413.

17. Gwinn JL, Lewin KW, Peterson HG. Roentgenographic Manifestations of Unsuspected Trauma in Infancy. *JAMA* 1961; 176:926–929.

18. Kempe CH, Silverman FN, Steele BF, et al. The Battered Child Syndrome. *JAMA* 1962; 181:105–112.

19. Zollinger RW, Creedon PJ, Sanguily J. Trauma in Children in a General Hospital. *Am J Surg* 1962; 104:855–860.

20. Barta RA, Smith NJ. Willful Trauma to Young Children: A Challenge to the Physician. *Clin Peds* 1963; 2:545–554.

21. Griffiths DL, Moynihan FJ. Multiple Epiphysial Injuries in Babies: "Battered-Baby" Syndrome. *BMJ* 1963; 2:1558–1561.

22. Fontana VJ, Donovan D, Wong RJ. The Maltreatment Syndrome in Children. *NEJM* 1963; 269:1389–1394.

23. McHenry T, Betram BR, Elmer E. Unsuspected Trauma with M. Injuries During Infancy and Childhood. *Pediatrics* 1963; 31:903–908.

24. Fairburn AC, Hunt AC. Caffey's "Third Syndrome"—A Critical Evaluation. *Med Sci & Law* 1964; 4:123–126.

25. Bain K. The Physically Abused Child (commentary). *Pediatrics* 1963; 31:895–897.

26. Fontana, VJ. Recognition of Maltreatment and Prevention of the Battered Child Syndrome. *Pediatrics* 1966; 38:1078.

27. American Academy of Pediatrics Committee on Infant and Pre-school Children. Maltreatment of Children: The Physically Abused Child. *Pediatrics* 1966; 37:377–382.

28. Gilkes MJ, Mann TP. Fundi of Battered Babies (letter). *Lancet* 1967; 2:468.

29. Holzer A, Tobin JO. Fundi of Battered Babies (letter). *Lancet* 1967; 2:723.

30. Breinin G. Personal communication, August 1998.

31. Bray PF. *Neurology in Pediatrics.* Chicago: Year Book Medical Pub.; 1969.

32. Bray PF. Personal communication, November 2000.

33. American Academy of Pediatrics Committee on Infant and Pre-school Children. Maltreatment of Children: The Physically Abused Child. *Pediatrics* 1973; 50:160–162.

34. Kempe CH. A Practical Approach to the Protection of the Abused Child and Rehabilitation of the Abusing Parent. *Pediatrics* 1973; 51:804–809.

35. Anonymous. Physicians Told How to Deal with Child Abuse. *JAMA* 1970; 211:35.

36. Fontana VJ, Robison E. A Multidisciplinary Approach to the Treatment of Child Abuse. *Pediatrics* 1976; 57:760–764.

37. Guthkelch AN. Infantile Subdural Hematoma and Its Relationship to Whiplash Injuries. *BMJ* 1971; 2:430–431.

38. Guthkelch AN. Personal communication, June 1998.

39. Ommaya AK, Faas F, Yarnell P. Whiplash Injury and Brain Damage. An Experimental Study. *JAMA* 1968; 204:285–289.

40. Carty H, Ratcliffe J. The Shaken Infant Syndrome (review). *BMJ* 1995; 310:344–345.

41. Guthkelch AN. Serious Effects of Shaking Were Described in 1971. *BMJ* 1995; 310: 1600.

42. Editors. Whiplash Injury in Infancy. *Med J Australia* 1971; 2:456.

43. Caffey J. On the Theory and Practice of Shaking Infants. *Am J Dis Child* 1972; 124: 161–169.

44. Showers J. "Don't Shake the Baby": The Effectiveness of a Prevention Program. *Child Abuse & Neglect* 1992; 16:11–18.

45. O'Neill JA, Meacham WF, Griffin PP, Sawyers JL. Patterns of Injury in the Battered Child Syndrome. *J Trauma* 1972; 13:332–339.

46. Caffey J. The Whiplash-Shaken Infant Syndrome: Manual Shaking by the Extremities with Whiplash-Induced Intracranial and Intraocular Bleedings, Linked with Residual Permanent Brain Damange and Mental Retardation. *Pediatrics* 1974; 54:396–403.

47. Collins C. On the Dangers of Shaking Young Children. *Child Welfare* 1974; 53:143–146.

48. Oliver JE. Microcephaly Following Baby Battering and Shaking. *BMJ* 1975; 2:262–264.

49. Hussey HH. The Battered Child Syndrome: Unusual Manifestations (letter). *JAMA* 1975; 234:856.

50. Ellison PH, Tsai FY, Largent JA. Computed Tomography in Child Abuse and Cerebral Contusion. *Pediatrics* 1978; 62:151–154.

51. Zimmerman RA, Bilaniuk LT, Bruce D, et al. Interhemispheric Acute Subdural Hematoma: A Computed Tomographic Manifestation of Child Abuse by Shaking. *Neuroradiology* 1978; 16:39–40.

52. Taylor L, Newberger EH. Child Abuse in the International Year of the Child. *NEJM* 1979; 301:1205–1212.

53. Bennett HS, French JH. Elevated Intracranial Pressure in Whiplash-Shaken Infant Syndrome Detected with Normal Computerized Tomography. *Clin Peds* 1980; 19:633–634.

54. Benstead JG. Shaking as a Culpable Cause of Subdural Haemorrhage in Infants. *Med Sci Law* 1983; 23:242–244.

55. Ludwig S, Warman M. Shaken Baby Syndrome: A Review of 20 Cases. *Ann Emerg Med* 1984; 13:104–107.

56. Editors. Child Abuse by Whiplash. *Emerg Med* 1984; 16:71–72.

57. Billmire ME, Myers PA. Serious Head Injury in Infants: Accident or Abuse? *Pediatrics* 1985; 75:340–342.

58. Frank Y, Zimmerman R, Leeds NMD. Neurological Manifestations in Abused Children Who Have Been Shaken. *Devel Med Child Neuro* 1985; 27:312–316.

59. Dykes LJ. The Whiplash Shaken Infant Syndrome: What Has Been Learned? *Child Abuse & Neglect* 1986; 10:211–221.

60. Alexander RC, Schor D, Smith WL. Magnetic Resonance Imaging of Intracranial Injuries from Child Abuse. *J Ped* 1986; 109:975–979.

61. Duhaime AC, Gennarelli TG, Thibault LE, et al. The Shaken Baby Syndrome: A Clinical, Pathological, and Biomechanical Study. *J Neurosurg* 1987; 66:409–414.

62. Hanigan WC, Peterson RA, Njus G. Tin Ear Syndrome: Rotational Acceleration in Pediatric Head Injuries. *Pediatrics* 1987; 80:618–622.

63. Vowles GH, Scholtz CL, Cameron JM. Diffuse Axonal Injury in Early Infancy. *J Clin Patholog* 1987; 40:185–189.

64. Kleinman PK. *Diagnostic Imaging of Child Abuse.* Baltimore: Williams & Wilkins; 1987.

65. Bruce DA, Zimmerman RA. Shaken Impact Syndrome. *Ped Annals* 1989; 18:482–494.

66. Hadley MN, Sonntag VK, Rekate HL, Murphy A. The Infant Whiplash-Shake Injury Syndrome: A Clinical and Pathological Study. *Neurosurg* 1989; 24:536–540.

67. Alexander RC, Crabbe L, Sato Y, et al. Serial Abuse in Children Who Are Shaken. *Am J Dis Child* 1990; 144:58–60.

68. Alexander RC, Sato Y, Smith WL, Bennett T. Incidence of Impact Trauma with Cranial Injuries Ascribed to Shaking. *Am J Dis Child* 1990; 144:724–726.

69. Spaide RF, Swengel RM, Scharre DW. Shaken Baby Syndrome. *Amer Fam Phys* 1990; 41:1145–1152.

70. American Academy of Pediatrics Section on Radiology. Diagnostic Imaging of Child Abuse. *Pediatrics* 1991; 87:262–264.

71. Showers J. Shaken Baby Syndrome: The Problem and a Model for Prevention. *Children Today* 1992; 21:34–37.

72. American Academy of Pediatrics. Shaken Baby Syndrome: Inflicted Cerebral Trauma. *Pediatrics* 1993; 92:872–875.

73. Brown JK, Minns RA. Non-Accidental Head Injury, with Particular Reference to Whiplash Shaking Injury and Medico-Legal Aspects. *Devel. Med. & Child. Neuro.* 1993; 35: 849–869.

74. Fischer H, Allasio D. Permanently Damaged: Long-Term Follow-Up of Shaken Babies. *Pediatrics* 1994; 33:696–698.

75. Starling SP, Holden ITR, Jenny C. Abusive Head Trauma: The Relationship of Perpetrators to Their Victims. *Pediatrics* 1995; 95:259–262.

76. Bonnier C, Nassogne MC, Evrard P. Outcome and Prognosis of Whiplash Shaken Infant Syndrome: Late Consequences after a Symptom-Free Interval. *Dev Med Child Neurol* 1995; 37:943–956.

77. Duhaime AC, Christian C, Moss E, Seidl T. Long-Term Outcome in Infants with Shaking-Impact Syndrome. *Ped Neurosurg* 1996; 24:292–298.

78. Gilliland MGF, Folberg R. Shaken Babies—Some Have No Impact Injuries. *J For Sci* 1996; 41:114–116.

79. Lazoritz S, Baldwin S, Kini N. The Whiplash Shaken Infant Syndrome: Has Caffey's Syndrome Changed or Have We Changed His Syndrome? *Child Abuse & Neglect* 1997; 21: 1009–1014.

80. Duhaime AC, Christian C, Rorke LB, Zimmerman RA. Nonaccidental Head Injury in Infants: The "Shaken-Baby Syndrome." *NEJM* 1998; 338:1822–1829.

81. Alexander RC, Smith WL. Shaken Baby Syndrome. *Inf & Young Child.* 1998; 10:1–9.

82. Chadwick DL, Chin S, Salerno C, et al. Deaths from Falls in Children: How Far Is Fatal? *J Trauma* 1991; 31:1353–1355.

83. Lancon JA, Haines DE, Parent AD. Anatomy of the Shaken Baby Syndrome. *New Anatomist* 1998; 253:13–18.

84. Conway EE. Nonaccidental Head Injury in Infants: The Shaken Baby Syndrome Revisited. *Ped Ann* 1998; 27:677–690.

85. Dias M, Backstrom J, Falk M, Li V. Serial Radiography in the Infant Shaken Impact Syndrome. *Ped Neurosurg* 1998; 29:77–85.

86. Jenny C, Hymel KP, Ritzen A, et al. Analysis of Missed Cases of Abusive Head Trauma. *JAMA* 1999; 281:621–626.

87. Reece R, Sege R. Childhood Head Injuries: Accidental or Inflicted? *Arch Ped Adolesc Med* 2000; 154:11–15.

88. DiScala C, Sege R, Guohua L, Reece R. Child Abuse and Unintentional Injuries: A 10-Year Retrospective. *Arch Ped Adolesc Med* 2000; 154:16–22.

CHAPTER SIX

✧   ✧   ✧

Intracranial Injuries

HEAD INJURY IS THE MOST COMMON INJURY in child abuse cases. It is also the most common cause of death.[1] Norman and colleagues listed four ways that head injury causes death: cerebral anoxia and edema caused by cardiorespiratory arrest; increased intracranial pressure; severe concussion injury; and skull fracture with brain/scalp laceration.[2]

Infants are born with softer craniums than adults. Their sutures, or fontanelle, are open and protect the brain from excessive trauma during birth within the pressure-inducing vaginal canal. An infant's brain is gelatinous in texture and is proportionately smaller than an adult's brain. Because of this, there is extra intracranial space to allow the brain to grow as a child ages. Finally, the nerve fibers, or axons, which connect the infant's brain together at its major sections, are not protected by the insulating myelin sheath. This means these young, weak, and growing axons are especially liable to tearing and stretching. Axons carry brain messages to outer parts of the body and receive information as well. (See figure 6.1.)

The human brain is composed of blood, cerebrospinal fluid, and brain matter. This substance is divided into gray and white matter. During shaking, these two elements shift to and fro, rapidly pulling away from each other. When the brain expands afterward from cerebral edema, the gray and white matter can lose their individual densities and become blended.

When an infant is shaken, several things occur within the cranium. Sudden acceleration and deceleration of the infant head is the type of movement that causes the intracranial injuries seen in SBS. This whiplash motion forces the brain to rotate within the skull, elongate, and careen against the skull wall. This rota-

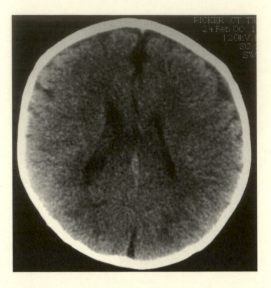

FIGURE 6.1   *Normal infant head CT. Normal brain in a three-month-old.*

tional movement is key in the biomechanics that cause severe intracranial injuries. In accidental injuries, such as a fall, there will not be the dramatic effects as seen in shaking injuries. Falls produce translational forces—a straight-line effect without rotation of the brain. These are impact or contact injuries and are usually minimal, whereas acceleration or rotational forces tear brain matter and shear blood vessels.

One of the main arteries in the human brain is called the sagittal sinus, which carries blood away from the cortex. This can be severed and torn during an episode of shaking, leading to the production of subdural hematoma and subarachnoid hemorrhage. Other, smaller blood vessels and axonal nerves attached to the brain are torn as well.

Besides such major bleeding, smaller intracranial injuries can occur. For example, less traumatic shaking can often accomplish the goal perpetrators of shaking crimes are seeking—the quieting of the child. In actuality, the child may have sustained some degree of concussion and become unconscious. The perpetrator then believes that shaking is a way to achieve their desired good, and the shaking may subsequently become harder and longer the next time the child cries. The infant may even be thrown onto a bed, floor, or against a wall, which results in further, more extensive damage. There has been considerable controversy in recent years over the question of whether a sudden striking force is needed at the end of a shaking incident to cause such injuries in SBS.

Below, listed alphabetically, are various intracranial processes that can occur when an infant is shaken.

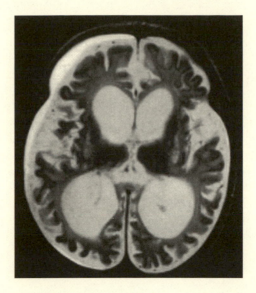

FIGURE **6.2**   *T2 weighted axial MRI obtained three months after shaking injury in a four-year-old child reveals severe atrophic changes.*

INTRACRANIAL INJURIES THAT MAY OCCUR IN SBS

Cerebral Anoxia

Shaking typically produces cerebral edema. The swelling from the edema makes it difficult for oxygen to reach the brain.[3] As a result, the brain is starved of oxygen and other vital nutrients, a condition known as cerebral anoxia, which causes permanent loss of function to affected areas. The more widespread the anoxia, the greater the loss.

Cerebral Atrophy

When brain cells die, they are eventually scavenged away, so there is a net loss of brain tissue, which is called cerebral atrophy. A brain scan will show that the ventricles and the spaces around the brain have enlarged because of diffuse cerebral atrophy. (See figure 6.2.) Sometimes the atrophy is limited to one side; this focal atrophy produces unilateral shifting of the brain, so that over time, a scan may show one hemisphere may be smaller than the other.[4]

Cerebral Edema

Edema is one of the three "hallmarks" of SBS, along with subdural hematoma and retinal hemorrhaging. This condition, which is a buildup of fluid in the brain tissue and is one of the earliest and most serious consequences of injury, may develop soon after a shaking episode. It commonly reaches a maximum in two to four days. It can be diffuse (widespread) or focal (targeting one area of the brain).

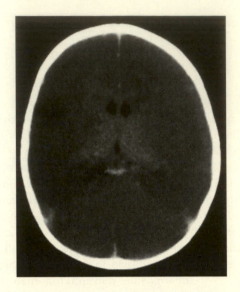

FIGURE **6.3**   *CT scan without contrast in a four-year-old child reveals diffuse cerebral edema, which caused a loss of the distinction between grey and white matter, obliteration of cortical sulci, and diffuse low density.*

Diffuse effects of edema compress the brain's ventricles, and there is a loss in ventricle size. Focal effects, more easily identified on CT or MRI scans, may appear as an area of increased blood flow. Focal edema can cause a shift of the cerebral hemisphere across the midline, which can distort the anatomy of the blood vessels supplying it. If there is not significant ventricular or venous compression, the effects of edema can be reversible.[5] Hyperemia, which is increased blood flow, is thought to be the initial physiological response to injury that precedes edema.[6,7] It causes an infant's brain to swell and produces increased intracranial pressure (ICP).

Edema occurs from a buildup of sodium and water in the cerebral tissues, which can lead to further edema. This pattern of repeated accumulation needs to be controlled, or death can become imminent. Because the skull of the very young child has the ability to expand, his or her ICP may rise more slowly than that of an adult, who has a rigid cranium. This may allow for a greater chance of improved outcome in tolerating ICP.[8]

On a normal CT or MRI scan, the infant brain is clearly defined and symmetrical, with a clear differentiation of gray and white matter. Edema diminishes or obliterates this difference, and a diagnostic scan shows a patchy covering over the brain, called hypodensity. (See figure 6.3.) Cohen and associates coined the term "reversal sign" to describe a state in which severe edema and tissue destruction make the white matter of the brain stem, thalamus, and cerebellum appear as of higher density than the surrounding gray matter portions of the brain.[9] This has also been termed "the black brain" and carries a poor prognosis, with irreversible brain damage.[10,11]

When ICP is uncontrollable, death is likely to follow. Normal ICP ranges between 0 and 15 mm Hg (a measure of mercury pressure). Traumatic injury to the head can lead to moderate and dangerous ICP levels of 20 mm Hg and greater.[12] ICP may be monitored through various mechanisms: an intracranial bolt, a device inserted into the skull; a ventricular catheter, a tube inserted directly into the brain; or a fiber-optic probe, inserted into the epidural space. Intracranial swelling, by edema or by vein swelling, is dangerous and can lead to occlusion of cerebral arteries, thereby cutting off cerebral circulation and oxygenation needed to sustain life. Such a complication is known as hypoxia.[13]

Edema can be controlled through steroid therapy and hyperosmolar medication, which, through the process of osmosis, allows excess fluid to be pulled away from the inner recesses of the brain, thereby controlling edema. It can also be managed through hyperventilation and oxygenation. Carbon dioxide causes veins in the brain to constrict, which will increase a child's ICP. A mask or nasal cannula (short nose tubes) providing a constant intake of oxygen can help keep carbon dioxide levels down. Shunts are often inserted in an infant's brain to drain excess blood and fluid.

Correct management from nursing staff is important for infants with severe head injuries. Elevating the bed thirty degrees at the head to increase blood return from the brain and maintaining proper head–neck alignment are important ways to manage such an injury.[14] Though edema may not be seen on a normal CT scan, this should not be interpreted as a normal brain. There can be elevated ICP without abnormal CT findings.[7]

Concussion

Concussion is a sudden neurological response to a traumatic event. Contact injury has typically occurred prior to the onset of a concussion where there is partial or complete loss of functioning with impaired consciousness. Consciousness will usually be regained within minutes if there are no other medical complications. It is also interesting to note that the biomechanics of concussion—impact injury—do not match the Latin origin of the word, which means "shaken violently."

Ommaya studied the effects of impact injuries, directly or through whiplash, in primates in the 1960s and 1970s, and determined that the rotational effects of whiplash movement (shaking) with impact will produce a concussive injury more frequently than impact alone.[15] It was also concluded that in order for a human to sustain concussion from whiplash, the rotational acceleration would have to be in excess of 1800 rad/sec^2.

Contusional Hemorrhage and Tearing

Contusions are bruises that develop on the brain at the point of impact after an infant is slammed against a surface after being shaken. Contusions can be cortical or cerebellar. Cortical contusions, the more common entity, are usually associated with edema and subdural hematoma.

Adams and colleagues found that "gliding contusions," those associated with shearing injuries and diffuse axonal injury, were less likely to produce intracranial bleeding.[16] Such a contusion occurs when the brain is pulled forward, often seen in impact injuries from automobile accidents, and the brain stem and basal ganglia at the opposite side are damaged. Generally, contusional hemorrhage appears as a small, white patch or large dot on a CT or MRI scan, primarily in the frontal area. The resultant neurological effects correlate with the part of the brain that was injured. Over the course of weeks or months, a child may experience focal seizures, hemiplegia, or eye deviations.

Tearing can occur when the brain experiences shearing forces from the whiplash motion of shaking and impact. Tears appear as slits or gaps in the brain's white matter and are typically found in the frontal and temporal lobes.[17] Usually there is little bleeding around the tears, yet tears can extend to the brain's gray matter and into major arteries and spaces, such as subdural and subarachnoid. Several authors believe that the younger the brain (less than five months), the more easily torn in trauma, because of the softness of the unmyelinated infant brain.[18,19]

Diffuse Axonal Injury

Axonal nerves, or pathways, connect the various areas of the brain. An infant's myelination, or connectedness, of the axonal nerves is in a very fragile state and is much more vulnerable to injury than an adult brain—especially in the first few postnatal months of life.[20]

During an episode of shaking, the axonal nerves can actually be sheared apart from the tissue to which they are connected. This occurs from the rotational, accelerational shearing forces applied to the brain during an incidence of shaking. Brain messages are lost or severely slowed, making simple processes, such as limb movement, difficult or impossible. An infant with diffuse axonal injury (DAI) may be in a deep coma, and prognosis for full recovery is usually poor.[21]

DAI produces tiny lesions, known as focal lesions, scattered throughout the brain's white matter.[22] When sheared apart, axons will usually swell at one end, producing what are appropriately known as retraction balls. This injury results from the brain having been accelerated, and not from hypoxia or swelling.[23] Often there are associated contusional tears and a low rate of intracranial bleeding.[24] Over time, the axonal nerves either repair themselves by new growth or degenerate. Axonal lesions are a main reason why cerebral atrophy occurs and why there are resultant neurological deficits in survivors of SBS.

DAI has only recently been described in infants and is more common than was previously known. Vowles et al. emphasized microscopic examination of the brain as an important tool in suspected child abuse cases.[24] The majority of cases of DAI can be confirmed at autopsy, though such lesions can be noted on MRI scans.[25]

Finally, Shannon and colleagues found that spinal cord injury seemed to correlate with DAI findings in seven of eleven cases of infants who were shaken.[26] They stated that axonal chemical response in the cervical spinal area of infants appeared to be a direct measure of DAI, which would later develop.

Epidural, or Extradural, Hematoma

Epidural means outside the dura mater, the membranous lining that covers the brain just underneath the skull. Thus an epidural hematoma is a collection of fluid or clotted blood from ruptured arteries within the brain that occurs *outside* the dura membrane. Epidural hematomas are rare occurrences and are present in only about 3 percent of pediatric head injuries.[27] Such a hematoma appears as a large, lens-shaped area on CT or MRI scans and is frequently associated with a skull fracture or impact injury.[28]

After the hematoma develops, there is a kind of "yo-yo" response within the brain. After the initial trauma, there is a loss of consciousness, though this may be gradual; then a moment of lucidity, as the brain recovers (seen as drowsiness in infants); and finally, a rapid clinical decline of the patient as ICP rises. Ingraham and colleagues stated that associated symptoms of an epidural hematoma include scalp swelling, hemiparesis, stupor, unequal pupils, vomiting, and possible shock due to the blood loss of intracranial bleeding.[29]

Epidural hematoma produces cerebral compression, especially if there is accompanying edema. Pressure on the brain's tentorium will cause pupil dilation on the side where the hematoma is located. Hemiparesis occurs on the opposite side of the body from the hematoma and appears in the form of limb rigidity. Immediate neurosurgical intervention to evacuate the hematoma usually leads to good recovery in infants and children.[30] Prognosis is thought to be somewhat better for infants than for children with epidural hematoma.[31]

Hypoxia

Hypoxia refers to a deficiency in the amount of oxygen reaching the brain. There are four classes. Hypoxic hypoxia occurs when the arterial blood supplying the brain is not fully oxygenated, as when a child cannot breathe freely. Anemic hypoxia occurs when sufficient oxygen reaches the lungs, but there is insufficient hemoglobin in the blood to carry this oxygen to the body tissues. Ischemic hypoxia occurs when oxygen and hemoglobin supplies are adequate, but either the blood pressure is low or the arteries supplying the brain are constricted to the point that blood flow is insufficient. Finally, histotoxic hypoxia occurs when oxygen, hemoglobin, and blood flow are all adequate, but some defect in the metabolism of the brain cells prevents them from using available oxygen.[7] Since brain cells can survive only a few minutes in the absence of oxygen, any form of hypoxia is a potentially life-threatening complication of head trauma.

Interhemispheric Hemorrhage

This is subdural or subarachnoid blood lying along the midline fold of the dura mater of the brain. It can cause extensive ICP. This is unique to SBS and appears on a CT or MRI scan as a thick-to-thin white line cleaving the brain's halves.[4,32,33] Because its presence indicates that the veins draining the adjacent parts of the cerebral hemispheres have been torn off the sagittal sinus, it is often considered to be indicative of a shaking injury. (See figure 6.4.)

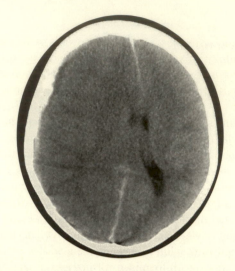

FIGURE **6.4** *Interhemispheric subdural hemorrhage with an acute right-sided sub-dural hematoma. There is ventricular effacement and midline shift.*

Intracerebral, or Intraparenchymal, Hematoma

Shaking injuries can produce bleeding in and around the parenchyma, which is the actual substance of the brain matter. This bleeding is seen frequently in the temporal and frontal regions. These types of hemorrhages are rare and relate to an area of direct injury, such as a contusion.[13] They are best viewed on a CT scan one to two days after a shaking incident.

Intracranial Hypertension

Accumulation of extra fluid, as from bleeding or edema, puts an extraordinary amount of pressure on an infant's growing, delicate brain. Initially, the body compensates by secreting less cerebrospinal fluid and absorbing more back into the bloodstream. Blood is also squeezed out of the veins of the brain. The compression of the veins reduces the drainage of blood. This stagnation of blood within the brain causes intracranial hypertension. Fontanelle bulge as a result of such pressure.

The end result of intracranial hypertension is increasing coma, seizures, or death. When possible, treatment is to remove or reverse the condition caused by ICP. Diuretics, such as Mannitol, are used to draw water away from the brain substance. Another therapy is induced hypothermia, in which an infant or child's body temperature is maintained between 90 and 93 degrees F (32 and 34 degrees C) for a period of several days to reduce the body's demands on the brain and subsequently reduce pressure.[6] Anticonvulsants, such as Phenobarbital or Carbamazepine, are used to control seizures.

Intraventricular Hemorrhage

An intraventricular hemorrhage (IVH) is associated with the shearing action of small blood vessels during a shaking episode and can be isolated within any of the brain's ventricles. Hemorrhages often will appear at the base of the occipital horns of the brain on CT scans. In its acute stage, intraventricular hemorrhage is of high density and is seen as a white shadow with a flat upper surface on a brain scan.[34] It is related to massive intracranial injury and is often an extension of an intraparenchymal hemorrhage.

Lesions

A brain lesion is defined as a small, visible injury, such as a wound, in any area of the brain. Bonnier and colleagues described two types of brain lesions in infants: those occurring from a shaking incident, and those due to head impact.[35] The latter can be related to a shaking incident but may also result from battery, automobile accidents, major falls, and so on. Depending on the type of injury a child withstands, lesions may appear in any section of the brain.

Microcephaly

Microcephaly means "small head." There can be many medical reasons for this to occur in infants and children, of which shaking is one. In response to a traumatic injury, the damaged brain often goes through dramatic changes. One such change is atrophy, where the ventricles of the brain pull together and shrink in size. If the brain retains this shape and size, the skull may also fail to grow.

Oliver did one of the first studies on microcephaly as a result of shaking and "battering" and proposed that physical child abuse be considered by physicians when faced with a child with this condition.[36] Head circumference measurements at regular pediatrician visits can determine whether a child's head size falls within normal limits. Nothing medically can be done to affect head growth, and shaking victims often have small heads for the remainder of their lives.

Petechial Hemorrhage

Petechial hemorrhages are small, pinpoint effusions of blood found on the surface of the brain or in its substance after a traumatic event. Usually they are noted on autopsy. Petechial spots are caused from blood being traumatically pushed into other regions outside its normal limits.[37] Besides brain matter petechiae, such marks can be found on the skin (see chapter 3).

Subarachnoid Hemorrhage

The arachnoid membrane is a loose cell covering just below the dura mater membrane. Normally, clear cerebrospinal fluid (CSF) flows freely within this network of cells. Subarachnoid hemorrhage (SAH) occurs after violence sufficient to contuse or lacerate the brain causes blood from nearby leaking veins to enter the subarachnoid space.

Bloody CSF during a lumbar puncture is one way to diagnose SAH. The condition of hydrocephalus, wherein CSF accumulates within the brain, leading to enlarged head size, can often be a consequence of SAH, as the normal flow of CSF is disrupted.[34] For the purpose of confirming the presence of SAH, the CT scan is the method of choice in the realm of diagnostic imaging. When a large SAH develops, it can be seen as a bright area surrounding the brain stem. Because of the hemorrhage's mix with CSF and the oxygen content, it will often be difficult to see on an MRI scan.[38] The ongoing presence of blood in the subarachnoid space can cause significant neurological deficits and tissue breakdown.[34]

Subdural Effusion, or Hygroma

The dura mater is the first membrane below the skull to act as a covering for the brain. When a fluid-containing sac develops in the brain in response to a traumatic event, it can be known as a subdural effusion, based on its location. Subdural means "below the dura." Cerebrospinal fluid often escapes from its normal areas of the brain after traumatic injury and goes into the space under the dural cavity, where a sac of the fluid develops. Subdural effusions most often develop concurrently with intracranial bleeding. Any increase in size or bleeding around a subdural effusion makes for a poor prognosis.[39]

For the purpose of diagnosis, subdural effusions will show up more clearly on an MRI than on a CT scan. They create a widening of the brain's interhemispheric fissure and enlargement of the ventricles.[40] Small effusions usually reabsorb spontaneously, but larger ones occasionally require surgical drainage.

Subdural Hematoma

A subdural hematoma (SDH) is a collection of blood, or clot, within the subdural space. Though this condition can develop from accidental injury, it most typically results from physical child abuse and may cause permanent brain damage or death.[41–43] This hematoma typically develops when the bridging veins, which cross the cerebral hemispheres to the sagittal sinus, are stretched, torn, and leak blood by an acceleration–deceleration injury, such as from shaking.

Many authors question whether shaking alone is sufficient to cause SDH in infants and contend that there must be associated impact.[44–46] The violence of an infant head whipping back and forth can shear intracranial veins, however, producing subdural hematomas. Research and witnessed accounts have identified shaken infants that were not impacted but developed intracranial complications, including SDH.[47,48]

Symptoms of SDH usually develop within a short time after blood collects within the brain. These can include bulging or tense fontanelle, failure to thrive, focal or generalized seizures, a high-pitched cry, increased head circumference, irritability, lethargy, setting-sun sign (the eyes are downturned, showing a small amount of white sclera visible above the iris, easiest to see when the infant is lying face up), and vomiting. Symptoms, such as ongoing seizures, may persist for several months, even after treatment has been given.

Medications can be given according to the type and severity of symptoms that

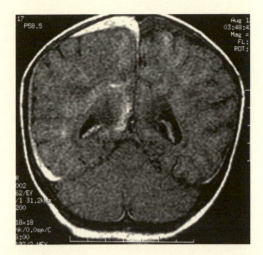

FIGURE **6.5** *An example of bilateral subdural hematomas of different ages. (Two different episodes of trauma.)*

accompany SDH. Corticosteroid medications and diuretics are commonly used to reduce swelling of the brain. Anticonvulsant medications may be used to control or prevent seizures.

The time it takes for these hematomas to develop ranges from hours to months and depends on the rate of blood accumulation. There are several types of SDH that may be identified. Silverman listed five: hyperacute, acute, early subacute, late subacute, and chronic.[49] *Acute SDH* develops and progresses rapidly, with symptoms usually appearing within twenty-four hours of the injury. Rapid deterioration occurs thereafter, due to an uncontrollable increase in ICP. In *subacute SDH*, leakage of blood into the subdural space is slightly slower, and symptoms usually are not seen until two to ten days after injury. In *chronic SDH*, there is ongoing pooling of intracranial blood. A membrane will form around the collection, and it appears as a large clot.[50] ICP develops and presses on the brain, causing symptoms and loss of brain function that may worsen as the hematoma enlarges. This pressure causes inflammation of the brain tissues and leads to cerebral edema, which further increases ICP.

SDH can be seen on radiographs and CT or MRI scans in a unilateral or bilateral position in the brain. (See figure 6.5.) An interhemispheric SDH (see *interhemispheric hemorrhage* above) is a bleed typically seen in SBS. Subdural hematomas may be completely reabsorbed into the brain and disappear over a period of weeks to months.[51] Subdural hematomas appear as crescent-shaped on CT or MRI scans. Such bleeding can be missed on initial CT scans, as the collection of blood has yet to form. Radiologists should look for image subtleties in the process of diagnosing, especially in the early hours and days following an injury. An SDH will appear as old or new based on the density (or brightness) of the bleeding on a radiograph or scan image. Fresh bleeding usually appears as high-density and older blood as low. Changes in a chronic SDH can also be seen diagnostically as blood is reabsorbed and a new layer is produced under the hematoma closest to the brain. The age of a subdural hematoma can be dated by the changes seen while the brain repairs itself.[4]

When an infant with an underlying SDH is brought to the emergency room, initial examination may show neurological deficits and abnormal reflexes, though symptoms may be less pronounced. In years past, it was regular practice to perform subdural tapping, wherein needles were inserted into an infant's head to see if blood or fluid was present. Today several diagnostic techniques are available to confirm the presence of SDH. First, a CT scan will display the location of intracranial bleeding. Follow-up MRI scans will detail the SDH more completely.[13,52] Examination may also reveal a need for emergency surgery to relieve pressure within the head without taking time for further diagnostic testing to establish the location of an SDH. One such surgical method involves drilling small burr holes in the skull to relieve pressure and allow drainage of the hematoma. Subdural shunts are often placed within the cranium to drain blood and fluid. These shunts may need to be maintained to manage chronic SDH. Craniotomies, which involve the temporary removal of a section of skull, are the most invasive type of treatment for SDH and still may be done when other treatments for chronic SDH fail. These operations were performed more regularly decades ago. In the late 1960s, Till found that infants did better in terms of follow-up intelligence when given shunts as compared with craniotomies.[53] There was also a much lower death rate.

Subdural hematoma can also occur from the pressures or trauma experienced at birth. This should be considered when an infant with SDH is brought to a hospital emergency room. Usually, SDH received from birth injuries resolves within three to four weeks and should have been documented in a child's medical record.[54] If a two- or three-month-old infant is found to have a "spontaneous" SDH with an inconclusive history, then child abuse should be suspected.

Children usually recover quickly and completely from SDH, yet the complexities of abusive head trauma go beyond isolated intracranial bleeding. When there is incomplete recovery, it is the result of permanent brain damage.

Subgaleal Hematoma

This is a collection of blood that lies between the galeal lining of the scalp and the periosteum covering of the skull. This type of hematoma has been described as occurring from hair pulling, but it can also result from an impact after an episode of shaking or other types of physical child abuse.[55] A noticeable bump may occur, due to the bleeding under the scalp, and can easily be seen on a CT scan. If the hematoma is not reabsorbed or surgically evacuated, it may form a thin layer of calcification, pressure on which produces a characteristic crackling sensation, like pressure on a cracked egg shell. This hematoma will typically slowly disappear spontaneously.

Tin Ear Syndrome

Hanigan and colleagues first detailed this syndrome in 1987.[56] Tin Ear Syndrome occurs when an infant or child is hit on the side of the head, usually on the ear. The torsional motion of the impact violently rotates the brain, causing intracranial bleeding and nerve damage. Brain swelling is usually more prominent on the side of the head that was struck, known as ipsilateral cerebral edema. There will likely be bruising on or behind the child's ear that was struck, altered neurological symptoms, and radiological findings.

DIFFERENTIAL DIAGNOSES OF SBS HEAD INJURY

Ehlers-Danlos Syndrome

This genetic condition is a collagen vascular disease that affects the connectivity of an individual's tissues and blood vessels. Signs of this disease include hypermobility of joints, soft, stretchable skin, and a tendency for increased bleeding.

One report in the medical literature described an infant with Ehlers-Danlos, who was initially thought to have been a victim of SBS.[57] She had a seizure at home at age thirteen weeks. Upon admission to the hospital, she was found to have had bilateral retinal hemorrhaging, intracranial bleeding, and chronic subdural fluid collection. The medical team believed that the injuries were related to shaking.

Bleeding times and counts were obtained, and most were normal, though a Simplate bleeding time while the infant was held still was abnormal. Her family was interviewed, and the girl was placed in foster care for three months, after which she was returned to her family.

At three years of age, the family had the girl reevaluated for bleeding times. It was found that she bruised easily and had hypermobile joints, soft skin, and two areas of fine, wrinkled scarring. The girl's mother was examined for similar symptoms. Once the bleeding times over the past three years were reviewed, which were all prolonged, the diagnosis of Ehlers-Danlos Syndrome was made.

The authors of this report suggested birth trauma as the cause for the chronic subdural fluid collections but were perplexed by the acute intracranial and retinal hemorrhaging noted. They suggested that this might have been nonaccidental injury in an infant with a genetic disorder. Finally, they encouraged taking care in diagnosis and when interviewing families to consider the possibility of inherited conditions.

Glutaric Aciduria Type 1

Glutaric Aciduria Type 1 (GA-1) is a rare genetic disorder in which there is a deficiency in the metabolism of the basal ganglia, causing progressive central nervous system degeneration, leading to developmental delay, dystonia (poor muscle control), and epilepsy.[58] GA-1 manifests between seven and eighteen months of age, as the brain develops and grows.[59] Intracranial bleeding can easily occur as the subarachnoid space is widened due to cerebral atrophy, making the brain susceptible to minor trauma.

If the disorder is discovered when an infant is asymptomatic, there can be successful treatment. GA-1 is confirmed through urine organic acids and carnitine levels in the blood.[2] One team of doctors suggested that the only true method to establish the diagnosis of GA-1 with certainty is urinary analysis of the enzyme glutaryl-CoA dehydrogenase (GCDH) and GCDH mutation analysis.[60]

GA-1 is often referred to as the "Amish Syndrome," as the disorder affects only one in fifty thousand births in the general population, but one in five hundred in the Amish population of Pennsylvania.[61]

GA-1 has been misdiagnosed as SBS due to similar signs and symptoms, and a handful of cases have been wrongly prosecuted in the name of abuse. If this and other types of genetic disorders are ruled out, then SBS can be confirmed. This is one of the responsibilities of health-care providers in accurate diagnosis of any medical condition.

NEUROLOGICAL EVALUATIONS OF HEAD INJURY

Below are several examples of neurological tests used when an infant is brought to a hospital emergency room in critical condition. These tests are revised versions of the well-known Glasgow Coma Scale used in adults. Such tests give medical providers an idea of a child's current condition and potential for recovery.

The first scale presented (table 6.1)[62] can be used with children of any age; the second (table 6.2)[63] primarily targets young infants. Both depend on accurate observation of a child's responses to certain standard forms of stimulation. Each response is assigned a numerical value and the combined score is then compared with an expected "normal" score. The lower the total score, and the longer the child remains on that level, the worse the outcome.

TABLE **6.1**   *Pediatric Coma Scale*

Eyes open		*Best motor response*	
spontaneously	4	obeys commands	5
to speech	3	localizes pain	4
to pain	2	flexion to pain	3
not at all	1	extension to pain	2
		none	1

continued

TABLE **6.1**   *(continued)*

Best verbal response			Normal aggregate score	
oriented	5		birth to 6 months	9
words	4		6 to 12 months	11
vocal sounds	3		1 to 2 years	12
cries	2		2 to 5 years	13
none	1		over 5 years	14

$$\mathbf{E + V + M = 3\ to\ 15}\ (\text{less than or equal to 7 defines coma})$$

BEST SCORE[64]

	Good Recovery	Moderate Disability	Severe Disability
6 hours	10	8	6
24 hours	12	10	8
2 to 3 days	14	12	8

TABLE **6.2**   *Revised Infant Glasgow Coma Scale*

Eye opening			Best verbal response	
spontaneous	4		coos and babbles	5
to speech	3		irritable cries	4
to pain	2		cries to pain	3
none	1		moans to pain	2
			none	1

Best motor response

normal spontaneous movement	6
withdraws to touch	5
withdraws to pain	4
abnormal flexion	3
abnormal extension	2
none	1

NOTES

1. Bruce DA. Neurosurgical Aspects of Child Abuse. In: Ludwig S, Kornberg AE, eds. *Child Abuse: A Medical Reference*. 2nd ed. New York: Churchill Livingstone; 1992:117–129.

2. Norman MG, Newman DE, Smialek JE, Horembala EJ. The Postmortem Examination on the Abused Child: Pathological, Radiographic, and Legal Aspects. *Perspec Ped Path* 1984; 8:313–343.

3. Walker ML, Storrs BB, Mayer TA. Head Injuries. In: Mayer TA, ed. *Emergency Management of Pediatric Trauma*. Philadelphia: W.B. Saunders Co.; 1985:272–286.

4. Kleinman P. Head Trauma. In: Kleinman P, ed. *Diagnostic Imaging of Child Abuse*. Baltimore: Williams & Wilkins; 1987:159–199.

5. Harwood-Nash DC. Abuse to the Pediatric Central Nervous System. *Amer J Neuroradiol* 1992; 13:569–575.

6. Raphaely RC, Swedlow DB, Downes JJ, Bruce DA. Management of Severe Pediatric Head Trauma. *Ped Clin NA* 1980; 27:715–727.

7. Bruce DA, Alavi A, Bilaniuk L, et al. Diffuse Cerebral Swelling Following Head Injuries in Children: The Syndrome of Malignant Brain Edema. *J Neurosurg* 1981; 54:170–178.

8. Reynolds EA. Controversies in Caring for the Child with a Head Injury. *Mater Child Nurs* 1992; 17:246–251.

9. Cohen RA, Kaufman RA, Myers PA, Towbin RE. Cranial Computed Tomography in the Abused Child with Head Injury. *AJR* 1986; 146:97–102.

10. Han BK, Towbin RB, Courten-Myers GD, et al. Reversal Sign on CT: Effect of Anoxic/Ischemic Cerebral Injury in Children. *AJR* 1990; 154:361–368.

11. Duhaime AC, Bilaniuk L, Zimmerman R. The "Big Black Brain": Radiographic Changes after Severe Inflicted Injury in Infancy. *J Neurotrauma* 1993; 10 (abstract 1):S59.

12. Johnson DL. Head Injury. In: Eichelberger MR, ed. *Pediatric Trauma Care*. Rockville, MD: Aspen Pub.; 1988:87–99.

13. Vollmer DG, Dacey RG, Jane JA. Craniocerebral Trauma. In: Joynt RJ, Griggs RC, eds. *Clinical Neurology*. Vol. 3. Philadelphia: Lippincott–Raven; 1996:1–71.

14. Whaley LF, Wong DL. The Child with Cerebral Dysfunction. In: Whaley LF, Wong DL, eds. *Nursing Care of Infants and Children*. 3rd ed. St. Louis: Mosby; 1987:1617–1674.

15. Ommaya AK, Hirsch AE. Tolerances for Cerebral Concussion from Head Impact and Whiplash in Primates. *J Biomech* 1971; 4:13–21.

16. Adams JH, Doyle D, Graham DI, et al. Gliding Contusions in Nonmissile Head Injury in Humans. *Arch Pathol Lab Med* 1986; 110:485–488.

17. Case M. Head Injury in Child Abuse. In: Monteleone JA, Brodeur AE, eds. *Child Maltreatment: A Clinical Guide and Reference*. St. Louis: G.W. Medical Pub.; 1994:75–87.

18. Lindenberg R, Freytag E. Morphology of Brain Lesions from Blunt Trauma in Early Infancy. *Arch Path* 1969; 87:298–305.

19. Calder IA, Hill I, Scholtz CL. Primary Brain Trauma in Non-Accidental Injury. *J Clin Path* 1984; 37:1095–1100.

20. Davison AN, Dobbing J. Myelination as a Vulnerable Period in Brain Development. *Brit Med Bull* 1966; 22:40–44.

21. Wilkins B. Head Injury—Abuse or Accident? *Arch Dis Child* 1997; 76:393–397.

22. Gultekin SH, Smith TW. Diffuse Axonal Injury in Craniocerebral Trauma. A Comparative Histologic and Immunohistochemical Study. *Arch Pathol Lab Med* 1994; 118: 168–171.

23. Hymel KP, Faris AB, Parthington MD, Winston KR. Abusive Head Trauma: A Biomechanics-Based Approach. *Child Maltreatment* 1998; 3:116–128.

24. Vowles GH, Scholtz CL, Cameron JM. Diffuse Axonal Injury in Early Infancy. *J Clin Patholog* 1987; 40:185–189.

25. Adams JH, Doyle D, Ford I, et al. Diffuse Axonal Injury in Head Injury: Definition, Diagnosis and Grading. *Histopath* 1989; 15:49–59.

26. Shannon P, Smith CR, Deck J, et al. Axonal Injury and the Neuropathology of Shaken Baby Syndrome. *Acta Neuropathol* 1998; 95:625–631.

27. Schutzman SA, Barnes PD, Mantello M, Scott RM. Epidural Hematomas in Children. *Ann Emer Med* 1993; 22:535–541.

28. Shugerman RP, Paez A, Grossman DC, et al. Epidural Hemorrhage: Is it Abuse? *Pediatrics* 1996; 97:664–668.

29. Ingraham FD, Campbell JB, Cohen J. Extradural Hematoma in Infancy and Childhood. *JAMA* 1949; 140:1010–1013.

30. Beni-Adani L, Flores I, Spektor S, et al. Epidural Hematoma in Infants: A Different Entity? *J Trauma* 1999; 46:306–311.

31. Dhellemmes P, Lejeune JP, Christiaens JL, Combelles G. Traumatic Extradural Hematomas in Infancy and Childhood: Experience with 144 Cases. *J Neurosurg* 1985; 62:861–864.

32. Merten DF, Osborne DRS, Radkowski MA, Leonidas JC. Craniocerebral Trauma in the Child Abuse Syndrome: Radiological Observations. *Pediatr Radiol* 1984; 14:272–277.

33. Zimmerman RA, Bilaniuk LT, Bruce D, et al. Interhemispheric Acute Subdural Hematoma: A Computed Tomographic Manifestation of Child Abuse by Shaking. *Neuroradiology* 1978; 16:39–40.

34. Menkes JH. Perinatal Asphyxia and Trauma. In: Menkes JH, ed. *Textbook of Child Neurology*. 4th ed. Philadelphia: Lea & Febiger; 1990:284–326.

35. Bonnier C, Nassogne MC, Evrard P. Outcome and Prognosis of Whiplash Shaken Infant Syndrome: Late Consequences after a Symptom-Free Interval. *Dev Med Child Neurol* 1995; 37:943–956.

36. Oliver JE. Microcephaly Following Baby Battering and Shaking. *BMJ* 1975; 2:262–264.

37. Monteleone JA, Brodeur AE. Identifying, Interpreting and Reporting Injuries. In: Monteleone JA, Brodeur AE, eds. *Child Maltreatment: A Clinical Guide and Reference*. St. Louis: G.W. Medical Pub.; 1994:1–26.

38. Sklar EML, Quencer RM, Bowen BC, et al. Magnetic Resonance Applications in Cerebral Injury. *Emerg Dept Radiol* 1992; 30:353–365.

39. Aoki N. Extracerebral Fluid Collections in Infancy: Role of Magnetic Resonance Imaging in Differentiation between Subdural Effusion and Subarachnoid Space Enlargement. *J Neurosurg* 1994; 81:20–23.

40. Tsubokawa T, Nakamura S, Satoh K. Effect of Temporary Subdural-Peritoneal Shunt on Subdural Effusion with Subarachnoid Effusion. *Child's Brain* 1984; 11:47–59.

41. Klein DM. Central Nervous System Injuries. In: Ellerstein NS, ed. *Child Abuse and Neglect: A Medical Reference*. New York: Wiley; 1981.

42. Lloyd B. Subdural Haemorrhages in Infants. *BMJ* 1998; 317:1538–1539.

43. Jayawant S, Rawlinson A, Gibbon F, et al. Subdural Haemorrhages in Infants: Population-Based Study. *BMJ* 1998; 317:1558–1561.

44. Duhaime AC, Gennarelli TG, Thibault LE, et al. The Shaken Baby Syndrome: A Clinical, Pathological, and Biomechanical Study. *J Neurosurg* 1987; 66:409–414.

45. Howard MA, Bell BA, Uttley D. The Pathophysiology of Infant Subdural Haematomas. *Brit J Neurosurg* 1993; 7:355–365.

46. Wrightson P. The Shaken Infant Syndrome. *New Zealand Med J* 1995; 108:278.

47. Starling SP, Holden ITR, Jenny C. Abusive Head Trauma: The Relationship of Perpetrators to Their Victims. *Pediatrics* 1995; 95:259–262.

48. Gilliland MGF, Folberg R. Shaken Babies—Some Have No Impact Injuries. *J For Sci* 1994; 41:114–116.

49. Silverman FN, Byrd SE, Fitz CR. Trauma. In: Silverman FN, Kuhn JP, eds. *Caffey's Pediatric X-Ray Diagnosis*. Vol 2. 9th ed. St. Louis: Mosby; 1985:247–257.

50. Lagos JC, Siekert RG. Intracranial Hemorrhage in Infancy and Childhood. *Clin Peds* 1969; 8:90–97.

51. Duhaime AC, Christian C, Armonda R, et al. Disappearing Subdural Hematomas in Children. *Ped Neurosurg* 1996; 25:116–122.

52. Sato YS, Yuh WTC, Smith WL, et al. Head Injury in Child Abuse: Evaluation with MR Imaging. *Radiology* 1989; 173:653–657.

53. Till K. Subdural Hematoma and Effusion in Infancy. *BMJ* 1968; 2:400–402.

54. Sinal SH, Ball MR. Head Trauma Due to Child Abuse: Serial Computerized Tomography in Diagnosis and Management. *South Med J* 1987; 80:1505–1512.

55. Hamlin H. Subgaleal Hematoma Caused by Hairpull. *JAMA* 1968; 205:314.

56. Hanigan WC, Peterson RA, Njus G. Tin Ear Syndrome: Rotational Acceleration in Pediatric Head Injuries. *Pediatrics* 1987; 80:618–622.

57. Nuss R, Manco-Johnson M. Hemostasis in Ehlers-Danlos Syndrome. *Clin Peds* 1995; 34:552–556.

58. Menkes JH. Metabolic Diseases of the Nervous System. In: Menkes JH, ed. *Textbook of Child Neurology*. 4th ed. Philadelphia: Lea & Febiger; 1990:56–57.

59. Hoffman GF, Naughten ER. Abuse or Metabolic Disorder? (letter). *Arch Dis Child* 1998; 78:399.

60. Baric I, Zschocke J, Christensen E, et al. Diagnosis and Management of Glutaric Aciduria Type 1. *J Inher Metab Dis* 1998; 21:326–340.

61. Childs ND. Genetic Disorder Culprit in Some Shaken Baby Cases. *Ped News* 1998; 32:1.

62. Simpson P, Reilly D. Pediatric Coma Scale (letter). *Lancet* 1982; 2:450.

63. Raimondi AJ, Hirschauer J. Head Injury in the Infant and Toddler. *Child's Brain* 1984; 11:12–35.

64. Davis RJ, Dean M, Goldberg AL, et al. Head and Spinal Cord Injury. In: Rogers MC, ed. *Textbook of Pediatric Intensive Care*. Vol. 1. Baltimore: Williams & Wilkins; 1987: 649–699.

CHAPTER SEVEN

History of Intracranial Injuries and Shaken Baby Syndrome

BESIDES CAFFEY'S CLASSIC 1946 DESCRIPTION of subdural hematoma in infants, many other articles have been written over the years detailing pediatric cases of intracranial injury. The writers of these articles have left both an interesting history and an important legacy in terms of the evolution of pediatric neurosurgery. This body of work is summarized below.

THE EARLY YEARS

In 1930, David Sherwood of the Infants and Children's Hospital in Boston detailed and summarized an unfortunate condition that occurred too frequently in infancy—chronic subdural hematoma.[1] He outlined cases he had found while researching the topic and stated that the condition caused "enlargement of the head [hydrocephalus], vomiting, irritability, hemorrhages in the eyegrounds [retinal hemorrhaging], downward displacement of the eyes [setting-sun sign] and symptoms of the central nervous system." He reviewed many citations from Germany that appeared during the first two decades of the 1900s. The first article to describe the injuries seen in SBS was written in 1904.[2] The author was perplexed at the findings of a seven-month-old with "pachymeningitis" [subdural hematoma], retinal hemorrhaging, bulging fontanelle, and spasticity. Syphilis, regularly included in differential diagnoses of the time, was ruled out. No reason was given for the infant's condition. All the other German authors whose work was reviewed described the combination of subdural hematoma and retinal hemorrhaging in infancy—without apparent cause.

Sherwood highlighted the 1914 work of British physician Wilfred Trotter, who wrote in the *British Journal of Surgery* that trauma was always the cause of subdural hematoma, with the accurate description of the source of the bleeding being "the cerebral veins that pass from the brain to the tributaries of the superior longitudinal sinus through the dura."[3] Sherwood also identified the first American to call attention to subdural hematomas in infants as Gordon, who reported two cases, one of whom also had retinal hemorrhaging, in his 1914 article.[4]

Sherwood detailed nine of his own cases in this groundbreaking paper. He agreed with Trotter's theory that trauma was directly responsible for "many cases," though histories of trauma were not forthcoming from caretakers. The nine infants described came from varying backgrounds. Five of the nine came from "dubious home conditions," being cared for in foster homes or by charitable institutions. Seven of the nine infants received ophthalmologic checks during examination, and 57 percent had retinal hemorrhaging. The cases are summarized as follows:

Case 1

E.F., a four-month-old female, admitted with irritability and convulsions. Mother had a positive Wassermann reaction for syphilis, father and E.F. were negative. Bilateral subdural hematomas were tapped. Large retinal hemorrhages were found. Two weeks after discharge, E.F. had a bloody lumbar tap at another hospital. Seven months after discharge, no symptoms were noted.

Case 2

C.R., an eleven-month-old male, admitted with loss of weight and a three-week course of vomiting. Unmarried twenty-three-year-old mother; father living and well. C.R. boarded with a foster mother. Three weeks prior to admission, convulsions were noted. Upon exam, bilateral subdural hematomas tapped and right optic disk blurred about the margins. C.R. gained weight in the hospital and continued to have slightly bloody subdural taps one month after discharge.

Case 3

C.E., a seven-month-old male, admitted with hydrocephalus and convulsions. Described by mother as "sick and colicky." Three weeks prior to admission, a ten-minute convulsion occurred. Spread cranial sutures, subarachnoid and subdural hematomas, and marked retinal hemorrhages with disk atrophy were noted soon after admission. After two months in the hospital, C.E. was discharged. At age two years, his development was normal, though he"tired rather easily."

Case 4

R.M., a seven-month-old male, was admitted with convulsions. He was cared for by a charitable institution. Upon admission, R.M. was semicomatose and spastic. Bilateral subdural hematomas and retinal hemorrhaging were found. He remained hospitalized for two months and gained four pounds. As there was some question about impaired vision, he was sent to the Nursery for Blind Babies. Four years after discharge, he "was living in an institution for feeble-minded children."

Case 5

E.B., a nine-month-old female, was admitted with hydrocephalus and recurrent convulsions beginning two months prior. She was being cared for as a ward of the state, and "her father knew little about the course of her illness." Examination showed retinal hemorrhaging with disk atrophy, spread cranial sutures, bilateral subdural hematomas, and a healing radial fracture. E.B. was discharged one month later. At age fifteen months, she showed retarded development and strabismus.

Case 6

A.A., a ten-month-old male, was admitted with hydrocephalus and fever. The mother stated that she did not have syphilis, but A.A. did. He was living with a foster mother. Twice-a-week projectile vomiting had started at age five months and continued to age eight months. Two weeks prior to admission, A.A. became irritable and refused food. Upon examination, he was pale and comatose, with clubbing of the toes. Ophthalmological exam was normal. Wassermann reaction for syphilis was positive, and cultures showed B. coli. Bilateral subdural hematomas were tapped. A.A. died forty-eight hours after admission, with a temperature of 105 degrees F at the time of death. Autopsy was performed.

Case 7

J.S., an eleven-month-old male, was admitted with convulsions. His biological mother was dead, and he was cared for by a foster mother. Seizures before admission had caused a rise in temperature, as high as 103 degrees F. Examination of the eyes revealed pallor of the disks, but no hemorrhages. J.S. had a left subdural hematoma. He was readmitted two more times over the next nine months, with recurrent subdural hematomas. At age two years, he showed retarded development.

Case 8

C.G., a ten-month-old female, was admitted with vomiting and "loss of weight." She had an admission weight of thirteen pounds, eleven ounces, down from nineteen pounds, five ounces six weeks earlier. Eye exam was not performed. Her anterior fontanelle was slightly bulging, and a lumbar puncture *showed bloody fluid. A right subdural hematoma was identified as well. At age three years, she was seen as an outpatient and had normal development.*

Case 9

N.R., a one-month-old female, was admitted to the private ward with "twitch-ing" and a history of vomiting. Examination showed a bulging fontanelle, generalized convulsions, and eyes displaced downward. She had a history of a heart murmur. A lumbar puncture showed bloody fluid, and bilateral subdural hematomas were found. Her eyes were not examined. N.R.'s family requested a discharge two days after admission. Follow-up at age five months revealed that she was developing normally.

In none of these cases was trauma identified, nor was the possibility explored at any depth. The combinations of injuries indicate many early cases of SBS that were not diagnosed as abuse. Sherwood's contribution to the study of subdural hematoma in infants is significant, as he paved the way for medical providers to question such findings.

Another early review of intracranial bleeding in infants was by Peet and Kahn in 1932.[5] An early name for subdural hematoma was pachymeningitis hemor-rhagica, and this term was used as a formal diagnosis in many of the nine cases the authors presented. The infants ranged in age from three to thirteen months. All had subdural hematoma and associated symptoms, such as vomiting, lethargy, or convulsions, as well as ophthalmological changes, including "diffuse choroiditis," "neuroretinitis with edema of the nerve heads," "large hemorrhages," "bilateral choked disks," "early optic atrophy," and "optic pallor." Most of the children were "illegitimate," and one infant was "syphilitic" by a positive Wassermann test.

The process for diagnosis and treatment was outlined. The physicians often used "percussion," tapping on the head of a patient to hear either a dull or tym-panic resonance. Diagnosis was confirmed once the fontanelle was "pierced." Colorless ventricular fluid indicated hydrocephalus; straw-colored fluid or blood meant acute or chronic subdural hematoma.

Craniotomies were the surgical procedure of choice to evacuate the collec-tions of blood. Peet and Kahn referred to this process as making an "osteopathic flap." Of these cases, five of the nine infants died postoperatively. In many, respi-ration suddenly ceased, but the "pulse could be felt for several minutes." In those days, resuscitation and critical care were primitive, to say the least.

THE 1940s

One of the most thorough records of subdural hematoma in infancy was pub-lished in the *Journal of Pediatrics* in 1944.[6] Ingraham and Matson featured actual admission photographs of about fifteen cases of infants brought to their hospital with subdural hematomas and other physical problems. Some appeared normal; others had experienced obvious abuse and neglect, with bruises, signs of malnu-trition, swollen fontanelle, or hydrocephalus.

Ninety-eight infants who had been brought to Children's Hospital in Boston in the previous six years were studied. Eleven had skull fractures, twenty-one showed retinal hemorrhaging (though not all infants' eyes may have been checked), and fifty-five were noted to have convulsions. Causative agents, such as birth trauma, were highlighted. Twenty-eight children were known to have experienced "severe trauma at birth," yet subdural hematomas were not noted at the time of birth. The authors described falls from beds or tables as a reason for the development of subdural hematoma in infants. They inaccurately stated: "It is well known that the head injury which gives rise to subdural hematoma need not be a severe one. The fact that only eleven of these ninety-eight patients had skull fractures visible by x-ray is evidence of this fact."

Some of the children had symptoms for weeks or months before being brought to the hospital. Fifty-seven of the infants were tracked for follow-up (nine had died upon admission or postoperatively). Of these, 25 percent were mentally retarded or "grossly deficient"; the others were developing normally and were asymptomatic.

This was a rare documentation of abused and shaken children, an issue only hinted at in the following suggestion by the authors:

> It seems justifiable to us to conclude that some form of trauma is practically a constant etiologic factor. In malnourished and diseased infants it may take less injury to produce this lesion, and in poor economic surroundings the exposure rate to adequate trauma is undoubtedly higher, but the common denominator probably remains the same. We should like to emphasize again, however, the inadequacy of a history of trauma should never influence the diagnosis against subdural hematoma.

Interestingly, in June 1947, an article by Govan and Walsh describing subdural hematoma in infants and adults appeared in an ophthalmology journal.[7] Their purpose was to compare the way intracranial bleeding differently affects the brains of infants and adults. Little did they realize they were detailing many cases of SBS. Much of the information that was outlined is useful even today. For example, they noted that convulsions due to the presence of subdural hematoma were found in 91 percent of infant patients and only 4 percent of adults. Vomiting occurred in half the infants and approximately one-third of the adults, but 50 percent of the infants studied had retinal hemorrhaging, compared with 0.6 percent of the adults. This was an obvious finding by today's standards, but the authors found it difficult to explain: "It is generally believed that subhyaloid bleeding is venous in origin, but the exact mechanism responsible for the production of pre-retinal hemorrhage is unknown."

F. D. Ingraham continued his studies on the infant brain and joined forces with two other physicians, Campbell and Cohen, in 1949 to study epidural hematoma.[8] In those years, such intracranial findings were regularly called extradural hematomas, a name that continued throughout the 1980s. These authors were the first to fully explain the details of this rare condition occurring in infants and children. They explained the need for "prompt neurosurgical treatment" to reduce the mortality of such cases. Symptoms accompanying epidural hematoma were detailed and included progression of drowsiness to stupor or coma, positive Babinski's reflex (see glossary), swelling of the scalp at or near the site of the injury, hemiparesis, and dilation of the pupil on the side of the lesion. Skull fractures were commonly found, as a blow to the head was considered the mechanism "chiefly responsible" for such hematomas. The authors also discussed the physiology of the infant cranium and its potential for expandability, and outlined the surgical procedure for removing the hematoma via burr hole or craniotomy.

That same year, Elvidge and Jackson produced a comprehensive review of fifty-four cases of "subdural hematoma and effusion" in infants.[9] They divided this group into four categories: definite birth injuries, probable birth injuries, postnatal head injuries, and unclassified. From today's vantage point, only the first category seemed likely to substantiate a viable reason for the presence of intracranial injury. All other categories appear questionable.

Category two included infants (average age five months) with symptoms such as hydrocephalus, seizures, spasticity, poor feeding, respiratory difficulties, and other neurological abnormalities. Within this group, there was a 19 percent mortality rate. The authors commented, "The fact that the symptomatology of some of the infants in this group had been present since birth would most likely indicate that they had sustained a cerebral injury at birth, in spite of the absence of a history of a difficult labor or delivery."

Category three included nine infants (average age fourteen months) "whose complaints definitely followed a severe postnatal head injury." Six infants were brought to the hospital unconscious, the other three several weeks after their head injury. Thirty percent had skull fractures, and all had subdural collections. There was a 78 percent mortality rate.

Finally, the unclassified category four was made up of ten infants (average age twelve months) who were brought to the hospital as chronically ill but who had experienced normal birth. This stumped the authors, but they provided an implicit consideration: "Perhaps the reason for the existence of this etiologic group is the lack of pertinent facts obtained in the history from the parents." Eight of the infants had either hydrocephalus or seizures. Another finding in 30 percent of this group was papilledema, swelling of the optic nerve area. The delay in seeking medical attention for the onset of symptoms was rather telling—two days to sixteen months (a six-month average). There was a 20 percent mortality rate, due to complications during or after operation. Of the surviving infants, four were followed over a several-year period, and all were mentally retarded.

Elvidge and Jackson provided an important glance at the treatment and management possibilities for head-injured infants, though they failed to consider abuse as a factor in the production of such injuries. They instead centered on "the stress and strain of the fetal head" during the molding of birth as the culprit for subdural effusion.

THE 1950s

In 1950, Pickles described his experience with cerebral edema ("acute focal edema of the brain") in infants and children.[10] His presentation of eight cases of pediatric head injury (ages one to twelve years) substantiated his belief that many cases with "middle meningeal hemorrhage" and the "rapid disappearance of these indications" are actually cases of cerebral edema. Because edema is a significant finding in cases of SBS, this article was an important link to the general understanding of head injury and how the brain responds to swelling caused by edema.

Pneumoencephalography was one of many invasive procedures early diagnosticians used to enhance their view of head radiographs. This process filled a patient's cranium with air by way of the spinal column. Air could be seen on a radiograph, and the findings would show the medical provider the extent of bleeding or brain alteration. It was often a dangerous procedure and was widely used. Many physicians felt that the use of pneumoencephalography might actually *cause* subdural hematoma in infants.[11] Surgeons often considered "dry taps" to indicate that no subdural hematoma was present, when actually infants suffering from abusive head trauma had collections of blood in the process of developing.

Another procedure believed to cause subdural hematoma was the treatment of hydrocephalus.[12] If a cranium was drained too quickly of cerebrospinal fluid, via shunts or during craniotomy, many surgeons thought the sagittal sinus and other veins would pull away from the dura and cause a subdural hematoma. Guthkelch reported that this happened mostly during the time of uncontrolled drainage.[13] He also stated that Holter's and Pudenz's valved systems put an end to this problem. Low-pressure shunts could even cause young brains to simply fold up, which would leave a large subdural space into which cerebrospinal fluid would escape.

Intracranial cysts and other manifestations develop in infants, yet "trauma" as a cause for bulging fontanelle, hydrocephalus, and other anomalies was never addressed in the majority of early cases. Often, science was in the forefront of a clinician's mind, rather than social issues. Writers in medical journals even went so far as to state such things as the following (emphasis added): "The present study is concerned with the mechanisms responsible for the persistent accumulation of fluid in a posttraumatic subdural effusion and *not with its initial formation*."[14] One case presented by Rabe and associates was a five-month-old boy with "apnea and paleness," multiple fractures, and subdural hematoma who was initially diagnosed with osteogenesis imperfecta but later identified as a victim of trauma.

At a New York City clinical conference in 1956, Ransohoff detailed his procedure for the management of chronic subdural hematoma in infants.[15] He described the use of shunting to drain large subdural collections. In a step-by-step process, he showed how the majority of infants with chronic subdural hematomas had successful outcomes. Two ends of his T shunt went into the subdural spaces, and the other end was placed in the pleural cavity of the lungs. He explained that sometimes the tubing became collapsed or infected. There was no monitoring system in place for infants with shunts, since Ransohoff believed they would eventually fall out as the brain grew in size. He concluded his presentation at the conference with a statement about the cause of the hematoma: "Whether it occurs at birth or shortly after birth, I cannot decide. The history of trauma has not been available in all instances. I also don't know whether prematurity is a factor."

THE 1960s

The 1960s brought more detailed studies of the brains of both infants and adults in relation to specific types of trauma: blunt and whiplash.

The blunt type of trauma was first described by Lindenberg and Freytag.[16] They coined the term "contusional tearing" to explain the injuries found in white matter tearing of the brain after impact. Sixteen infants were autopsied following death from "head injury," falls, and maltreatment. All were twelve months old and younger. The authors illustrated the character of the tears as "sharply outlined, slit-like, or irregularly shaped clefts," found occasionally beneath the site of impact. Fresh tears contained small amounts of blood, whereas older tears had a brownish stains on their walls. "In some cases, they contained a small amount of fresh blood from a second injury suffered shortly before death." These authors also were the first to describe what is known today as diffuse axonal injury, which they referred to as "diffuse astrocytic fibrosis." This article was an important addition to the greater understanding of what the pediatric brain experiences in the aftermath of traumatic events, such as shaking.

Yashon and colleagues looked at the long-term effects in infants with "traumatic" subdural hematoma.[17] Of ninety-two patients with such hematomas, they reported a 27 percent fatality rate, 13 percent living but "unable to function adequately, and 60 percent living "socially acceptable" lives. Of the "well" group, 91 percent had residual effects from their injuries, such as mild hemiparesis or occasional seizures. The others in this group had moderate hemiparesis, frequent seizures, or loss of visual acuity. The "fair" group had some amount of "mental deficiency" or neurological deficit.

One of the first instances of the term "battered baby" in the neurological literature was in 1964, when O'Doherty wrote several paragraphs in *Developmental Medicine and Child Neurology* about physically abused children with subdural hematomas.[18] He felt that retinal hemorrhaging was an important diagnostic sign of subdural hematoma, as such ocular abnormalities were present in nearly 90 percent of the infants that he saw. He unknowingly saw a great deal of shaken infants.

For the management of chronic subdural hematoma, a plethora of interventions were being utilized by the late 1960s, including subdural-pleural, subdural-peritoneal, and subdural-jugular shunting. This was an important historical portrayal of accepting disability due to the long-term effects of head injury.

Prior to the advent of the technological advances in diagnostic imaging, early studies included the use of radioactive mercury. Hawkes reported the use of the mercury 203 brain scan in infants and children to detect intracranial bleeding.[19] A less toxic method of understanding traumatic brain injuries was to become available the following decade, with the creation of the CT scan.

In 1968, Rabe and colleagues studied the prognosis of sixty-two infants with subdural hematomas. In the article, they compared which method fared better as treatment.[20] Repeated subdural taps were found to be slightly more efficacious over burr holes and craniotomy in order for study infants to be placed in an "excellent" category at follow-up.

Ommaya and Yarnell detailed whiplash injuries in adults during this same time, giving future researchers and medical providers an idea of what an infant may experience during an incident of shaking.[21] Here, neurosurgery combined forces with the field of biomechanics. They reviewed two cases of nonimpact vehicular whiplash in adults, which brought on subdural hematomas. Rotational effect, velocity, and acceleration were all described as physical components making up the foundation for such brain injury caused by whiplash—all aspects of traumatic brain injury that foreshadowed the ones later studied in relation to SBS.

THE 1970s

The 1970s began with standard features of evaluating intracranial trauma. Subdural taps, burr holes, craniotomies, and shunting made up the listing of surgical interventions. Carotid arteriogram, or angiography, was included in the brief listing of diagnostic interventions.[22] And then came the new technology of computed tomography (CT), which now provided scientists and radiologists with a new view of the brain. Various processes were now able to be more completely studied and understood.

The clinical picture of the subdural hematoma was studied for the first time in this new way, without dramatic intervention (surgery) or autopsy. In a landmark article describing CT imaging, Scotti and colleagues showed that density patterns in CT scans were important factors to help establish the chronology of brain injuries.[23] New terms were used: hyperdense, referring to hematomas with a higher attenuation than the brain; isodense, hematomas with the same attenuation as the brain; and hypodense, hematomas with a lower attenuation than the brain. Though archaic by today's standards, the initial technology of CT was the most accurate way of determining the age of a subdural hematoma and for its treatment and management.

THE 1980s

In light of this new technology and the subsequent improvements to the diagnostic images, the dawn of magnetic resonance imaging (MRI) brought significant changes to the way pediatric medicine and neurosurgery were performed throughout the 1980s and beyond.

As the art of CT scanning advanced, Bruce and associates showed in 1981 what Pickles could only have imagined in 1950.[24] Cerebral edema was now more thoroughly understood, and its management more secure. The authors believed that hyperemia, and not edema, was the cause of cerebral swelling following acceleration–deceleration injury of the brain. Through CT scanning, they were able to follow the progression of the shape, size, and position of the brain's ventricular system.

Throughout the 1980s, biomechanical research on head injury was continued, as begun by Ommaya and associates in the 1960s. Gennarelli and Thibault focused their efforts on the biomechanics of subdural hematoma.[25] They compared clinical cases of subdural hematoma with their own experimental observations of laboratory primates fitted into helmets attached to a pneumatic actuator. The head of the monkeys were rotated sixty degrees between five and twenty-five milliseconds. They studied the results of cerebral concussion, "diffuse brain injury," and acute subdural hematoma (ASDH). They confirmed that sagittal veins were subject to tensile strains and will rupture, as the brain and skull moved in different directions during angular acceleration. They also decided that "nothing need strike the head in order for ASDH to occur." The authors concluded that the formation of a subdural hematoma in the human brain was dependent upon three factors: magnitude of acceleration; rate of acceleration onset; and duration of the acceleration. Granted, studies like this were focused on the adult brain, but they were extremely important nonetheless in their application to pediatric head injury.

Adams and associates continued their research into the deep recesses of the brain and contributed greatly to the medical field's understanding of the concept of diffuse axonal injury (DAI).[26] They defined such an injury as "diffuse damage to the axons in the cerebral hemispheres, in the corpus callosum, in the brain stem, and sometimes also in the cerebellum resulting from a head injury." They developed a ranking system in the study of DAI based on its location and severity; for example, focal lesions in the corpus callosum are grade 2. The authors explained that in cases where DAI was present, there was often poor prognosis. Death could occur within days to weeks. Many other individuals existed in comas or vegetative states. They believed that the classic retraction balls (axonal swelling) seen in cases of DAI required approximately twelve to eighteen hours to develop.

They reported their conclusions on the mechanism of injury in cases of DAI, as a substantial amount of force was required for the condition to occur. In doing so, they made a case for today's findings in SBS injuries:

> We have still to encounter a case of diffuse axonal injury in anyone who has simply fallen from his or her own height . . . this type is insufficient to produce the severe shear and tensile strains in the brain required to produce axonal disruption. Thus, if Diffuse Axonal Injury is found in a patient who appears to have died as a result of such a fall, the pathologist must be alerted to the fact that the original injury must have been much more severe, e.g., as a result of an assault when the head may have been forcibly propelled onto the ground or a solid wall.

THE 1990s

Two studies in the early 1990s compared abusive and accidental head injury cases. These were critical, because they helped in the emergency room, as well as the courtroom, to more accurately identify and treat children in abusive environments and ultimately help protect them from further injury.

In 1992, Duhaime and associates reported on the findings of one hundred head-injured children under the age of two years.[27] This was the first effort on the part of medical personnel to actively identify head-injured children as either abused or accidental cases through the use of a profile questionnaire, which was administered when a child was admitted to the hospital or entered the study. Parents, caretakers, and other witnesses were interviewed and police records and emergency medical technician reports were also used. The profile included questions such as the following: "What time did the accident occur?" "Was the accident witnessed?" "What did the baby do immediately after the accident?" and "Was the baby manipulated in any way after the accident (shaking, resuscitation, etc.)?" The majority of the children studied had skull fractures. Most of the injuries sustained were reportedly due to falls, and 24 percent of the cases were "inflicted," with a 4 percent death rate. The authors confirmed the hypothesis that simple falls (less than four feet) do not produce significant brain injury, as can falls from greater heights. This was an important conclusion, as parents or caretakers who bring a child to a hospital emergency room with a brain injury often report a low-height fall. All head-injured children with an inconsistent history by the parent or caretaker upon admission were found to have inflicted injuries. Both intracranial and retinal hemorrhaging were significant findings in the inflicted group only. The latter was found in three cases: a motor vehicle accident, a fatal three-story fall, and a (questionable) fall down stairs in a walker. The authors reiterated their view that impact is required not only to sustain head injury, but also to be considered SBS.

Another team of researchers also found that an inconsistent history given by a child's parent or caretaker was pathognomonic for abuse cases.[28] To the intracranial injury findings, Goldstein and colleagues added the combination of physical findings on examination and the presence of retinal hemorrhaging. Any two of these three diagnoses were representative of physical abuse. The Glasgow Coma Scale was administered to all cases, and the severity of neurological injury was worse in the group with inflicted injuries. Other significant findings that separated the inflicted from the accidental group included subdural hematoma (especially interhemispheric) and blindness as a result of the injuries.

The topic of epidural hematoma, originally studied by Ingraham in the late 1940s, was further examined in the 1990s by several authors in regard to its association with child abuse injuries. In 1993, Schutzman and her colleagues examined fifty-three children diagnosed with traumatic epidural hematoma.[29] They found that twenty-four of these children had sustained this injury in falls less than five feet. Forty percent were alert and then had "neurologic deterioration before surgery," which is common in this type of injury. Skull fractures were found in 68 percent of the children, another common finding. The team emphasized that although epidural hematomas are rare (3 percent of all pediatric head trauma), they are "critical to identify because they are life-threatening and readily treated surgically."

Shugerman and his group concurred with Schutzman's findings, though they added a comparison twist: child abuse injuries.[30] They found a dramatic difference when comparing subdural hematoma and epidural hematoma in children. Of ninety-three head-injured children, abuse was diagnosed in 47 percent of the children with subdural hematomas and in 6 percent of those with epidural hematomas. This group reviewed the physiology of both types of intracranial injury. Epidural hematoma occurred from linear impact injuries. In an abrupt deceleration, between the skull and a hard surface, "the arteries and veins that are adherent to and tightly encased in the potential space between the skull and the dura may be sheared. The bleeding that results accumulates as an EDH." Subdural hematoma, on the other hand, was caused from the shearing effects of rotational acceleration–deceleration of shaking, twisting blows to the head, and motor vehicle accidents. "Such forces result in disconjugate motion of the brain and skull."

In 1996, Sargent and associates wrote an article in the *Journal of Forensic Sciences* about a concept that was embraced by the defense team at the au pair trial in Boston the following year.[31] The authors gave the "rebleed theory" as an explanation for the finding of recurrent subdural hematomas on CT scans. The basis for this theory was that a minor injury, as from a slight hit on the head or a fall to the floor, might reinjure an old collection of intracranial blood (the rebleed) and cause the brain to swell. The authors believed that different densities of blood seen on a head CT scan signified different stages of bleeding, one of these being a rebleed (or hyperacute hematoma): "Rebleeding within a chronic subdural hematoma is thought to involve the tearing of pathologically fragile neovascular structures within the organizing hematoma." The problem with actual rebleed cases ultimately is that children do not suffer a catastrophic injury, get better without anyone observing that there is a problem, suffer another slight injury, and then rapidly decline. In the Boston au pair case of 1997, this issue was brought to light. The Woodward defense team tried to use the rebleed theory because of a finding at Matthew Eappen's autopsy, which made the pathologist consider that the infant's intracranial bleeding was not new. Many physicians across the country signed a letter to the editor of *USA Today* and *Pediatrics*, stating that the concept was "inaccurate, contrary to vast clinical experience and unsupported by any published literature."[32]

Another boost to the clinical understanding of SBS, and legal recourse afterward, was a 1997 article by Willman and colleagues that discussed the premise of timing in fatal inflicted injuries.[33] Often, in abusive head trauma cases, defense teams contend that their client could not have been the perpetrator, as such a head injury could have happened at any time during the day, and that the child's parents may even have been the abusers. The writers of this article evaluated ninety-five children with traumatic fatal head injuries, both accidental and nonaccidental. They found only one case of a "lucid interval" prior to death, in an eleven-year-old boy. All the other children had no lucid moments in any way, especially in cases of subarachnoid or subdural hemorrhage. Cerebral edema was found to have occurred as quickly as one hour after an injury. The presence of edema using head CT scans was not useful as a determinant for identifying the timing of an injury.

Their conclusions will help medical and legal personnel decide whether the histories given in SBS cases are accurate or false: "Except in cases of epidural hematomas, the time of injury in a fatal head injury case can be restricted to after the last confirmed period of normal consciousness for the child."

RECENT STUDY

In the March 2000 edition of the journal *Pediatrics*, Morris and associates reviewed nine cases of infants who had subdural hematomas but no other injuries, such as retinal hemorrhaging, fractures, or bruising.[34] They found that such a finding alone may be difficult for child protection workers. Thorough review of past medical records, prompt investigation by law enforcement officials, and coordination by a multidisciplinary child-protection team was imperative to help bring case resolution. The authors concluded that infants with cerebral trauma in the absence of severe accidental trauma have likely sustained inflicted trauma, and child abuse investigation should be quickly initiated.

CONCLUSIONS

Research on the pediatric aspects of intracranial trauma has improved knowledge considerably over the past one hundred years. Studies continue in this specialized field to determine not only the functionality of the pediatric brain, but also the recovery potential. This type of research is essential to the lives of survivors of SBS and their families. In fact, ongoing research can lead to lifesaving techniques for shaken children not expected to live. Understanding the complexities of the pediatric brain is essential to the well-being of all children.

NOTES

1. Sherwood D. Chronic Subdural Hematoma in Infants. *Amer J Dis Child* 1930; 39: 980–1021.

2. Finkelstein. *Berl klin Wchnschr* 1904; 41:403.

3. Trotter W. *Brit J Surg* 1914; 2:271.

4. Gordon A. *J Nerv and Ment Dis* 1914; 41:383.

5. Peet MM, Kahn EA. Subdural Hematoma in Infants. *JAMA* 1932; 98:1851–1856.

6. Ingraham FD, Matson DD. Subdural Hematoma in Infancy. *J Peds* 1944:24:1–37.

7. Govan CD, Walsh FB. Symptomatology of Subdural Hematoma in Infants and Adults. *Arch Ophthal* 1947; 37:701–715.

8. Ingraham FD, Campbell JB, Cohen J. Extradural Hematoma in Infancy and Childhood. *JAMA* 1949; 140:1010–1013.

9. Elvidge AR, Jackson IJ. Subdural Hematoma and Effusion in Infants. *Am J Dis Child* 1949; 78:635–657.

10. Pickles W. Acute General Edema of the Brain in Children with Head Injuries. *NEJM* 1950; 242:607–611.

11. Smith HV, Crothers B. Subdural Fluid as a Consequence of Pneumoencephalography. *Pediatrics* 1950; 5:375–389.

12. Anderson FM. Subdural Hematoma, a Complication of Operation for Hydrocephalus. *Pediatrics* 1952; 10:11–17.

13. Guthkelch AN. Personal communication, December 18, 1998.

14. Rabe EF, Flynn RE, Dodge PR. A Study of Subdural Effusions in an Infant: With Particular Reference to the Mechanisms of Their Persistence. *Neurol* 1962; 12:79–92.

15. Ransohoff J. Chronic Subdural Hematoma Treated by Subdural-Pleural Shunt. *Pediatrics* 1957; 41:561–564.

16. Lindenberg R, Freytag E. Morphology of Brain Lesions from Blunt Trauma in Early Infancy. *Arch Path* 1969; 87:298–305.

17. Yashon D, Jane JA, White RJ, Sugar O. Traumatic Subdural Hematoma of Infancy. *Arch Neurol* 1968; 18:370–377.

18. O'Doherty NJ. Subdural Haematoma in Battered Babies. *Devel Med & Child Neuro* 1964; 6:192–193.

19. Hawkes CD. Craniocerebral Trauma in Infancy and Childhood. *Clin Neurosurg* 1964; 11:66–75.

20. Rabe EF, Flynn RE, Dodge PR. Subdural Collections of Fluids in Infants and Children: A Study of 62 Patients with Special Reference to Factors Influencing Prognosis and the Efficacy of Various Forms of Therapy. *Neurology* 1968; 18:559–570.

21. Ommaya AK, Yarnell P. Subdural Hematoma after Whiplash Injury. *Lancet* 1969; 2: 237–239.

22. James HE, Schut L. The Neurosurgeon and the Battered Child. *Surg Neurol* 1974; 2: 415–418.

23. Scotti G, Terbrugge K, Melancon D, Belanger G. Evaluation of the Age of Subdural Hematomas by Computerized Tomography. *J Neurosurg* 1977; 47:311–315.

24. Bruce DA, Alavi A, Bilaniuk L, et al. Diffuse Cerebral Swelling following Head Injuries in Children: The Syndrome of Malignant Brain Edema. *J Neurosurg* 1981; 54:170–178.

25. Gennarelli TA, Thibault LE. Biomechanics of Acute Subdural Hematoma. *J Trauma* 1982; 22:680–686.

26. Adams JH, Doyle D, Ford I, et al. Diffuse Axonal Injury in Head Injury: Definition, Diagnosis and Grading. *Histopath* 1989; 15:49–59.

27. Duhaime AC, Alario AJ, Lewander WJ, et al. Head Injury in Very Young Children: Mechanisms, Injury Types and Ophthalmologic Findings in 100 Hospitalized Patients Younger than 2 Years of Age. *Pediatrics* 1992; 90:179–185.

28. Goldstein B, Kelly MM, Bruton D, Cox C. Inflicted versus Accidental Head Injury in Critically Injured Children. *Crit Care Med* 1993; 21:1328–1332.

29. Schutzman SA, Barnes PD, Mantello M, Scott RM. Epidural Hematomas in Children. *Ann Emer Med* 1993; 22:535–541.

30. Shugerman RP, Paez A, Grossman DC, et al. Epidural Hemorrhage: Is it Abuse? *Pediatrics* 1996; 97:664–668.

31. Sargent S, Kennedy JG, Kaplan JA. Hyperacute Subdural Hematoma: CT Mimic of Recurrent Episodes of Bleeding in the Setting of Child Abuse. *J Foren Sci* 1996; 41:314–316.

32. Chadwick DL, et al. Shaken Baby Syndrome: A Forensic Pediatric Response (letter). *Pediatrics* 1997; 101:322–323.

33. Willman KY, Bank DE, Senac M, Chadwick DL. Restricting the Time of Injury in Fatal Inflicted Head Injuries. *Child Abuse & Neglect* 1997; 21:929–940.

34. Morris M, Smith S, Cressman J, Ancheta J. Evaluation of Infants with Subdural Hematoma Who Lack External Evidence of Abuse. *Pediatrics* 2000; 105:549–553.

CHAPTER EIGHT

✧ ✧ ✧

Ocular Injuries

JAMES PEINKOFER and ALEX V. LEVIN, MD

E YE INJURIES DUE TO ABUSE in infants have been well recognized in the medical literature over the past three decades. Caffey originally combined
intracranial and intraocular manifestations into the first complete description of SBS.[1,2] However, his description of retinal hemorrhages in infants was not
new. Earlier authors had made the association of eye trauma relating to Battered
Child Syndrome and other variants of abuse (discussed in chapter 9), some of
which were clearly SBS before Caffey's landmark characterization.[3,4]

As in other types of physical child abuse, physicians confronted with ocular
injuries, such as retinal hemorrhages, in an infant need to rule out other diagnoses, such as birth trauma, leukemia, and bleeding disorders. When ocular
injuries are coupled with intracranial trauma and fractures, child abuse becomes
evident. A discrepancy between ocular findings and a caretaker's history of the
injuries is a particularly strong indicator of abuse.[5]

Various types of intraocular injuries may occur when an infant is shaken,
though the most outstanding is retinal hemorrhaging (RH). The mechanism that
causes RH is becoming better understood. Originally, it was thought that pressure
from a perpetrator's hand around the thorax of an infant during shaking increased the venous return (return of blood) to the infant's head, thus causing
RH.[6] Increased intracranial pressure (ICP) was also once thought to play a major
role in causing RH in infants. But much of the current medical research on this
topic now refutes these claims. Instead, it is the acceleration–deceleration forces
of the shaking itself that are believed to cause significant damage to the retina and
other parts of the eye.[7]

OCULAR CONDITIONS

Listed below, alphabetically, are descriptions and treatments of ocular conditions that may result from shaking injuries. They are *not* listed in order of frequency or importance. The most common ocular manifestations of SBS are RH (including traumatic retinoschisis), cortical visual loss, and optic atrophy.

Amblyopia

This term refers to a reduction of vision in an eye due to a failure of normal visual development brought on by a preference of the brain for one eye over the other. This may occur because one eye is disadvantaged by excess refractive error (farsightedness, nearsightedness, or astigmatism), misalignment (strabismus), malformation, or injury. Amblyopia is sometime referred to as "lazy eye" in lay language, although this term may also be applied for a misaligned eye. Amblyopia occurs when the disadvantaged eye does not receive enough visual stimulation.

Shaken children may develop amblyopia due to asymmetric injury of the eyes, particularly if hemorrhage or retinoschisis involves one macula and fovea more than the other.[8] As hemorrhaging is healing, the brain will prefer to use the less-injured eye; as a result, visual development will fail to continue properly in the more injured eye, even if it only takes days or weeks for the hemorrhage to resolve. The presence of more long-standing obstruction to vision, such as cataract, vitreous hemorrhage, or optic atrophy, heightens the chance that more serious amblyopia will occur. Correction of amblyopia requires the child to wear a patch over the "good" eye to force the use of the affected eye until normal vision is restored.

Cataract

Often thought of as a disease of the elderly population, cataracts, though quite rare in SBS, can result from shaking and other types of physical child abuse. In SBS, cataract is rarely present unless there has been blunt trauma directly to the eyeball or the shaking has caused a severe disruption of the intraocular contents. Cataracts can be difficult to diagnose by the nonophthalmologist but may be suspected on the basis of an abnormal red reflex. Visual inspection alone is likely to miss all but the most severe total white cataracts.

Treatment for cataract involves surgical removal of the lens of the eye, with or without insertion of a plastic lens implant. When cataract is seen in conjunction with other types of ocular trauma, however, the outcome for proper visual functioning may be poor.

Cortical Blindness

The most frequent cause of permanent visual loss in SBS is damage to the visual cortex of the brain. When extreme, this results in total blindness or only light perception. Injury to the occipital region of the brain, the most important area for vision, can be visualized on CT or MRI scans and has been found to be a determinant for profound visual loss.[10] The occipital cortex may be injured by ischemia or infarction, contusion (coup or contra coup), laceration, or hemorrhage. Less commonly, intraparenchymal brain injury can affect other parts of the vision pathways. Diffuse axonal injury and cerebral atrophy are also predictors of potential vision loss. Swelling caused by ICP can also negatively affect the visual cortex, though when swelling is reduced, vision can return. With cortical visual loss, pupillary reactions to light usually remain normal unless there is also damage to the optic nerves or severe disruption of the intraocular contents.[11]

Glaucoma

Glaucoma, another condition typically associated with the elderly, can very rarely develop in infants who are shaken, particularly when there is severe disruption of the intraocular contents or direct blunt impact injury to the eyeball. Glaucoma is due to raised intraocular pressure that results in optic nerve damage. Signs and symptoms may include photophobia (intolerance to light), tearing, an enlarging eye size, or hazy cornea, but the condition may be present with no symptoms or signs. For this reason, after severe intraocular injury, such as retinal detachment, cataract, or hyphema, patients should be monitored by an eye doctor. After direct blunt trauma to the eye, if the drainage angle is damaged (angle recession), glaucoma may even be delayed until adulthood. Treatments include topical or systemic medication and surgery. A successful outcome is more likely when there has been a quick response to the elevated pressure, thus halting further degeneration of the optic nerve.

Hyphema

In 1971, Mushin and Morgan described two cases of Battered Baby Syndrome with hyphema.[12] Hyphema occurs when there is bleeding in the anterior (front) chamber of the eye, in front of the iris and behind the cornea. It develops from a stretching of the ocular tissues.[9] This is rarely seen in SBS and occurs only when there is severe disruption of the eye contents or direct blunt trauma to the eyeball. Treatment for hyphema needs to be aggressive to prevent complications and save eyesight. Usually eyedrops are sufficient, but occasionally surgery may be needed.

Macular Scarring

The retina is the inner lining of the eyeball. It acts like film in a camera, recording what we see and then sending image messages to the brain. The macula is an area of the retina, lateral to the optic nerve, that is located straight back in the line of sight (figure 8.1). The fovea is a tiny spot in the center of the macula that is specialized to allow for normal straight-ahead vision (20/20). When the retina is damaged, the macula can also be significantly damaged. The macula may not heal evenly, and scarring can occur that will drastically affect vision, especially if the fovea is involved. Harcourt and Hopkins originally described the condition of macular scarring and its relation to Battered Baby Syndrome in 1971.[13] Scarring can also be the result of traumatic retinoschisis.

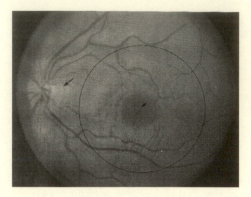

FIGURE 8.1   *Normal retina. Area within circle is the macula. Short arrow points to fovea. Long arrow points to normal optic nerve.*

Optic Nerve Atrophy

The optic nerve is the second of twelve pairs of nerves that originate in various parts of the brain. Optic nerve atrophy is a common occurrence in SBS and, less commonly, in other types of physical child abuse.[14] Atrophy occurs when the fibers in the optic nerve die in response to trauma. When the optic nerve head in the eye is then examined (figure 8.1), it appears pale. In SBS, the optic nerve may be damaged either by forces transmitted along the skull following blunt trauma or by shaking of the orbital contents behind the eye, where the optic nerve runs on its way to the brain.

One or both optic nerves may experience atrophy. Vision loss is usually proportional to the amount of atrophy present. Even when central vision is not affected, there may be changes in color perception or peripheral vision. Optic nerve atrophy is a long-term consequence of shaking and may take weeks or months to develop. There is no effective treatment.

Optic Nerve Sheath Hemorrhage

The optic nerve is covered with a sheath that protects the important nerve fibers that carry messages of sight to the brain. After an episode of shaking, there may be bleeding within this sheath. Although ICP or blood tracking directly from the brain may play some role, the primary factor appears to be the acceleration–deceleration forces of shaking, which cause direct injury to bridging blood vessels between the sheath and the optic nerve tissue.[15,16] Hemorrhaging within the sheath may affect only part or all of the length of the optic nerve in the orbit.

Pale- or White-Centered Hemorrhage

Any retinal hemorrhage, from any disease or cause, may have a pale or white center. They are entirely nonspecific and may result from central resolution of the hemorrhage, infectious emboli in sepsis, infiltrates in leukemia, ischemia, or even light reflexes on a hemorrhage that is elevated.

Papilledema

Papilledema is a swelling of the optic nerve secondary to elevated ICP. This condition is uncommon in SBS, despite the high prevalence of increased ICP. It is typically bilateral and can develop due to any cause of increased ICP, including brain tumors, cerebral trauma, or hemorrhage. On examination, the optic nerve head appears enlarged and elevated. The optic nerve tissue becomes opaque, so that the course of the blood vessels over the nerve head is obscured. There may also be small splinter or flame-shaped superficial hemorrhages in the area immediately around the nerve, known as peripapillary hemorrhages. If hyperemic, the nerve may appear more pink, although usually the appearance is whiter. The retinal veins may be engorged and tortuous. In severe papilledema, there may be exudation of fluid from the retinal blood vessels, forming a star-shaped pattern in the macula, but this not been reported to our knowledge in SBS. Prolonged papilledema can lead to optic atrophy.

Purtscher Retinopathy

Extremely forceful chest compression, as from safety belt straps in a major motor vehicle accident, can produce a small number of RH in association with large, white retinal patches, the etiology of which is not well understood. These retinal abnormalities are due to a dramatic acute increase in intrathoracic pressure, which is transmitted to the veins of the head and neck, as well as the eye.

This condition was initially described in the early 1900s. It was implicated as the cause of RH in children in the 1960s and 1970s, but in retrospect, these children had most likely been shaken. Tomasi and Rosman showed that Purtscher retinopathy could indeed occur in SBS.[17] The infants in their study had experienced seizures and were found to have increased ICP. Unfortunately, the nature of the abuse was not described. Although chest compression in SBS may be so severe that the child sustains rib fractures, Purtscher retinopathy remains very uncommon and is therefore not a major factor in the generation of RH after shaking. It has also never been described following cardiopulmonary resuscitation with chest compression, further underscoring that resuscitation does not cause hemorrhagic retinopathy.

Retinal Detachment

When an infant is shaken, the vitreous gel that fills the eye is also shaken. The abrupt movement of the vitreous, which is attached to the retina, can cause tears to the retina, which can ultimately lead to retinal detachment, resulting in the loss of retinal function. Surgical reattachment is possible, but eyes with such damage, fortunately rare in SBS, have a poor prognosis.

Retinal Folds

The vitreous in children is particularly attached to the macula. Traction from the shaking vitreous can raise a circumlinear fold that may or may not form a complete circle in the macula. Gaynon and associates believed that when such a feature was seen in an infant, it was a hallmark of SBS, especially when other

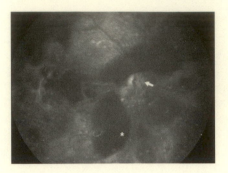

FIGURE **8.2**   *Severe retinal hemorrhages in Shaken Baby Syndrome.*

diagnoses had been ruled out.[18] Such folds have never been reported in any other entity in the SBS age range. They frequently occur at the edges of traumatic retinoschisis. No treatment is necessary, as the folds rarely run through the fovea. Over time, the area under the fold may become depigmented, leaving an indicator that shaking previously occurred.

Retinal Hemorrhage

Retinal hemorrhaging (RH) occurs in 50 to 100 percent of infants who are shaken.[5,19,20] Shaking is second only to normal birth as a cause for RH in infants. Beyond the first two weeks of life, the condition is so rare in infants that when identified, and other diagnoses are ruled out, diffuse retinal hemorrhaging—with hemorrhages in front of (preretinal), within (intraretinal), and under (subretinal) the retina, and extending out to the edges of the retina behind the iris, particularly when the hemorrhages are too numerous to count—it should be considered diagnostic of SBS (figure 8.2). The mechanism for the cause of this injury has been debated for many years. Recent research indicates that the most likely mechanism is the extreme repetitive acceleration-deceleration motion of the infant's head during shaking. The tractional pull between the retina and vitreous is significant enough to cause bleeding, particularly since the vitreous is attached to retinal blood vessels.[8] In addition, shaking of the orbital contents behind the eye may injure blood vessels on their way to the eye, as well as the autonomic nerves, which are responsible for vascular autoregulation.[21]

Shaking typically creates superficial flame-shaped (also called splinter) intraretinal hemorrhages and dot/blot deeper intraretinal hemorrhages that are more circular in shape.[18] These hemorrhages may be few in number and confined to the macula or more widely distributed with diffuse involvement of the entire retina. Preretinal hemorrhages are also common and appear as elevated, dome-shaped areas obscuring the blood vessels that run underneath them. Subretinal hemorrhages are distinguished by the blood vessels that run over them. RH may occur asymmetrically between the two eyes, or even unilaterally. RH that is noted to extend to the peripheral edge of the retina, the ora serrata, is particularly important in distinguishing SBS from accidental head trauma or other causes of RH (except leukemia), although few studies have been done to determine the statistical specificity and sensitivity of this finding.

When a child brought to a hospital emergency room exhibits lethargy, irritability, tense or bulging fontanelle, stupor, or any of the signs and symptoms of potential brain injury, particularly when the diagnosis is not apparent, the history is unclear, or SBS is suspected, ophthalmological consultation should be included in the clinical work-up. The infant's eyes should be dilated with mydriatic drops to optimize the view of the retina, unless there are strong neurological indicators not to do so. Consultation with professionals from larger institutions should be considered if smaller hospitals do not have the services of an ophthalmologist familiar with SBS.

Failure to search diligently for RH, and therefore make the diagnosis of SBS, may leave the child open to repeat injury if returned to an unsafe environment and hence failure to prosecute the perpetrator of the shaking.

RH can also occur as a result of the normal birth process, by any route. Superficial flame hemorrhages always resolve within two weeks (usually by one week), and dot/blot hemorrhages by six weeks (usually four weeks). RH within these time windows may be indistinguishable from SBS. However, subretinal hemorrhaging is very rare after normal birth, and macular folds and traumatic retinoschisis have never been reported. Of course, the fractures and intracranial injuries of SBS are not seen due to normal birth. Birth-related RH should be documented in the infant's medical record.[22,23]

In less than 3 percent of pediatric accidental head trauma, RH may occur. Such accidents are very traumatic, such as falls from several stories or motor vehicle accidents, and would rarely leave the clinician with a concern about SBS.[24] Home-related accidents that produce RH are extremely rare events and do not include "simple falls" from the arms of an adult or rolling off a bed or couch. When RH is identified and the cause cannot be explained adequately, shaking should be viewed as the culprit. Reece and Sege reviewed 287 head-injured children seen at the Rainbow Babies Hospital in Cleveland over a ten-year period.[25] In that paper, 18 out of 54 children with head injuries caused by abuse had RH, compared with 5 out of 233 with accidental injuries. The accidental injuries causing RH included a fall from great height, a motor vehicle collision, and a gunshot wound to the face. Riffenburgh and Sathyavagiswaran have stated that RH found in unexplained infant deaths should be attributed to trauma rather than SIDS.[26] Retinal hemorrhages due to accidental injury are usually few in number, confined to the macula or just beyond (not to the ora serrata), unilateral or bilateral, and most often intra- or preretinal.

RH has rarely been noted in infants and children after CPR with chest compressions, usually after an extended time.[27–29] However, with the exception of one of the patients reported by Goetting and Sowa in each of the few reported cases there is not an adequate explanation to rule out child abuse, or there are other factors that independently may have caused the RH, such as coagulopathy or sepsis. Research by several authors has now conclusively shown that RH rarely results from CPR, and when it does the hemorrhages tend to be very few in number and confined to the macula or peripapillary areas (posterior pole).[9] Diffuse, bilateral retinal hemorrhaging is *not* caused by CPR chest compressions.[9,30]

A computer model to research RH has been a topic of study in Australia. The model, in the form of a simulated shaken infant's head, was developed by pediatric ophthalmologists in conjunction with civil engineers at the University of Queensland, Australia, for use in a two-year project. A study of children suspected to be victims of abuse with RH at four hospitals will be followed to study the mechanisms for causing RH and the outcomes of the children. Animal models, including the woodpecker and the rat, are also being developed. In the research of the authors (AVL), it appears that woodpecker eyes are protected from the effects of shaking and impact by being rigidly encased in the skull with no true orbital tissue, closing of the eyelids to firm up the system, and intrascleral bone and cartilage. These findings highlight the susceptibility of the human infant eye to the forces of shaking.

The long-term prognosis of RH is actually quite good, provided that there is not concomitant brain injury to the occipital cortex or optic nerve. Retinal hemorrhages themselves, even traumatic retinoschisis, rarely result in vision loss after they resolve, unless amblyopia sets in from a fovea blocked by hemorrhage. A child may experience complete recovery and normal vision once the hemorrhages clear. As it is difficult to predict the visual outcome with certainty, clinical follow-up with an eye doctor maximizes the chances of early identification of children who need visual assistance or intervention.

Retinal Ischemia

Ischemia refers to a deficiency in blood flow, and the accompanying oxygen supply it brings, to an area of the body. Retinal ischemia, when seen after shaking, is thought to have occurred from local shearing forces or vascular damage. It is a very uncommon manifestation of shaking and is usually confined to the macula. Ischemia can cause long-term vision loss.

Retinoschisis

The retina has ten layers. Retinoschisis refers to the splitting of the layers, one from another. Traumatic retinoschisis results from the acceleration–deceleration forces of shaking, whereby a tractional pulling occurs between the vitreous and the retina, usually in the macula (figure 8.3). As a result, a cyst appearing as an elevated dome, develops acutely between retinal layers. Blood may accumulate in the intervening space. Most often, only the most superficial layer of the retina, the internal limiting membrane, is stripped away. If so, the prognosis for good visual recovery is excellent, provided there is no concomitant damage to the visual cortex or optic nerves. However, if deeper layers of the retina are split, the prognosis is guarded. At the edges of the circular or somewhat circular area involved in schisis, retinal folds, hemorrhagic folds, or depigmentation may occur (see figure 8.3).[14,24] Traumatic retinoschisis was first recognized by Greenwald and co-workers, who found

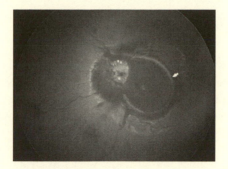

FIGURE **8.3**   *Traumatic retinoschisis. Note the hypopigmented border at edge of the schisis cavity. The marker indicates blood within the schisis.*

that it may be associated with delayed vitreous hemorrhage or abnormal electroretinogram.[31] Because the attachments between the vitreous and retina are particularly strong in childhood, traumatic retinoschisis has never been reported from any cause other than SBS in young children.

Treatment is usually not required but has been attempted, often with unfavorable results. The blood in the cavity may take weeks or even months to resolve, although sometimes it clears up within days. There is no clear answer as to when intervention should be considered to prevent amblyopia.

Subhyaloid Hemorrhage

The vitreous is also known as the hyaloid body. Blood can accumulate in the potential space between the retina and vitreous, where it is known as a subhyaloid hemorrhage. In SBS, this is usually blood that has extended from bleeding into the retina or a traumatic retinoschisis cavity. The blood may have a crescent-shaped ("boat-shaped") appearance. Careful ophthalmological examination should be done to differentiate subhyaloid hemorrhage from superficial retinoschisis, as the latter is so specific for SBS.[21] Identification of the edges of a schisis cavity can be a key distinguishing feature. If a subhyaloid or vitreous hemorrhage is lying over the macula, and therefore possibly obscuring a schisis cavity, it is advisable to examine the child again one to two weeks later to see if a schisis, which would be diagnostic of SBS, has been revealed as the hemorrhage resolves. Treatment is usually not necessary for subhyaloid blood.

Terson Syndrome

Terson Syndrome refers to the coexistence of intracranial blood and intraocular hemorrhage. The exact mechanism by which this occurs is unknown. Typically it is seen in adults with subarachnoid hemorrhage and RH following spontaneous subarachnoid hemorrhage, vascular malformation, or head trauma. There is often blood in the optic nerve sheath. Many authors in the past have attributed RH in SBS to Terson Syndrome.[32] Although Terson Syndrome is not uncommon in adults, it is rare in infants.[21] In shaken children, blood in the optic nerve sheath is thought to occur primarily from the tractional pull of shaking on the optic nerve.

Vitreous Hemorrhage

Bleeding into the vitreous gel, the viscous fluid that fills the majority of the eye, occurs as a result of migration of blood from retinal hemorrhaging out into the vitreous.[33] Although vitreous hemorrhages can appear immediately following a shaking event, they may also take a few days to develop, especially when due to blood spreading out of a traumatic retinoschisis cavity. Vitreous hemorrhages are slow to resolve, sometimes taking many weeks to clear.[21,24] Surgery may be needed to allow for clear vision and prevention of amblyopia.

Matthews and Das found that the presence of dense vitreous hemorrhages predicts both poor visual and neurological prognosis.[33] Three out of the five shaken infants they studied had significant vitreous hemorrhages. They were all left with neurological complications, such as spasticity and hemiparesis. Green and associates found that severe trauma is needed to cause vitreous hemorrhages, and that vitreous hemorrhages are often correlated with severe intracranial bleeding and/or cerebral lacerations.[8] Other studies have confirmed that the severity of intraocular hemorrhaging is positively correlated with the severity of brain injury. However, some patients may have severe eye injury but mild brain injury, and vice versa.

✧   ✧   ✧

Ocular injuries related to SBS have been researched in greater detail in recent years. It is therefore particularly important that physicians and ophthalmologists appropriately educate themselves on the implications of intraocular injury in the setting of possible child abuse. In doing so, they will be able to make a significant contribution as part of the interdisciplinary team that is needed to work with families and child victims.

NOTES

1. Caffey J. On the Theory and Practice of Shaking Infants: Its Potential Residual Effects of Permanent Brain Damage and Mental Retardation. *Am J Dis Child* 1972; 124: 161–169.

2. Caffey J. The Whiplash-Shaken Infant Syndrome: Manual Shaking by the Extremities with Whiplash-Induced Intracranial and Intraocular Bleedings, Linked with Residual Permanent Brain Damage and Mental Retardation. *Pediatrics* 1974; 54:396–403.

3. Friendly DS. Ocular Manifestations of Physical Child Abuse. *Am Acad Ophthalmol Otolaryngol* 1971; 75:318–332.

4. Kempe CH, Silverman FN, Steele BF, et al. The Battered Child Syndrome. *JAMA* 1962; 181:105–112.

5. Gilliland MGF, Luckenbach MW, Chenier TC. Systemic and Ocular Findings in 169 Prospectively Studied Child Deaths: Retinal Hemorrhages Usually Mean Child Abuse. *Foren Sci Int* 1994; 68:117–132.

6. Spaide RF, Swengel RM, Scharre DW. Shaken Baby Syndrome. *Am Fam Phys* 1990; 41:1145–1152.

7. Levin AV. Ocular Manifestations of Child Abuse. *Ophthalmol Clin N Am* 1990; 3: 249–264.

8. Green MA, Lieberman G, Milroy CM, Parsons MA. Ocular and Cerebral Trauma in Non-Accidental Injury in Infancy: Underlying Mechanisms and Implications for Paediatric Practice. *Br J Ophthalmol* 1996; 80:282–287.

9. Levin AV. Ophthalmologic Manifestations. In: Ludwig S, Kornberg AE, eds. *Child Abuse: A Medical Reference*. 2nd ed. New York: Churchill Livingstone; 1992:191–215.

10. Han DP, Wilkinson WS. Late Ophthalmic Manifestations of the Shaken Baby Syndrome. *J Ped Ophthalmol Strabismus* 1990; 27:299–303.

11. Young T, Levin AV. The Afferent Pupillary Defect. *Ped Emerg Care* 1997; 13:61–65.

12. Mushin A, Morgan G. Ocular Injury in the Battered Baby Syndrome: Report of Two Cases. *Br J Ophthalmol* 1971; 55:343–347.

13. Harcourt B, Hopkins D. Ophthalmic Manifestations of the Battered-Baby Syndrome. *Br Med J* 1971; 3:398–401.

14. Annable WL. Ocular Manifestations of Child Abuse. In: Reece RM, ed. *Child Abuse: Medical Diagnosis and Management*. Philadelphia: Lea & Febiger; 1994:138–149.

15. Elner SG, Elner VM, Amall M, Albert DM. Ocular and Associated Systemic Findings in Suspected Child Abuse: A Necropsy Study. *Arch Ophthalmol* 1990; 108; 1094–1101.

16. Lambert SR, Johnson TE, Hoyt CS. Optic Nerve Sheath and Retinal Hemorrhages Associated with the Shaken Baby Syndrome. *Arch Ophthalmol* 1986; 104:1509–1512.

17. Tomasi LG, Rosman NP. Purtscher's Retinopathy in the Battered Child Syndrome. *Am J Dis Child* 1975; 129:1335–1337.

18. Gaynon MW, Koh K, Marmor MF, Frankel LR. Retinal Folds in the Shaken Baby Syndrome. *Am J Ophthalmol* 1988; 106:423–425.

19. Zimmerman RA, Bilaniuk LT, Bruce D, et al. Computed Tomography of Craniocerebral Injury in the Abused Child. *Radiology* 1979; 130:687–690.

20. McClellend CQ, Rekate H, Kaufman B, Persse L. Cerebral Injury in Child Abuse: A Changing Profile. *Childs Brain* 1980; 7:225–235.

21. Levin AV. Retinal Haemorrhages and Child Abuse. In: David TJ, ed. *Recent Advances in Paediatrics 18*. London: Churchill Livingstone; 2000:151–219.

22. Cruz OA, Giangiacomo J. Ophthalmologic Manifestations of Child Abuse. In: Monteleone JA, Brodeur AE, eds. *Child Maltreatment: A Clinical Guide and Reference*. St. Louis: GW Medical Publ.; 1994:67–73.

23. Lyon TD, Gilles EE, Cory L. Medical Evidence of Physical Abuse in Infants and Young Children. *Pacific Law J* 1996; 28:93–169.

24. Buys YM, Levin AV, Enzenauer RW, et al. Retinal Findings after Head Trauma in Infants and Young Children. *Ophthalmol* 1992; 99:1718–1723.

25. Reece R, Sege R. Childhood Head Injuries: Accidental or Inflicted? *Arch Ped Adol Med* 2000; 154:11–15.

26. Riffenburgh RS, Sathyavagiswaran L. The Eyes of Child Abuse Victims: Autopsy Findings. *J Foren Sci* 1991; 36:741–747.

27. Goetting MG, Sowa B. Retinal Hemorrhage after Cardiopulmonary Resuscitation in Children: An Etiologic Reevaluation. *Pediatrics* 1990; 85:585–588.

28. Gayle MO, Kissoon N, Hered RW, Harwood-Nuss A. Retinal Hemorrhage in the Young Child: A Review of Etiology, Predisposed Conditions, and Clinical Implications. *J Emerg Med* 1995; 13:233–239.

29. Kramer K, Goldstein B. Retinal Hemorrhages Following Cardiopulmonary Resuscitation. *Clin Ped* 1993; June:366–368.

30. Odom A, Christ E, Kerr N, et al. Prevalence of Retinal Hemorrhages in Pediatric Patients after In-Hospital Cardiopulmonary Resuscitation: A Prospective Study (abstract). *Pediatrics* 1997; 99:861–862.

31. Greenwald MJ, Weiss A, Oesterle CS, Friendly DS. Traumatic Retinoschisis in Battered Babies. *Ophthalmol* 1986; 93:618–625.

32. Giangiacomo J, Barket KJ. Ophthalmoscopic Findings in Occult Child Abuse. *J Ped Ophthalmol Strabismus* 1985; 22:234–236.

33. Matthews GP, Das A. Dense Vitreous Hemorrhages Predict Poor Visual and Neurological Prognosis in Infants with Shaken Baby Syndrome. *J Ped Ophthalmol Strabismus* 1996; 33:260–265.

CHAPTER NINE

Historical
Ophthalmologic Reports

T HE FIELD OF PEDIATRIC OPHTHALMOLOGY has gone through dramatic changes since reports of physical child abuse first began appearing in the medical literature. This area of medicine in relation to trauma was slow to be addressed by clinicians on a regular basis. Not until the 1970s did intraocular aspects of abuse become the subject of research. Even today, there is some debate among ophthalmologists as to the physiology and mechanism of infant retinal hemorrhaging. One issue is that the finding of such hemorrhages in infants, when other pathologies and etiologies are ruled out, is unequivocal for a shaking injury. It has taken thirty years of inexact study to come to this conclusion. The research described below summarizes these years of investigating how the young eye deals with sustained trauma of abuse.

THE EARLY YEARS

When Statten reported retinal hemorrhaging in 75 percent of the infants and children he saw suffering from subdural hematoma in the late 1940s, little did he realize that most were probably shaken.[1] He made no attempt to identify the cause of his patients' injuries, but rather sought to identify the symptoms that were present.

Guthkelch, too, noted retinal hemorrhaging in cases of infants with subdural hematomas and effusions in the 1950s.[2] He saw such hemorrhages as part and parcel of children with traumatic brain injury. It was a finding that no one thought to question.

Then, Hollenhorst and Stein of the Mayo Clinic wrote an article in 1958 devoted to the question of ocular abnormalities found in combination with intracranial bleeding in forty-seven cases of infants and children.[3] While 60 percent had retinal hemorrhaging or papilledema, the authors also followed the prognosis of these children. Of the twenty who had not sustained retinal hemorrhaging, none had died and only two had permanent physical deficits, but of the twenty-seven retinal hemorrhage cases, three had died and nine were disabled; the difference is significant ($p < 0.01$). Thirty-five percent of the group with retinal hemorrhaging had "permanent visual handicaps," which concurs with today's statistics on the aftereffects of shaking injuries. Finally, Hollenhorst and Stein reported on the causes of the injuries sustained by the children, which included skull fracture, auto accident, birth trauma, falls, and "unknown." This was an article written during a time of "don't ask, don't tell."

During the 1960s, only one article was written on the ocular injuries of abuse. Kiffney detailed the unfortunate case of a "Negro male infant," whom he first saw at age seven months.[4] The boy had bilateral detached retinas, and one eye needed to be removed. The infant also had a history of sustaining multiple skull fractures with bilateral subdural and subarachnoid hemorrhages (age two months); a broken leg "while having his diaper changed by the mother" (age three months); and "poor vision" (age five months). This infant's injuries were initially noted by a public health nurse, who made the recommendation that his nineteen-year-old mother seek immediate medical attention for the boy, "Two months later she brought the patient to our clinic." The outcome of the case is unknown though it was deemed a "battered child" case. This is classic documentation of a shaken infant who was caught up in a pattern of abuse by a young mother.

THE 1970s

In 1971, David Friendly completely detailed what was known about ocular findings of child abuse.[5] His article, "Ocular Manifestations of Physical Child Abuse," was initially presented in October 1970 at the annual meeting of the American Academy of Ophthalmology and Otolaryngology. This contribution was significant in paving the way for medical providers to see the great variety of physical child abuse injuries. Friendly used tables to demonstrate the association of ocular injuries with other injuries of the body. To the listing of ocular injuries that had been previously noted in abuse cases, such as retinal hemorrhaging and detachment, he added orbital edema, periorbital ecchymoses (bruising), cataracts, vitreous hemorrhage, esotropia (crossed eyes), and papilledema (optic nerve swelling). He reported that of fifty-four child abuse cases he studied, the most common ocular abnormality was the presence of retinal hemorrhaging with intracranial bleeding. Friendly stayed active in child abuse issues throughout the next two decades.[6,7] He worked as an ophthalmologist at the Children's Hospital of Washington, D.C. He died in the mid-1990s and remains an icon in his field.

He helped guide the medical field in child abuse injuries and made significant contributions to our understanding of SBS as it is known today.

Three more significant articles were published in 1971 reporting the ophthalmologic manifestations of "the battered-baby syndrome," which now can be viewed as classic SBS.[8–10] Mushin and Morgan specifically outlined the clinical history of a three-month-old who had been strangled with a blanket by his father; "the parents spent the rest of the night shaking the child to revive him." Harcourt and Hopkins presented tables that showed the multitude of injuries experienced by the children in their case histories. They reiterated Gilkes and Mann's hypotheses of chest constriction and "being swung by the feet" as the cause for cranial injury and intraocular hemorrhaging. Jensen and associates found that the most common ocular condition in their group of forty-eight "battered children" was retinal hemorrhaging. They provided case examples of two infants who, by today's standards, were obviously shaken. The injury histories given by the parents of two sisters were reported as "bed falls." A seventeen-month-old girl, who was malnourished with a weight below the third percentile, had multilayered retinal hemorrhaging with papilledema, bilateral subdural hematoma, and epiphyseal fractures of both humeri. One year later, her eleven-month-old sister was found to have leg bruises, retinal hemorrhaging with papilledema, linear skull fracture, cerebral edema, left tibial fracture, and bilateral subdural hematoma. The complications of these injuries led to this girl's death and "legal proceedings against her father." Her sister on follow-up had severe ocular complications, which included optic and choroidal atrophy. She was eventually admitted to a school for the blind.

Harcourt and Hopkins described the condition of chorio-retinal lesions in "battered" children in 1973.[11] They found that permanent lesions and scarring were typical findings among abused children and referred to Gilkes and Mann's 1967 article to suggest a possible mechanism for injury. Though the authors did not describe specific cases of abuse, they outlined important steps for physicians to follow when faced with a child with "any disorder of possible traumatic origin in which the history is inadequate to explain the physical findings." This included a detailed ocular examination, as well as a complete interview with a child's parents or caretakers.

Purtscher retinopathy was first proposed as a cause for abusive injuries in the eyes in 1975.[12] This ophthalmological anomaly occurs in adults who experience some kind of sudden chest trauma (as from seat-belt injury) that causes retinal hemorrhaging. Because the two infants in the cases described in this article had pre-retinal and retinal hemorrhaging, bruising about the thorax, and minimal intracranial involvement, Tomasi and Rosman concluded that the syndrome must be Purtscher retinopathy. Using the diagnosis of Purtscher retinopathy was an attempt to suggest an *adult* process, however, which has very rarely been seen in children.

In the United States' bicentennial year, an article was written that described an eight-week-old boy who was "battered" and developed bilateral retinal detachment.[13] The authors initially did not believe that physical abuse was the source of the infant's injuries and sought a congenital cause. Yet the boy had a subdural hematoma and a diagnosis of failure to thrive three weeks earlier. His mother was seventeen years old and lived with the boy's father, who ultimately was found to have caused the abuse. As shaking can produce retinal detachment, especially bilateral, this detailed an undiagnosed case of SBS five years after the condition was initially described in the medical books.[14]

The 1970s concluded with an article by Eisenbrey, who reviewed ocular findings of Battered Child Syndrome.[15] He had seen a significant number of abused children at the Children's Hospital of Detroit and emphasized that retinal hemorrhaging in a child with multiple injuries and an inconsistent history was "pathognomonic of battering." He was also one of the first authors to discount "short falls" from chairs or beds as the cause for injuries sufficient to result in retinal hemorrhaging.

THE 1980s AND BEYOND

As the new decade progressed, so did the skills of medical professionals in their understanding, treatment, and reporting of child abuse and shaking injuries. Two disturbing cases of sexual abuse were reported by San Martin and associates in 1981.[16] Both victims (ages thirteen months and fifteen months) were found to have significant retinal hemorrhaging. One boy subsequently died. The authors proposed that anal penetration caused "Purtscher's retinopathy" in these infants. They also suggested that "overvigorous manipulations" of these infants could have compounded the retinopathy. They did not realize the effects of shaking and retinal hemorrhaging at that time and, though they diagnosed these cases inaccurately, they brought attention to a new issue in the complexities of SBS—sexual abuse.

Toward the middle of this decade, ocular injury attributed to shaking took a new turn. Lambert and associates examined the eyes of children who had been shaken and suggested that optic nerve sheath hemorrhage occurred in tandem with retinal hemorrhaging more frequently than previously considered.[17] They supported the growing belief that retinal and optic nerve sheath hemorrhaging occurred from a rise in intracranial pressure, and dismissed the consensus of previous years that Purtscher or Valsalva hemorrhagic retinopathy was the cause of such injury.

During this same time, several other authors considered other types of intraocular injury—traumatic retinoschisis and retinal folds—as pathognomonic of shaking. First, Greenwald and colleagues observed the perplexing anomaly of a "cystic or crater-like configuration" in the retinas of shaken infants.[6] They later determined this to be an actual splitting of the retina. The authors stated that repetitive acceleration–deceleration forces of shaking would not only create a disruption of the veins in the infant's "relatively spacious cranium," but would act similarly on the eyes as well:

> One of their effects would be to make the relatively dense [eye] lens move forward
> and back within the ocular fluids. In infancy, firm attachments exist between the

lens, the vitreous gel, and the retina, especially the macular region. Transmission of force through these connections could result momentarily in significant traction on the retina, particularly in the posterior pole. This abrupt tugging on the retina could create a separation along some plane within tissue, possibly more than one.

Two years later, Gaynon and others confirmed Greenwald's findings and reported on two cases of shaken infants with "retinal folds."[18] A four-month-old girl, shaken by a babysitter, arrived at the hospital comatose, with bilateral hemorrhaging throughout the retinas and "elevated ring-shaped white retinal or subretinal ridges noted surrounding both maculae." The authors stated that the retinas appeared to have "folded over themselves." The vitreous hemorrhages never cleared, and the girl remained quadriplegic. The other case was of a ten-month-old girl who was also admitted in a comatose state after having "fallen five feet" while being carried downstairs by her stepfather. There was not only intracranial bleeding, but significant intraocular bleeding and edema as well. She, too, had the white retinal or subretinal ridges, which did not clear, and she remained quadriplegic. The authors suggested that during shaking there is a "rupture of the retinal pigment epithelium," as the retina is displaced by "vitreous traction."

Kanter led the way in 1986 with a topic that continued to draw controversy throughout the following years: retinal hemorrhaging associated with cardiopulmonary resuscitation (CPR) of children.[19] The author was often confronted with the claim that retinal hemorrhaging had occurred because of the trauma of chest compression during CPR, so he studied fifty-four pediatric patients who had received CPR. Nine children had trauma preceding cardiorespiratory arrest. Five of these children had retinal hemorrhaging. A sixth child also had retinal hemorrhaging, but this was found to be due to hypertension after seizures. Kanter concluded that "when retinal hemorrhage is detected in the pediatric patient after CPR, prior trauma should be assumed . . . [and] should not be attributed to the mechanical effects of cardiopulmonary resuscitation." This was a significant finding, as it led medical providers to a greater understanding of the uniqueness that retinal hemorrhages have in SBS.

Ocular injuries in autopsy findings were primarily described in 1988 by a joint U.S.–China team led by Rao, who examined the eyes of fourteen fatally abused children and sixteen control cases who died over a two-year period.[20] They found that ten of the fourteen abuse cases showed such ocular changes as retinal hemorrhage, retinal detachment, papilledema, vitreal hemorrhage, and optic nerve hemorrhage. The team believed that five of the ten infants had been shaken. In their conclusion, they proposed "concussion" as an important cause of retinal hemorrhaging. A mechanism for causing such hemorrhage was suggested as occurring when the globe of the eye is thrust against the orbital contents, thus producing a wave of forces great enough to cause hemorrhage. An additional force occurs when the retina impacts against the sclera. This study was important, as it helped shape today's understanding of the mechanism of how retinal hemorrhages are produced.

In 1989, Wilkinson and colleagues proposed a new slant on intraocular injuries in SBS.[21] They found a correlation between the severity of retinal hemorrhaging and the severity of neurological injury. The authors studied the ocular injuries in fourteen cases of SBS. Those children with "vitreous hemorrhage, subhyaloid hemorrhage [equal to or greater than two disc areas], or diffuse involvement [hemorrhage in all three fundus regions] had a significantly higher risk of severe acute neurologic injury." Using a scale of the author's design, children with a higher initial neurological score (having such problems as motor or cognitive delay or seizures) would follow this trend, having significant, long-term neurological problems.

The following year, Han and Wilkinson continued to report on long-term effects of SBS on the eyes of the abused infants.[22] They studied six children from a group of fourteen shaken over five-year period. All the children initially had either unilateral or bilateral retinal hemorrhaging in conjunction with other ocular injury, such as macular fold or occipital lobe injury. At the time of shaking, the children ranged in age from three months to twenty months. At follow-up, their ages were between two and six years. The authors found that three of the six survivors had profound visual loss due to occipital lobe atrophy as a result of intracranial trauma at the time of the initial injury. This injury affected the visual pathways of the brain, causing cortical blindness. Two other children had macular folding, which caused mild-to-moderate "reduction of visual acuity." The article concluded with a call for ophthalmologists to carefully examine the eyes of shaken children, and then carefully document their findings "in the medical, legal, and psychosocial management of the abused child."

Also in 1990, Elner and associates wrote an article about their findings of ocular manifestations in seven of the ten children they autopsied who died of alleged child abuse.[23] All seven had optic nerve, retinal, and vitreous hemorrhaging; 54 percent had retinoschisis; 43 percent had macular retinal folds. All had intracranial injuries, especially subdural and subgaleal hemorrhage (found in 86 percent of the cases). The authors noted that injuries to the anterior section of the eye may or may not be attributed to shaking injuries. They also agreed with previous findings that blunt trauma seemed to be necessary for severe intraocular injuries when a child was shaken, and retinal hemorrhaging "may be the only clinical sign of covert child abuse and . . . may be a more sensitive indicator of early subdural hematoma than is CT." They, too, called for careful ocular examination to detect intraocular hemorrhage in cases of suspected child abuse and in postmortem exams, including staining of the eyes, saying this "may aid in the establishment of evidence of nonaccidental injury."

A short but significant abstract published in 1990 in the *American Journal of Diseases in Children* showed that, other than motor vehicle accidents, accidental injuries do not cause retinal hemorrhaging.[24] The authors evaluated fifty children who were brought to the emergency department with head trauma *without* a suspicion of physical child abuse. Though skull fractures and intracranial injuries did occur, not one child experienced retinal hemorrhaging. It was concluded that "retinal hemorrhages are not regularly found in young children who sustain mild-to-moderate head trauma as a result of common accidental injury." This finding assisted in questioning the trauma history when parents or other caretakers assert that a child has had "a fall."

In the early 1990s, two books on child abuse featured the writings of experts in the field of pediatric ophthalmology. First was Levin, with a chapter on ophthalmological manifestations in the book *Child Abuse*, edited by Ludwig and Kornberg.[25] He mapped the physiology of the eye for the reader and showed the types of findings that occurred in cases of abuse, including everything from cataracts to retinal detachment. He also outlined the various ways that the retina might hemorrhage, including dot, flame-shaped, and preretinal. Levin suggested that vitreous hemorrhage can occur in infants at the time of the shaking incident or days to weeks following the assault. He outlined differential diagnosis for ocular injuries and follow-up management.

The next book, which featured a chapter on ocular manifestations as a result of child abuse, was also titled *Child Abuse*, edited by Reece.[26] Annable, the chapter's author, took an innovative approach. He began by describing external injuries to the eye, and then led the reader progressively back through the inner layers of the eye through the lens, vitreous, optic nerve, and finally to the cerebral cortex. The author also thoroughly reviewed ocular injuries that directly related to SBS. For example, he discounted previous citations that retinal hemorrhaging was caused by syndromes such as Terson, Valsalva hemorrhagic retinopathy, and Purtscher retinopathy. Finally, he described laboratory and imaging studies both to "rule out etiologies of lesions that can be confused with nonaccidental injuries" and to confirm the "presence of the associated central nervous system lesions" when there is a finding of retinal hemorrhaging in an infant.

In 1993, Munger and associates examined the eyes of twelve infants who had died as a result of SBS injuries.[27] They correlated intracranial injuries with intraocular injuries and found that all the victims had retinal hemorrhaging: 91 percent had either subarachnoid hemorrhage or subdural hematoma, 83 percent had cerebral edema, and 75 percent had subarachnoid hemorrhage or subdural hematoma of the optic nerve. The authors also provided a well-made schematic representation of what occurs in the human retina and the location of various hemorrhages. They confirmed that hemorrhages can be found not only in the superficial layers of the retina, but also in the middle and deep layers. Their findings of retinal folds, indicative of a shaking injury, were not as frequently detected as in other studies (50 percent of their cases).

Betz and associates conducted a study of retinal hemorrhaging in cases of physical child abuse and compared these with injuries in children reported by other means, such as severe head injury or SIDS.[28] They actually measured the size of the retinal hemorrhages that they discovered. In cases of physical child abuse, retinal hemorrhaging was found in 19 to 73 percent of the entire retinal area. In comparative nonabuse cases, there was either no retinal hemorrhaging or hemorrhaging took up a minimal area of the retina (1 to 3 percent). The two cases of accidental retinal hemorrhaging occurred in adults, injured in a fall and in a traffic accident. The authors concluded that "massive retinal hemorrhages exceeding 20–30% of the entire retinal area cannot be explained by a single traumatic event and must be regarded as a very strong indicator for violent shaking."

In the same year as the Betz article, Green et al. set out to show that different levels of trauma to infants and children will produce different levels of intraocular injury.[29] They looked at the eyes of twenty-three children who had died as a result of nonaccidental injury. They then focused on those children who had central nervous system (CNS) involvement. Higher correlation was found between head-injury death and subdural hemorrhage. Eighty-one percent of those children with a head-injury death had "traumatic ocular lesions." It was interesting to note that the team found no scalp hematomas or soft tissue contusions in the heads of the children, which seems to indicate a lack of impact after shaking. They looked within the eye at the precise site where intraocular injuries had developed. They also looked at what CNS injuries were found. They concluded that there was a progressive increase in the amount of trauma a child sustained in relation to his or her injuries. Severe trauma to the head caused subdural hemorrhage as an initial finding. Slightly higher levels of trauma produced subhyaloid and intraretinal hemorrhages and optic nerve sheath hemorrhages. More trauma produced retinal detachment. And the most severe trauma produced choroidal and vitreous hemorrhages, which coincided with massive intracranial bleeding and/or cerebral lacerations. The authors concluded that when examined children were found to have intraocular lesions and/or retinal detachment, intracranial abnormalities should be suspected and evaluated.

In 1997, a short article by Tyagi and colleagues detailed the findings of unilateral retinal hemorrhaging in nonaccidental injury cases.[30] The authors said that even though such hemorrhaging is typically bilateral in SBS, unilateral cases did occur, and they supported this assertion with three cases of their own. They also stated that even when retinal hemorrhaging occurred in one eye, "a good prognosis can not be assured." Two years later, Drack and colleagues reaffirmed that unilateral retinal hemorrhaging occurred in shaken children, and speculated that this was because an adult abuser had a dominant hand, which ended up twisting the infant to one side during shaking.[31]

Three separate SBS cases presented in the 1999 medical literature showed unique ophthalmological findings. Lin and Glasgow described a case of a six-month-old male who died at home as a result of physical abuse by a babysitter.[32] Pathological examination of the infant's eyes found bilateral optic nerve hemorrhages, along with widespread retinal and vitreal hemorrhages. Another finding that had not been documented before was hemorrhages within the sclera of the eyes near the optic nerve. The authors concluded that such findings aid in the support of forensic evidence for child abuse in cases of traumatic head injury.

In the next case, Gonzales and associates found a latent case of SBS in a seven-year-old.[33] According to the boy's father, he "bumped into things and sat close to the television." Upon ophthalmoscopic examination, the boy was found to have bilateral retinal detachments and peripheral vitreous base avulsion in the left eye. No hemorrhages were seen, but child abuse was ultimately confirmed upon obtaining further history. The authors concluded that retinal hemorrhages most likely had been present but resolved due to the delay in seeking ocular treatment. They encouraged medical providers to consider child abuse when such unique ocular signs are found.

The condition of optic disc neovascularization was reported in the last of these unique SBS cases. Brown and Shami described[34] a four-month-old infant who was admitted to the hospital for lethargy and seizures and was found to have intracranial bleeding, edema, and infarction. An ophthalmological consultation found massive hemorrhagic retinoschisis cavities. After hospitalization, the infant had frequent follow-up visits with an ophthalmologist because of caregiver concern. At the four-month follow-up, the left optic disc showed a line of new faulty blood vessel formation (neovascularization). Laser surgery corrected this defect. The authors concluded that it was important that the infant's caregivers pressed for regular outpatient visits, and they suggested that infants diagnosed with massive retinoschisis should be followed monthly for several additional visits to monitor for neovascularization.

RECENT STUDIES

In 2000, an important study brought to light for the first time the prognostic indicators in SBS by both intraocular and intracranial findings. McCabe and Donahue reviewed[35] thirty cases of infants and children who had been diagnosed with SBS. They found that certain initial physical findings could accurately predict the outcome for SBS victims. The authors showed that 100 percent of "patients with nonreactive pupils on presentation died, while all patients with a pupillary light reaction lived ($p < 0.001$)." They also found that the majority of children (86 percent) who had a midline shift of the brain structures on neuroimaging studies died. Finally, the authors showed that all children who did *not* require ventilator support in the hospital had better vision at follow-up. All of these findings are very important in predicting both survival and visual acuity in shaken infants and children.

That same year saw the publication of a book chapter by Dr. Alex Levin that will become the gold standard for clinicians and legal professionals when examining retinal hemorrhaging in children: "Retinal Hemorrhaging and Child Abuse," in volume 18 of *Recent Advances in Paediatrics*.[36] The chapter contains over 280 references and quantifies each known reason why retinal hemorrhaging occurs in infants and children. By reviewing past medical literature as well as his own clinical cases, Levin explained why diffuse retinal hemorrhages do not occur from the causes that perpetrators of SBS typically claim, such as simple falls, CPR, or SIDS. This important chapter will help medical professionals reconsider old information about the formation of retinal hemorrhaging and the mechanisms behind them, and will allow prosecuting attorneys to present their cases in SBS-related trials more confidently.

CONCLUSION

The study of the pediatric eye has changed greatly over the years in light of physical child abuse identification. Research over this time has been vital in differentiating accidental from nonaccidental injury. Today, ophthalmologists trained in identifying ocular injuries of child abuse are key people in diagnosing, treating, and prosecuting cases of SBS. Ongoing research and discussion among professionals will broaden what has already been learned and may even help prevent further abuse. This is the charge to all medical professionals who have clinical contact with children.

NOTES

1. Statten T. Subdural Hematoma in Infancy. *Canad Med Assoc J* 1948; 58:63–65.

2. Guthkelch AN. Subdural Effusions in Infancy: Twenty-Four Cases. *BMJ* 1953; 1: 233–239.

3. Hollenhorst RW, Stein HA. Ocular Signs and Prognosis in Subdural and Subarachnoid Bleeding in Young Children. *Arch Ophth* 1958; 60:187–192.

4. Kiffney GT. The Eye of the "Battered Child." *Arch Ophthal* 1964; 72:231–233.

5. Friendly DS. Ocular Manifestations of Physical Child Abuse. *Am Acad Ophthalmol & Otolaryngol* 1971; 75:318–332.

6. Greenwald MJ, Weiss A, Oesterle CS, Friendly DS. Traumatic Retinoschisis in Battered Babies. *Opththalmol* 1986; 93:618–625.

7. Johnson DL, Braun D, Friendly D. Accidental Head Trauma and Retinal Hemorrhage. *Neurosurg* 1993; 33:231–235.

8. Mushin A, Morgan G. Ocular Injury in the Battered-Baby Syndrome: Report of Two Cases. *Brit J Ophthal* 1971; 55:343–347.

9. Harcourt BI, Hopkins D. Ophthalmic Manifestations of the Battered-Baby Syndrome. *BMJ* 1971; 3:398–401.

10. Jensen AD, Smith RE, Olson MI. Ocular Clues to Child Abuse. *J Ped Ophthal* 1971; 8:270–272.

11. Harcourt B, Hopkins D. Permanent Chorio-Retinal Lesions in Childhood of Suspected Traumatic Origin. *Trans Ophthal Soc UK* 1973; 93:199–205.

12. Tomasi LG, Rosman NP. Purtscher Retinopathy in the Battered Child Syndrome. *Am J Dis Child* 1975; 129:1335–1337.

13. Weidenthal DT, Levin DB. Retinal Detachment in a Battered Infant. *Am J Ophthal* 1976; 81:725–727.

14. Guthkelch AN. Infantile Subdural Hematoma and its Relationship to Whiplash Injuries. *BMJ* 1971; 2:430–431.

15. Eisenbrey AB. Retinal Hemorrhage in the Battered Child. *Child's Brain* 1979; 5:40–44.

16. San Martin R, Steinkuller PG, Nisbet RM. Retinopathy in the Sexually Abused Battered Child. *Ann Ophthal* 1981; 13:89–91.

17. Lambert SR, Johnson TE, Hoyt CS. Optic Nerve Sheath and Retinal Hemorrhages Associated with the Shaken Baby Syndrome. *Arch Ophthal* 1986; 104:1509–1512.

18. Gaynon MW, Koh K, Marmor MF, Frankel LR. Retinal Folds in the Shaken Baby Syndrome. *Am J Opththal* 1988; 106:423–425.

19. Kanter RK. Retinal Hemorrhage after Cardiopulmonary Resuscitation or Child Abuse. *J Pediatrics* 1986; 108:430–432.

20. Rao N, Smith RE, Choi J, et al. Autopsy Findings in the Eyes of Fourteen Fatally Abused Children. *Foren Sci Inter* 1988; 39:293–299.

21. Wilkinson WS, Han DP, Rappley MD, Owings CL. Retinal Hemorrhage Predicts Neurologic Injury in the Shaken Baby Syndrome. *Arch Ophthal* 1989; 107:1472–1474.

22. Han DP, Wilkinson WS. Late Ophthalmic Manifestations of the Shaken Baby Syndrome. *J Ped Ophthalmol Strabismus* 1990; 27:299–303.

23. Elner SG, Elner VM, Amall M, Albert DM. Ocular and Associated Systemic Findings in Suspected Child Abuse: A Necropsy Study. *Arch Opththal* 1990; 108:1094–1101.

24. Alario A, Duhaime A, Lewander W, et al. Do Retinal Hemorrhages Occur with Accidental Head Trauma in Young Children? (abstract). *AJDC* 1990; 144:445.

25. Levin AV. Ophthalmologic Manifestations. In: Ludwig S, Kornberg AF, eds. *Child Abuse: A Medical Reference*. 2nd ed. New York: Churchill Livingstone; 1992:191–211.

26. Annable WL. Ocular Manifestations of Child Abuse. In: Reece RM, ed. *Child Abuse: Medical Diagnosis and Management*. Philadelphia: Lea & Febiger; 1994:138–149.

27. Munger CE, Peiffer RL, Bouldin TW, et al. Shaken Baby Syndrome and Retinal Hemorrhages: Ocular and Associated Neuropathologic Observations in Suspected Whiplash Shaken Infant Syndrome. *Am J Foren Med Path* 1993; 14:193–200.

28. Betz P, Puschel K, Miltner E, et al. Morphometrical Analysis of Retinal Hemorrhages in the Shaken Baby Syndrome. *For Sci Inter* 1996; 78:71–80.

29. Green MA, Lieberman G, Milroy CM, Parsons MA. Ocular and Cerebral Trauma in Non-Accidental Injury in Infancy: Underlying Mechanisms and Implications for Paediatric Practice. *Br J Ophthal* 1996; 80:282–287.

30. Tyagi AK, Willshaw HE, Ainsworth JR. Unilateral Retinal Hemorrhages in Non-Accidental Injury. *Lancet* 1997; 349:1224.

31. Drack AV, Petronio J, Capone A. Unilateral Retinal Hemorrhages in Documented Cases of Child Abuse. *Am J Ophthal* 1999; 128:340–344.

32. Lin KC, Glasgow BJ. Bilateral Periopticointrascleral Hemorrhages Associated with Traumatic Child Abuse. *Am J Ophthal* 1999; 127:473–475.

33. Gonzales CA, Scott IU, Chaudry NA, et al. Bilateral Rhegmatogeous Retinal Detachments with Unilateral Vitreous Base Avulsion as the Presenting Signs of Child Abuse. *Am J Ophthal* 1999; 127:475–477.

34. Brown SM, Shami M. Optic Disc Neovascularization Following Severe Retinoschisis Due to Shaken Baby Syndrome. *Arch Ophthal* 1999; 117:838–839.

35. McCabe CF, Donahue SP. Prognostic Indicators for Vision and Mortality in Shaken Baby Syndrome. *Arch Ophthal* 2000; 118:373–377.

36. Levin AV. Retinal Hemorrhaging and Child Abuse. In: David TJ, ed. *Recent Advances in Paediatrics*. Vol. 18. London: Churchill Livingstone; 2000:151–219.

CHAPTER TEN

Myths and Controversies

THERE ARE MANY MYTHS SURROUNDING SBS that are argued in hospitals, police stations, and courtrooms. Injuries of child abuse have been well documented over many decades and have now become an exact science. Due to the complexities of the brain's response to traumatic injury, SBS is one form of child abuse more difficult to understand and draw conclusions about.

Simulation studies on shaking obviously cannot be performed on infants, living or deceased. So instead, the medical community bases its conclusions about what happens to an infant who is shaken on such things as autopsy results, perpetrator or witness accounts, and mechanical studies.

Kirshner and Wilson developed a listing of excuses that people use to escape culpability in child abuse cases, titled "Common Suspicious Stories (a Dirty Dozen)":[1]

1. Child fell from a low height (less than 4 feet), such as from a couch, crib, bed, or chair.

2. Child fell and struck head on floor or furniture, or hard object fell on child.

3. Unexpectedly found dead (age or circumstances not appropriate for SIDS).

4. Child choked while eating and was therefore shaken or struck on chest or back.

5. Child suddenly turned blue or stopped breathing, and was then shaken.

6. Sudden seizure activity.

7. Aggressive or inexperienced resuscitation efforts to a child who had suddenly stopped breathing.

8. Alleged traumatic event one day or more before death.

9. Caretaker tripped or slipped while carrying child.

10. Injury inflicted by sibling.

11. Child left alone in dangerous situation (as in a bathtub) for just a few moments.

12. Child fell down stairs.

The following discussion examines the excuses that are often proposed in SBS-related cases, including some of the above scenarios, as well as other myths that professionals working with shaken children have encountered. Depending on the source, such excuses are either strongly held beliefs or attempts to fabricate and confuse the medicolegal process. It is the hope of this author that readers will consider that these notions are typically false when rendering decisions.

MEDICAL AND LEGAL PROFESSIONALS' EXCUSES

Cardiopulmonary Resuscitation (CPR)

Although there have been claims that chest compressions of CPR cause diffuse retinal hemorrhaging in infants, many studies have been done over the years that discounted this claim.[2–4] Kanter was the first to study the mechanism of CPR in infants and found that retinal hemorrhaging was, instead, pathognomonic of the trauma of abuse.[5] Defense attorneys will often claim that clients of theirs should be viewed as heroes, because they attempted to save the life of a mysteriously unresponsive young child by using CPR. These attorneys may also claim that the finding of diffuse retinal hemorrhaging is a result of CPR compressions. Keen prosecuting attorneys will prove otherwise. After being shaken, infants may become limp and unresponsive. Perpetrators of such crimes may panic and perform CPR on such infants, who already have retinal bleeding from being shaken.

Weedn and colleagues presented a case of a four-month-old boy supposedly scalded by his two-year-old brother.[6] In critical condition at the hospital, the boy sustained a cardiac arrest and CPR was initiated. The boy died thirty hours after the initial injury and at autopsy was found to have cerebral edema and bilateral diffuse retinal hemorrhaging. The boy's mother was interviewed several times and was not considered a suspect. The authors attributed the infant's ocular injuries to the CPR, but it seems much more likely that this was a case of missed abuse with finger-pointing at an innocent brother.

Fackler and associates, in 1992, did a study on piglets wherein these animals were subjected to chest compressions.[7] No retinal hemorrhages were found as a result of the compressions. Levin reviewed six studies on infant CPR and retinal hemorrhaging and stated that in the absence of disease or traumatic injury, there is no such condition as CPR-induced diffuse retinal hemorrhaging.[8]

Two studies published in the 1990s described retinal hemorrhages in infants following prolonged CPR.[9,10] Goetting and Sowa proposed two cases for consideration and suggested that the rise in intrathoracic pressure during CPR produced a subsequent rise in retinal venous pressure, causing hemorrhage. One of these cases this author believes was nonaccidental (see chapter 11); the other was a SIDS case whereby the victim received CPR for seventy-five minutes, which produced a single retinal hemorrhage in one eye. Kramer and Goldstein's study found multiple retinal hemorrhages in a seventeen-month-old child after prolonged CPR. Prior to resuscitative efforts, funduscopic examination by a nonophthalmologist had revealed no retinal hemorrhaging. This particular case was not investigated, and autopsy following the girl's death diagnosed her as having adenoviral gastroenteritis. In hindsight, this now appears to be a case of missed SBS.

Retinal hemorrhages following CPR are present only in extremely rare cases; are commonly unilateral; stem from prolonged resuscitation efforts; and are limited to only one or two. The mechanism of shaking very often causes widespread bilateral hemorrhages, showing that extreme violence is required for such a condition, and there is an obvious difference in the anatomical nature of such hemorrhages from those produced by CPR.

Diphtheria/Pertussis/Tetanus (DPT) Vaccination

In years past and in very rare circumstances, some infants who received DPT vaccinations developed meningism (irritation of the lining membrane [meninges] of the brain). Infants with a marked reaction to the vaccination usually had a fever, became irritable, and cried inconsolably for many hours. There were even claims that infants died as a result of a reaction to the injection. Subsequent autopsy findings had been suggestive of SBS or may have been diagnosed as SIDS. Yet what medical and legal professionals often do not consider is that a crying, fussy baby, reacting to the effects of the vaccination, is more at risk of being shaken or suffocated.

There is a federal law that provides compensation for the parents of infants who have died as a result of any type of vaccination. This may or may not be supported by autopsy findings. A few parents of shaken infants have claimed compensation from the Federal Vaccine Injury Program, stating that the DPT injection caused "encephalopathy" with resultant convulsions and brain damage. However, there is no independent evidence (such as from countries where an issue of compensation does not arise) that the vaccination has ever caused subdural bleeding, brain swelling and bruising, or retinal hemorrhages.

In 1996, the American Academy of Pediatrics formed a consensus committee and verified that whole-cell pertussis vaccine has not been proven to be a cause of brain damage.[11] Activated pertussis in the vaccine is known to be contraindicated in children with seizure disorders, but for a healthy baby, a DPT vaccination is a safe, effective prevention measure. Nonetheless, in September 1998, an attorney successfully raised the defense that a DPT vaccination was responsible for signs of SBS in an infant. The prosecution in the case presented medical evidence that shaking was the only possible cause for retinal hemorrhaging found in a five-month-old male. Lawyers stated that injuries were caused by a preexisting medical condition that was not discovered until the infant had an adverse reaction to a DPT vaccination. The boy's father was found not guilty, regained custody of his son, was reinstated as a police officer, and received more than $100,000 in back pay.

Since 1998, pediatricians and family doctors routinely give the DPaT vaccination, in which the acellular form, rather than the whole-cell pertussis virus, is included. This rules out the possibility of any potential harm and can now put to rest this SBS myth that some have tried to legitimize in the courtroom.

External Bruising

Because a great majority of infants who have been shaken do *not* have external bruises, there can be a delay in the process of diagnosing SBS. Infants are brought to a hospital's emergency room with symptoms of lethargy, swollen fontanelle, and fever, and are worked up for a blood infection or some other cause. A shaken infant may appear healthy externally, yet have severe internal damage.

Often the only external bruising that does appear with SBS are fingertip markings on an infant's back and chest, or around the arms, where the perpetrator held the child during the shaking.[12,13] Close examination of an infant's entire body by medical providers may assist in properly diagnosing a shaken infant.

Lucid Interval

A "lucid interval" is the medical term for a period of apparent normality that may intervene between traumatic brain injury and unconsciousness. The argument is frequently put forth that a shaken child will appear normal after a traumatic injury, and therefore anyone who had access to the infant during a twenty-four- to forty-eight-hour period could be the perpetrator.

Infants who are shaken are shaken on a length-and-force continuum. Science does not know the length of time or amount of force required to cause even subtle intracranial alterations. What *is* known is that infants showing the signs and symptoms of SBS have been shaken extremely hard, for an extended period of fifteen seconds or more. Science also knows the severity required to produce a concussion.

In fatal cases of SBS, cerebral edema and intracranial bleeding often occur simultaneously. In other cases, there is intracranial pressure and a lack of oxygen and blood flow within the brain. Regardless, a child who has been shaken severely enough to cause injury to the brain will not be lucid or without symptoms. There will be unconsciousness immediately or within minutes.[1,14,15]

Children who experience less severe shaking, with mild-to-moderate injury to the brain, will display emotional or physical changes that a regular caregiver should question, such as irritability, poor feeding, lethargy, or vomiting. In these cases, there will typically be a loss of consciousness and a slowness to wake.

"Nice Parents"

It is well known that parents or caregivers who are most like their child's medical providers will be considered at least risk for child abuse, in the eyes of the provider. In early medical literature about injuries in young children, doctors viewed parents as being the last cause for trauma seen. Terms such as "spontaneous" and "unknown origin" graced journal pages. Cases continue today in hospitals, clinics, and courtrooms of parents who appear upstanding, confident, and loving, yet who are perpetrators of shaking and other child abuse crimes.

Physicians and other professionals may be hesitant to inquire about the possibility of abuse to avoid offending or wrongly accusing parents and caretakers.[16] If all pediatricians and emergency room doctors would consistently consider a differential diagnosis of child abuse for all injuries in children, then a more thorough examination, assessment, and interview could be accomplished, and a greater number of children protected.

"Shaken Baby Syndrome Does Not Happen"

Many medical professionals are skeptics when it comes to SBS. They believe it is not a syndrome because a minority of the cases recover "fully." Yet SBS is an appropriate diagnosis whenever an infant experiences intracranial and intraocular damage from being shaken, regardless of the outcome.

Some professionals believe that an adult cannot shake a baby hard enough to kill, even though this line of thinking counters a large body of evidence accumulated over the past two decades. They refer to the 1987 Duhaime study, which questioned the existence of pure SBS and concluded that "severe head injuries commonly diagnosed as shaking injuries require impact to occur and that shaking alone in an otherwise normal baby is unlikely to cause shaken-baby syndrome."[17] One of the shortcomings of this study was the model that was used. The hinge joint of the model infant could not duplicate the motion and rotation of a human infant head and neck and the damage that is caused within the cranium. The substance and myelination of an infant brain cannot be duplicated by science either.

There are well-documented cases of witnessed shaking without impact, perpetrator confessions (though such admissions are largely minimized), and cinematographically recorded animal studies. If no impact injuries are found at autopsy, then pure shaking should be considered to be the sole act that occurred.[18] Even if an infant was tossed onto a bed after shaking, the force of this type of impact is not thought likely to render significant injury.

Many parents and professionals affected by SBS believe that the *shaking* versus *shaking with impact* controversy is irrelevant. Shaking a baby is abusive, pure and simple, and is deserving of strict punishment. The fact that adults can seriously injure and kill a baby by shaking him or her is widely supported by medical professionals.

There are also individuals who believe that innocent people are imprisoned as perpetrators of shaking crimes due to findings of intracranial injuries and retinal hemorrhaging. Defense attorneys will often attempt to explain away such injuries as occurring from an infection or pressure in the brain, resulting from such innocent causes as accidental smothering or congenital seizures. SBS is a syndrome of a combination of injuries and should never be diagnosed or prosecuted in light of an isolated medical finding.

Shaken Baby Syndrome Resulting from Play or Roughhousing

When SBS was first identified and described in detail as a syndrome in 1972, Caffey proposed that swinging or bouncing a baby, along with a multitude of other play activities, might cause the associated injuries.[19] Chiocca echoed this warning in 1995, and then again in 1998.[20,21] But what is known today after years of research is that SBS occurs from violent whiplash motions in infants at the hands of adolescents or adults. While certain play activities can potentially injure an infant through careless handling, these activities do not cause SBS. Anyone playing with an infant to the point of questioning "Is this too rough?" should not be playing at all.

PARENTAL EXCUSES

Bed or Couch Falls

Over the past several decades, falls in infancy and childhood have been detailed in the medical literature.[22–25] Falls from short distances, such as couches or beds, do not produce significant injuries in infants, especially when a fall is onto a carpeted surface. And an infant placed in the middle of a bed or on a large couch can roll off only if he or she has the ability to turn over.

Over the years, falls have been widely used as an excuse for infant injuries by perpetrators of abuse.[26] Such innocuous injury histories given by caretakers were believed until the 1970s, when studies on infant falls finally began.[27] It is now known that shaking is the only *physical* mechanism that produces the combination of subdural hematoma and retinal hemorrhaging, other than falls from several stories or high-speed, unrestrained motor vehicle accidents.

Car Seat Injury

Several years ago, a letter to the editor described an infant who had the symptomatology of SBS "but was not shaken."[28] Instead, Mehl wrote, the infant was subject to the faulty driving of his mother, who was poorly versed in clutch control. Other passengers substantiated that the baby's head was jostled. Apparently the infant was not secured properly or was not rear-facing. The doctor who ruled out SBS and wrote this letter truly believed that such jarring arising from poor clutch control caused the infant's intracranial hemorrhaging. Substantial forces are required to produce the injuries seen in SBS. This doctor gave credence to the mother's story because she was from an upstanding community and the injury was substantiated by witnesses. (More details on this case appear in chapter 11.)

"I Didn't Know Shaking Would Hurt the Baby" or "I Didn't Mean to Hurt the Baby"

The force needed to cause SBS discredits these excuses. To cause and allow an infant's head, arms, and legs to whip violently back and forth is to breach one's responsibility as a positive, loving parent or caregiver. Perpetrators often resort to shaking as the first and only method to try to quiet an infant in their care.

According to Alexander, as stated in a 1997 *Woman's Day* magazine article, most shaking incidents last at least fifteen seconds, with as many as fifty shaking movements.[29] This time element coupled, with the ferocity of the act, surely discounts a claim of ignorance that the act would be harmful. Rather, this is an intentional deed used to knowingly inflict harm.

Chadwick has said that "an unintentional injury is one in which you know what occurred and inflicted injury is one where you won't always get the full story."[30] Three to 7 percent of all pediatric trauma admissions to hospitals are inflicted injuries.[31] With inflicted injury, there is also a delay in seeking care. The child may experience several episodes of shaking before the one that finally causes irreparable damage—that child was deliberately hurt, as is any child that is shaken. Physicians, as well as juries, often naively believe inflicted injury to be unintentional because of the need to believe in the goodness of parents and caretakers. This is a dangerous assumption and does not look toward protecting the child.

"I Just Snapped!"

Parents and caregivers typically have incredible feelings of frustration to the point of thinking, "I'm having a difficult time with this baby!" The difference that separates individuals, at that significant point, occurs when a loving parent or caregiver takes up the infant, holds him or her to a warm chest in comforting, protective arms, and says, "It's OK."

Sibling Abuse

Parents and caregivers have been known to blame other children in the home for inflicting SBS injuries. There have even been reports of two-year-old siblings accused by parents as perpetrators of shaking crimes. For SBS to occur, there needs to be sustained, significant force. This is something young children are incapable of producing.

Sleep Apnea

Apnea is rare in infants, especially if they were born healthy and are going for regular "well-baby" checkups to their pediatricians. This excuse is often used as a defense in the courtroom: "I found my baby not breathing, and I shook her to revive her." Certainly, loving parents may panic if they find their child not breathing, though it is hard to believe that such parents would severely shake their child to revive him or her. Light pats or rubs on an infant's back and gentle strokes on the face are techniques to be used if apnea occurs. In more severe cases, parents should call 911. If infant mouth-to-mouth resuscitation or CPR is known, it should be performed after calling for emergency assistance. Apnea as a *result* of

SBS has been studied and reported in the medical literature as indicating very severe brain injury with poor prognosis.[32,33] This condition is among a constellation of clinical indicators of trauma.

SOCIETAL EXCUSES

High-Risk Perpetrator

Although there are other reasons that may motivate a person to shake an infant, crying is by far the number one reason that leads to such an incident. Persistent crying occurs at all levels of our society, and perpetrators of shaking crimes come from all classes. Historically, child abuse and neglect have been more common in families with significant social problems; for example, low income or unemployment.[34] Some perpetrators are loving parents, some are child-care workers, some are drug addicts, and some are violent individuals. A crying infant can affect anyone—though not everyone shakes a crying infant. Concentrating on a group of individuals who are more "at risk" misses the need for prevention efforts across the board. Typically, SBS prevention efforts tend to be in response to highly publicized shaking cases, such as those occurring in daycare facilities or perpetrated by an au pair or stay-at-home dad. Instead, attention should be given to the syndrome itself, its causes, and how to prevent it from occurring within any part of society.

SBS Victims Are Poor, Minority Infants

In 1989, Brenner and colleagues reviewed 545 cases of abused infants seen over a period of five years.[35] They found twenty shaken infants, of which eight were Caucasian and twelve were African American. Yet of the total cases, 447 abused children were African American and 87 were Caucasian. So Caucasian infants represented a disproportionate number in the total cases of SBS (9 percent versus 2.7 percent). All social classes and races have shaken infants. It is a syndrome that does not discriminate. People, including physicians, whom society would think should know better, have been convicted of SBS crimes.[36]

UNUSUAL CASES OF SHAKEN BABY SYNDROME

Highlighted in the following paragraphs are five cases of SBS that do not follow the typical clinical course common to shaking injuries. These are presented to show the varieties of inflicted head injuries that may be seen. In all cases, medical personnel worked with law enforcement officials to verify abuse, thus adding to the understanding of the mechanisms of what actually caused each infant's injuries.

In 1997, Stephens and associates reported on the case of a newborn infant born with bilateral subdural hematomas.[37] Baby girl K was born after thirty-four weeks' gestation. The girl's mother had experienced high blood pressure throughout the pregnancy, and on the day prior to delivery, she noted a decrease in the movements of her unborn baby. Because of rising blood pressure, the child was subsequently delivered by cesarean birth.

At birth, the girl was cyanotic and in respiratory distress. After stabilization in the intensive care unit, the baby was weighed and measured. Her weight was in the twenty-fifth percentile and her head circumference in the ninety-fifth. An ultrasound of the head revealed large bilateral subdural hematomas. CT and MRI scans showed that the hematomas were of various ages. The blood collections were drained neurosurgically, and other intracranial abnormalities were noted.

The mother was questioned, and she admitted that her baby's father had frequently beat her throughout her pregnancy, approximately eight times over a six-month period. The beatings included abdominal blows, face and chest blows, kicks, and being shoved into furniture or onto the ground. When she experienced a reduction of fetal movement, she visited her doctor.

The authors proposed that due to recurrent acceleration–deceleration movements of the fetal cranium within the amniotic sac and the sudden impact of the mother landing on objects, the baby experienced symptoms equivalent to Shaken Impact Syndrome. They termed this condition Shaken Impact Fetus. They concluded that abuse should be considered when faced with a newborn infant with a similar condition, especially in the absence of birth trauma.

Piatt and Steinberg reviewed a case of a fifteen-month-old girl who had been left in the care of her mother's boyfriend.[38] The caretaker said that while he was in another room, the girl had fallen off a couch, landed on a popcorn tin, dented it, and was then unable to move after starting to crawl away. Two months previous to this incident, the girl had received medical treatment for facial burns after supposedly dipping her face into hot soup, also while in the care of the mother's boyfriend.

Examination of the young girl showed abrasions on her lip and tongue, linear contusions in front of her right ear and along her jaw, and petechiae across her neck, ears, jaw, arm, and upper chest. Fading bruises appeared over the girl's eyes and on her arms and right thigh.

Radiographs of the girl's cervical spine were normal, but MRI images showed a swelling of the spinal cord in the midcervical region with hematomyelia (hemorrhage in the spinal cord region). Further examination by nucleotide bone scan and radiography found an old fracture of the right clavicle. Skull radiographs were normal.

The infant had flaccid quadriplegia, and child abuse was highly suspected. The infant's grandmother made comments to implicate the mother's boyfriend, and there were also subsequent changes in the original story. A failed polygraph test led to the boyfriend's arrest.

As the girl had bruising on both arms, suggestive of shaking, and also had facial petechiae and jaw bruising, the authors proposed that the man grasped the infant "by the neck and, in distinction from the classical mechanism, whiplashed the body rather than the head." This child suffered no cerebral trauma, though she was left debilitated by a different form of shaking.

Piatt and Steinberg encouraged other medical providers to be careful in their examinations of infants brought in with unusual injuries, as were found in this child. They also stressed that thorough care histories should be taken. If they seem questionable in the presence of suspicious physical findings, child abuse should be highly considered.

Bird and associates detailed three cases of seven-month-olds originally diagnosed as being victims of strangulation.[39] CT scans showed intracranial bleeding, and two of the three infants had retinal hemorrhaging. None of the children had skull fractures or scalp swelling to suggest an impact injury. All had large cerebral infarctions associated with subdural hematomas. One child died, and the other two were left with severe hemiparesis.

Based on their findings, the authors concluded that all three infants were shaken while being held around their necks. These strangulation-shaking cases were the first of their kind to be described in the medical literature. The authors proposed that the infarct areas ("dead" tissue as a result of cessation of blood flow) identified in the infants' brains were caused by the obstruction of the common carotid artery during the strangulation and shaking. The midline shift of the brain caused by the infarct was unilateral in these cases. It was suggested that in each case the infant was held by one hand during the strangulation and shaking, with the perpetrator's thumb occluding one carotid artery, causing significant infarct damage to only one side of the infant brain.

The authors concluded that this form of SBS is underrecognized and that a complete examination is necessary for an infant with any intracranial injuries.

SBS AND FOLK MEDICINE

One variation of SBS that is a very rare occurrence is the Mexican folk medicine treatment of *caida de mollera*, or "fallen fontanelle." Two main articles from the medical literature, written twenty-five years apart, describe the features of this odd, deadly practice.[40,41]

The first case, by Guarnaschelli et al., illustrated a Mexican grandmother treating her two-month-old grandson for his "sunken" fontanelle. Because many Hispanic cultures believe that depressed fontanelle need to be raised, the grandmother held the infant upside down by the ankles, with his head partially submerged in a pot of boiling water. She then shook him, still upside down, while her assistant slapped the soles of his feet. The boy's fontanelle returned to a normal level and, in fact, began to bulge. He was brought to a local hospital near death and was found to have bilateral subdural hematoma and a subhyaloid hemorrhage in his right eye. He was left quadriplegic and never recovered, ultimately dying at age ten months.

Hansen reported[41] on two more recent cases of *caida de mollera*, involving a two-month-old and a five-month-old, both Mexican-American boys. One was brought to a hospital with new onset seizures and was found to have two different-aged subdural hematomas. The other boy was brought to a hospital with irritability and was found to have bilateral retinal hemorrhaging, both chronic and acute subdural hematomas, and two skull fractures. Both sets of parents reported taking their infants to folk healers several times for treatment of their boys' sunken fontanelle. A pan of warm water was described as being used in one case.

Caida de mollera may not be a true cause of SBS, as the biomechanics of shaking an infant upside down while being held by the ankles (a translational motion) would not appear to cause the acceleration–deceleration or rotational movements required to produce such dramatic injuries as seen in SBS. Hansen theorizes that these two infants were initially shaken; became dehydrated in response, causing the "fallen" fontanelle; taken to a folk healer for treatment; and then brought to a hospital. Or bulging fontanelle may have slowly appeared at the same time treatments were begun with the healer. In both instances, help was sought after injury.

Caida de mollera has only rarely been reported in the medical literature. If the practice is culturally based, then it would seem that there would be a vast amount of reports if this remedy generally caused SBS injuries. Guarnaschelli's case has been the only one to report the use of boiling water. This report so impressed John Caffey that he included it in his second essay on SBS.[42]

✧   ✧   ✧

Myths and controversies abound in the attempts to understand the true nature and effects of SBS.[43] With an improved understanding of the characteristics of SBS, these will be resolved, and when the true facts of SBS are more fully appreciated in our society, juries will not have such a difficult time deciding the fate of some accused persons. Research and prevention work need to be more amply supported in order to effect such change.

NOTES

1. Kirshner RH, Wilson HL. Fatal Child Abuse: A Pathologist's Perspective. In: Reece RM, ed., *Child Abuse: Medical Diagnosis and Management.* Philadelphia: Lea & Febiger; 1994:325–357.

2. Gilliland MGF, Luckenbach MW. Are Retinal Hemorrhages Found after Resuscitation Attempts?: A Study of the Eyes of 169 Children. *Am J Med Path* 1993; 14:187–192.

3. Levin AV. Retinal Hemorrhages after Cardiopulmonary Resuscitation or Child Abuse (comment). *Ped Emerg Care* 1986; 2:269–270.

4. Annable WL. Ocular Manifestations of Child Abuse. In: Reece RM, ed., *Child Abuse: Medical Diagnosis and Management.* Philadelphia: Lea & Febiger; 1994:138–149.

5. Kanter RK. Retinal Hemorrhage after Cardiopulmonary Resuscitation or Child Abuse. *J Pediatrics* 1986; 108:430–432.

6. Weedn VW, Mansour AM, Nichols MM. Retinal Hemorrhage in an Infant after Cardiopulmonary Resuscitation. *Amer J Forens Med Path* 1990; 11:79–82.

7. Fackler JC, Berkowitz ID, Green R. Retinal Hemorrhages in Newborn Piglets Following Cardiopulmonary Resuscitation. *Amer J Dis Child* 1992; 146:1294–1296.

8. Levin, AV. Retinal Hemorrhages in Shaken Baby Syndrome: What Have We Learned? Second National Conference on SBS. September 1998.

9. Goetting MG, Sowa B. Retinal Hemorrhage after Cardiopulmonary Resuscitation in Children: An Etiologic Reevaluation. *Pediatrics* 1990; 85:585–588.

10. Kramer K., Goldstein B. Retinal Hemorrhages Following Cardiopulmonary Resuscitation. *Clin Peds* 1993; 32:366–368.

11. American Academy of Pediatrics. The Relationship Between Pertussis Vaccine and Central Nervous System Sequelae: Continuing Assessment. *Pediatrics* 1996; 97:279–281.

12. Spaide RF, Swengel RM, Scharre DW. Shaken Baby Syndrome. *Am Fam Prac* 1990; 41:1145–1152.

13. Quirk P, Adelson PD. Shaken Baby Syndrome and the EMS Provider. *Emerg Med Services* 1997; 26:32,33,73,74.

14. Duhaime AC, Christian C, Rorke LB, Zimmerman RA. Nonaccidental Head Injury in Infants: The "Shaken-Baby Syndrome." *NEJM* 1998; 338:1822–1829.

15. Willman KY, Bank DE, Senac M, Chadwick DL. Restricting the Time of Injury in Fatal Inflicted Head Injuries. *Child Abuse & Neglect* 1997; 21:929–940.

16. Leventhal JM. The Challenges of Recognizing Child Abuse: Seeing Is Believing. *JAMA* 1999; 281:657–658.

17. Duhaime AC, Gennarelli TG, Thibault LE, et al. The Shaken Baby Syndrome: A Clinical, Pathological, and Biomechanical Study. *J Neurosurg* 1987; 66:409–414.

18. Gilliland MGF, Folberg R. Shaken Babies—Some Have No Impact Injuries. *J For Sci* 1994; 41:114–116.

19. Caffey J. On the Theory and Practice of Shaking Infants: Its Potential Residual Effects of Permanent Brain Damage and Mental Retardation. *Am J Dis Child* 1972; 124:161–169.

20. Chiocca EM. Shaken Baby Syndrome: A Nursing Perspective. *Ped Nurs* 1995; 21: 33–38.

21. Chiocca EM. Shaken Baby Syndrome. *Nursing 98* 1998 May:33.

22. Chadwick DL, Chin S, Salerno C, et al. Deaths from Falls in Children: How Far Is Fatal? *J Trauma* 1991; 31:1353–1355.

23. Joffe M, Ludwig S. Stairway Injuries in Children. *Pediatrics* 1988; 82:457–461.

24. Lyons TJ, Oates RK. Falling Out of Bed: A Relatively Benign Occurrence. *Pediatrics* 1993; 92:125–127.

25. Reiber GD. How Far Must Children Fall to Sustain Fatal Head Injury? Report of Cases and Review of the Literature. *Am J Forens Med Pathol* 1993; 14:201–207.

26. Kravitz H, Driessen G, Gomberg R, Korach A. Accidental Falls from Elevated Surfaces in Infants from Birth to One Year of Age. *Pediatrics* 1969; 44:869–876.

27. Helfer RE, Slovis TL, Black M. Injuries Resulting When Small Children Fall Out of Bed. *Pediatrics* 1977; 60:533–535.

28. Mehl AL. Shaken Impact Syndrome (letter). *Child Abuse & Neglect* 1990; 14:603–604.

29. Eberlein T. A Moment's Rage, a Baby's Life. *Woman's Day* October 7, 1997:120–123.

30. Chadwick DL. Shaken Baby Syndrome: Fact, Fiction and Controversy. Second National Conference on SBS, September 1998.

31. Brown JK, Minns RA. Non-Accidental Head Injury, with Particular Reference to Whiplash Shaking Injury and Medico-Legal Aspects. *Ped Ann* 1989; 18:482–494.

32. Rosen CL, Frost JD, Glaze DG. Child Abuse and Recurrent Infant Apnea. *J Ped* 1986; 109:1065–1067.

33. Swischuk LE. Apnea and Cyanosis in an Infant. *Ped Emerg Care* 1993; 9:241–243.

34. Gregg GS, Elmer E. Infant Injuries: Accident or Abuse? *Pediatrics* 1969; 44:434–439.

35. Brenner SL, Fischer H, Mann-Gray S. Race and the Shaken Baby Syndrome: Experience at One Hospital. *J National Med Assoc* 1989; 81:183–184.

36. Editors. Father Found Guilty of Shaking Infant Daughter to Death. *Jet Magazine* April 27, 1998:56.

37. Stephens RP, Richardson AC, Lewin JS. Bilateral Subdural Hematomas in a Newborn Infant. *Pediatrics* 1997; 99:619–621.

38. Piatt JH, Steinberg M. Isolated Spinal Cord Injury as a Presentation of Child Abuse. *Pediatrics* 1995; 96:780–782.

39. Bird CR, McMahan JR, Gilles FH, et al. Strangulation in Child Abuse: CT Diagnosis. *Radiol* 1987; 163:373–375.

40. Guarnaschelli J, Lee J, Pitts FW. "Fallen Fontanelle" (*Caida de Mollera*): A Variant of the Battered Child Syndrome. *JAMA* 1972; 222:1545–1546.

41. Hansen KK. Folk Remedies and Child Abuse: A Review with Emphasis on *Caida de Mollera* and its Relationship to Shaken Baby Syndrome. *Child Abuse & Neglect* 1998; 22: 117–127.

42. Caffey J. The Whiplash-Shaken Infant Syndrome: Manual Shaking by the Extremities With Whiplash-Induced Intracranial and Intraocular Bleedings, Linked with Residual Permanent Brain Damage and Mental Retardation. *Pediatrics* 1974; 54:396–403.

43. Krous HF, Byard RW. Shaken Infant Syndrome: Selected Controversies. *Ped & Devel Path* 1999; 2:497–498.

✧   ✧   ✧

CHAPTER ELEVEN

Missed Cases

P ROPOSED IN THE LATE 1960s and identified in the early 1970s, physical child abuse by shaking has been something in the medical literature that was often missed. Many factors played a role in medical providers' failure to identify SBS cases. Some providers were ignorant about obvious trauma inflicted on their patients. Others gave incorrect diagnoses, having believed the parents' or caretakers' stories. Still others did not perform comprehensive medical work-ups due to the absence of external trauma. Sometimes there was hesitancy on the part of the writer to name abuse due to the fear of litigation. One example of this was a case described in 1965 by O. James Staats, MD, and associates.[1] A five-month-old girl died in the hospital several hours after admission, having fallen out of her mother's arms and landed on her head on a hardwood floor. At autopsy, the girl was found to have an extensive skull fracture, a large epidural hematoma, subarachnoid hemorrhage, occipital lobe laceration, large intracortical hematoma, and pulmonary emboli consisting of brain tissue. By today's standards, the mechanism of the girl's death is greatly inconsistent with her injuries, and it would most likely be viewed as an incident of extreme physical abuse. This turned out to be the case, as Staats recounted thirty-six years later: "Her mother hit her in the head with a frying pan. I believe we knew at the time but could not write anything except the mother's original story for fear of a liability charge."[2]

The cases presented below are ones that have been gleaned from the medical literature as examples of missed cases of SBS. Most of the caretakers in these cases possess characteristics frequently seen in perpetrators of shaking and offered unlikely stories for the injuries typically seen in cases of abuse. Physicians can be fooled, as can any professional working with parents and caretakers. This was especially true in the days when physical child abuse was last on the list of considered causes for traumatic injury. Unfortunately, misdiagnosed cases of SBS continue to appear in today's medical journals.

CASES FROM THE MEDICAL LITERATURE

1942, Amsterdam, Netherlands

An early case of missed SBS appeared in an ophthalmology journal article written W. A. Manschot about "abnormalities of the fundus."[3] He detailed the case of a four-month-old female who supposedly fell from her dressing table onto her head. She soon afterward began to vomit and "became increasingly somnolent without complete loss of consciousness." At the hospital, the girl was found to have discoloration of the scalp, right-sided ptosis (drooping of the upper eyelid), a widened right pupil, left-sided paresis, and "in both fundi, numerous retinal haemorrhages." Operating, doctors found a skull fracture and a large epidural hematoma, which they removed. Areas beneath the dura were not fully explored. The girl's retinal hemorrhages disappeared after one month, and the paresis in her extremities disappeared within two months.

While a fall onto a hard surface producing an epidural hematoma and skull fracture is within the realm of possibility, numerous bilateral retinal hemorrhages are not seen after simple falls. Manschot attributed the retinal hemorrhages to increased intracranial pressure. Today, we know that this is insufficient to cause retinal hemorrhaging in infants.[4]

1959, Philadelphia

Jones and Shearburn described the case of one-month-old "L.M.," who was admitted to the hospital in September 1959 with seizures and tense fontanelle.[5] The girl's lumbar puncture "revealed grossly bloody cerebrospinal fluid which did not clear on drainage." Ventricular taps produced slightly bloody fluid. The baby was transferred to another hospital because of labored respiration. There, her "neurological findings were nuchal rigidity, slightly dilated pupils, retinal hemorrhages and stupor." An angiogram done six days later identified a "middle cerebral artery" aneurysm. Right frontal craniotomy surgery clipped the aneurysm, and the girl did clinically well and was discharged home in October. Several key factors show that this was a case of missed SBS: Spontaneous aneurysms in infants are rare; retinal hemorrhages were identified; and the caretaker's story focused on attempts to comfort the infant's crying. In a 1996 report, Lam and colleagues described a case of traumatic aneurysm that occurred from "clearly documented Shaken Baby Syndrome," lending support to the premise that shaking was the cause of this infant's aneurysm.[6]

1962, Manchester, England

Two infants and a young child with SBS were diagnosed in this Holzel, Smith, and Tobin study as having "Retino-Meningo-Encephalitis."[7] All three were brought to the hospital with seizures, vomiting, and bulging fontanelle.

Case 1

"D.T.," a five-month-old female, had a normal birth and development. In the hospital, she was found to have "extensive retinal hemorrhages, some close to the vessels, others in areas away from them." These hemorrhages had disappeared by the time of examination six weeks later. Her brain was never tapped to check for intracranial bleeding, but "it was suspected that she might have suffered some cerebral damage."

Case 2

"G.I.," a six-month-old male, had recently received a DPT vaccination. At the hospital, his temperature rose and his "optic discs showed slight temporal blurring and the retinal veins were congested." He soon became comatose. A week later, an ophthalmological exam revealed extensive retinal hemorrhages. These cleared after three weeks, but the nystagmus he developed in the hospital remained. "It seemed that the child's development had been delayed by his illness."

Case 3

"D.C.," a two-year-old male, was admitted to the hospital after three weeks of "listlessness," vomiting, and bronchiolitis. He supposedly had normal retinas. His muscle tone was "reduced." Two days later, he continued to be listless. His "fundi showed early papilloedema on the left side and small hemorrhages throughout both retinae, a third of these seemed to have a yellowish whitish centre lying in or on the wall of a vessel." He was ultimately discharged after a craniotomy and several ventricular taps. It is interesting to note that Dr. Norman Guthkelch, who was the first to describe the mechanism of SBS in 1971, was a consultant in this case.

Holzel and associates blamed these children's condition on a new type of encephalitis that produced retinal hemorrhaging. These were the days before computed tomography was available, hence no diagnostic imaging was performed. No subdural taps were performed, and intracranial bleeding was never mentioned. The authors truly believed that the rhinovirus they isolated in these three children caused the listlessness, vomiting, seizures, and retinal hemorrhaging they observed. Child abuse was never considered.

1965, London, England

Russell's article on subdural hematoma in infancy gave important clinical information but missed a significant number of infants now believed to have been shaken.[8] Of twenty-five cases studied of infants with subdural hematoma, 64 percent had retinal hemorrhaging and 28 percent had papilledema. The author described four case examples in clinical detail, but only one of these explains the cause of such an injury:

Case 3

A twenty-month-old initially was seen with bilateral hematoma, thought to be chronic from birth injury, which left him with an enlarged head and developmental delays. He was said to have had "a fall two weeks before admission." One month after surgery, he was walking and his speech was beginning to develop. At age five, the boy had an IQ of 74 and "had secondary optic atrophy with no perception of light in the left eye."

This case seems to be an early example of SBS with limited social explanation of the injury. In discussing the twenty-five cases, Russell suggests that some of the infants may have been subjected to "unadmitted trauma."

1967, Dallas

Watts and Acosta detailed the clinical course of an eight-month-old male who was admitted to their hospital with a history of a two-week cough, apneic episodes, and bulging anterior fontanelle.[9] Subdural taps revealed bilateral bloody fluid, and because of the nature of the cough and subsequent confirming fluorescent antibody studies, a diagnosis of pertussis was made. Over the course of his month-long hospital stay, the infant received many subdural taps and finally a craniotomy once his coughing subsided. The doctors determined that it was the forceful coughing from the pertussis that had caused the bilateral subdural hematomas. In this article, the authors included a statement that the boy was dropped by his mother one week prior to admission during an apneic episode. They believed that a small subdural hematoma was produced by the fall and was later exacerbated by increased intracranial pressure from the coughing. To their credit, the authors also wrote: "The etiology of the hematomas is obscured. In all such cases, trauma must be considered."

1968, Iowa City

Phelps described two cases of "pale-centered" retinal hemorrhaging in infants with intracranial bleeding—a very perplexing picture at the time.[10] He scoured the medical literature for information and came to the conclusion that the cause of these hemorrhages was unknown. He ruled out any sort of disease or blood disorder, but did not consider child abuse.

Case 1

A one-month-old girl was admitted after two days of irritability, progressing to poor eating and to "intermittent spells" in which she "drew up her knees, shook her arms, and grew rigid" (grand mal seizures). No history of trauma was given by the girl's parents. In the hospital, seizures progressed to every ten to fifteen minutes and lasted one minute in duration. She was unresponsive between seizures. Her fontanelle was tense. Funduscopic evaluation revealed unilateral "preretinal, retinal, and vitreous hemorrhages" in the left eye. A cerebrospinal fluid tap showed gross bloody fluid. Antibiotics were started. The second day of admission, the girl's right eye showed pale-centered retinal hem-

*orrhaging, and the left eye was now entirely hemorrhagic. A cerebral tap pro-
duced clotting blood. Her blood cultures came back normal. Seizures became
more frequent and uncontrollable, and the girl died on the third day of admission. "The final diagnosis was intraventricular cerebral hemorrhage. Her parents did not allow an autopsy."*

Case 2

*A seven-month-old girl was admitted after she "fell from a bed, striking her
head so severely that she was unconscious for a brief time." The girl had been
irritable and vomiting, and developed seizures, in addition to left-sided hemiparesis "between seizures." Ocular examination found bilateral white-centered
retinal hemorrhaging. Subdural taps produced blood-tinged fluid, and she was
treated with antiseizure medication. The girl's blood cultures were normal, as
was a third-day EEG. Subsequent intracranial taps produced little fluid. "By
the sixth day she seemed completely recovered, and two days later she was
discharged.... The final diagnosis was bilateral subdural hematoma."*

1968–72, Chicago

Gutierrez and Raimondi reported on six cases with delayed onset of "subdural effusion."[11] Four of these infants had retinal hemorrhaging, and all showed
classic signs of SBS.

Case 1

*An eight-month-old girl was brought to the hospital "after having fallen from
a bed." She was unconscious, had hematomas on her left jaw, bilateral retinal
hemorrhaging, a linear skull fracture, and bloody cerebrospinal fluid. Subdural
taps were negative, as were the findings of bilateral carotid angiogram. She
developed a right-sided seizure. After twelve days, she was discharged home.
Twenty-two days later, she was readmitted with lethargy, convulsions, and
recent retinal hemorrhaging. Subdural taps revealed bilateral bloody fluid.
Burr holes drained the fluid, and the girl was discharged after eighty-seven
days, "with residual motor and intellectual deficit."*

Case 2

*A nine-month-old girl was brought to the hospital after she had "fallen from
a bed and struck her head, without losing consciousness." She had soft tissue
swelling on the left side of her head and an underlying linear fracture. Subdural taps and cerebrospinal fluid were negative. She was discharged after six
days of observation. Two weeks later, she was admitted to a different hospital
with vomiting, left hemiparesis, and seizures. Her subdural tap was positive,
and her cerebrospinal fluid was bloody. Her subdural fluid was drained via
burr holes. She was discharged home one month later with "evidence of psychomotor retardation."*

Case 3

A four-week-old girl was brought to the hospital "with a history of twitching of the face and vomiting during the preceding twenty-four hours." On physical examination, she was found to be lethargic, seizing, with a full fontanelle and conjugate deviation of gaze. Bilateral subdural taps were negative, and cerebral angiograms showed no evidence of bleeding. Twelve days later she was discharged home. About a month later, she was readmitted with fever, bulging fontanelle, and vomiting—"without external signs of head or body injury." Bilateral subdural taps revealed blood-tinged fluid, and shunts were inserted. Prior to being discharged home, she had an exam that "showed evidence of brain atrophy."

Case 4

A two-month-old girl was brought to the hospital "with a skull fracture." Initial subdural taps were negative. She was discharged home after twelve days of observation. Soon afterward, she was brought back to the hospital with irritability, no appetite, and a new onset of seizures. Upon exam, she was lethargic and had a bulging fontanelle, bilateral retinal hemorrhaging, and hyperflexion. Bilateral subdural taps were positive, and a craniotomy was performed the following day. Surgery showed evidence of brain atrophy and persistent fluid. "Bilateral subdural-peritoneal shunts were recommended, but refused by the parents."

Case 5

A four-month-old girl was brought to the hospital "after having fallen from her bed." Soon after the injury, she developed right-sided seizures. Upon admission, she was lethargic and had acute retinal hemorrhaging and a linear skull fracture. Cerebral angiograms showed a cerebral contusion. She was discharged home when she had fully recovered. Two weeks later, she was brought to the hospital again with double hemiparesis, bulging fontanelle, acute retinal hemorrhaging, and seizures. Burr holes relieved the blood-tinged fluid that showed on repeat angiograms. Bilateral subdural shunts were placed. "A repeat cerebral angiogram, subsequent to that time, showed persistence of the subdural fluid, plus large ventricles."

Case 6

A ten-month-old boy was brought to the hospital "after having fallen from his parents' bed." He had immediate loss of consciousness. At the hospital, the boy was lethargic and had bilateral retinal hemorrhaging. Subdural taps showed blood-tinged fluid. After twelve days, he was discharged home alert and playful. One month later, at a visit to the neurosurgery clinic, the boy was found to have widened cranial sutures and bilateral papilledema. Admission to the hospital and subsequent cerebral angiograms found chronic subdural hematomas and increased pressure. "Bilateral burr holes were performed and bloody fluid was found."

The tragedy of these six cases was minimized because, like many medical professionals at the time, the authors never considered a diagnosis of child abuse. In June the following year, a letter written to the journal in which the article had appeared rebuked the authors for misdiagnosing these children, stating that they were all victims of child abuse, namely shaking injuries. The letter stated: "The authors report a mysterious occurrence; they do not propose a mechanism. A known mechanism for the same finding is violent shaking. . . . Down with 'mysterious events.'"[12] In reply, the authors of the original article reinforced their claims that the injuries were accidental: "Children do get themselves into some difficulties on their own, and accidents do happen."[13]

1970, New York

Sparacio and associates reported six cases of infants with acute subdural hematoma.[14] They accurately described the characteristics of subdural hematoma symptoms but unknowingly were portraying six cases of SBS.

Case 1

A three-month-old boy "fell from a crib and struck his head one day prior to admission." He had lost consciousness for one hour but awoke without difficulty. Having seizures the next day, he was brought to the hospital, where he was found to have bilateral retinal hemorrhaging and bilateral subdural hematomas (after subdural taps were performed). A craniotomy was ultimately done, and "the subdural collections eventually disappeared."

Case 2

A ten-month-old boy "fell from his father's arms two days prior to admission." Soon after, the boy developed left-sided seizures. Upon admission to the hospital, he was drowsy and irritable. He also had respiration difficulties, bulging fontanelle, and unilateral preretinal hemorrhaging. Bilateral subdural taps produced collections of liquid blood, and a subsequent craniotomy was performed, "following which the fluid did not reaccumulate significantly."

Case 3

A one-year-old female "with no history of trauma" began to vomit several days before hospital admission. She was found to be lethargic and irritable on admission and had preretinal hemorrhages in both eyes. Bilateral subdural taps showed collections of liquid blood, and a subsequent craniotomy was "only partially successful," though further subdural taps caused the collections to disappear.

Case 4

A ten-month-old male "fell from a couch three days prior to admission." The boy became lethargic, and ultimately seizures developed. Upon admission to the hospital, he was lethargic and very irritable, and had bilateral preretinal hemorrhages and bulging fontanelle. Subdural taps revealed liquid blood collections, which "disappeared after three taps on both sides."

Case 5

A six-month-old female was admitted with lethargy, respiratory distress, and irritability after no "known history of head trauma." Examination also found a bulging fontanelle and bilateral preretinal hemorrhaging. Subdural taps revealed a right-sided collection of blood, and subsequently the girl had a craniotomy. "No further fluid collection occurred."

Case 6

A nine-month-old boy "fell from his crib three days prior to admission." He subsequently developed vomiting, lethargy, and seizures. Admission examination revealed bulging fontanelle and bilateral preretinal hemorrhaging. Subdural taps showed bilateral liquid subdural hematomas. A craniotomy ultimately was performed. "After several more weeks of bilateral tapping, the collections were eliminated."

All the infants in these cases had the unique characteristics of what is known today as SBS: subdural hematomas, retinal (and preretinal) hemorrhaging, irritability, lethargy, a delay in seeking medical attention, and unlikely histories given.

1970, Jersey City, New Jersey

Curran and Wang described the medical complications and subsequent death of a six-week-old boy with undiagnosed hemophilia B.[15] The boy was brought to the hospital ER after he became limp and apneic at home. The only abnormality on physical examination was bilateral retinal and subretinal hemorrhaging seen through fixed and dilated eyes. The laboratory data showed abnormalities in the infant's bleeding times:

Plasma fibrinogen level was 860 mg/100 ml; prothrombin time, 13.5 seconds (control, 12.3 seconds); partial thromboplastin time, 73.5 seconds (control, 35.2 seconds); and thrombin time, 11 seconds (control, 10.2 seconds). Thromboplastin generated within 6 minutes produced plasma clotting in 20 seconds (control, less than 10 seconds).

The boy had a Factor IX bleeding study performed, which was 11.5 percent. He was classified as a "mild" hemophiliac. His mother's Factor IX level was 60 percent; however, his maternal grandfather's was 16 percent (though he had no history of bleeding difficulties).

Lumbar puncture (LP) revealed grossly bloody cerebrospinal fluid. Skull X-ray showed "marked widening of the cranial sutures." Four days later, ventricular taps produced a dark pink fluid that contained "homogenized brain tissue." On the fifteenth day of hospitalization, the boy died.

The boy's eighteen-year-old mother denied that he had suffered any kind of trauma prior to admission. She did state, though, that four days before admission, she had "slipped on a staircase while carrying the baby and fell to her right knee," without causing a direct head trauma to the infant. The authors of this paper believed that "sudden accelerating and decelerating forces could have brought about changes in intracranial dynamics sufficient to initiate bleeding."

Ironically, these are the kinds of biomechanical forces necessary to produce the injuries seen in SBS. There are many aspects that makes this particular case highly suspect for missed SBS. There was a timing conflict in the proposed mechanism of injury—the stairway fall—and the onset of symptoms—the infant was asymptomatic for three days afterward. Clinically, there are obvious questionable findings, including bilateral retinal hemorrhages, intracranial bleeding, and "homogenized" brain tissue, all indicative of trauma. There may also have been a missed occult skull fracture among the "widening . . . cranial sutures." It was not reported whether an autopsy was performed. An underlying bleeding disorder may, in fact, have been present in this infant, but there are many features in this case that lead to a conclusion that "hemophilia B" was not what initiated the boy's clinical downfall and ultimate death.

1972–83, Tokyo, Japan

In an article written about "infantile acute subdural hematoma," Aoki and Masuzawa failed to identify the twenty-six cases they presented as nonaccidental. Instead, the authors claimed the injuries in these cases were accidental, caused by simple falls to either a floor or a Japanese mat (78 percent of the cases), being hit with a toy, or falling against a table or shelf.[16] All of the infants, ranging in age from three to thirteen months, had subdural hematoma and retinal hemorrhages. Eighty-eight percent had some type of initial convulsion. There were no skull fractures present in any child. The authors even described these cases as "minor head trauma" and graded the subdural hematomas as mild (grade I), intermediate (grade II), or fulminant (grade III). Most cases were treated with subdural tapping.

Follow-up was done six months to eleven years later, with the following results: two children had died (one after unknown circumstances three months after discharge); one had epilepsy; one was mentally retarded; and twenty-two were "normal."

In a response to their article, Rekate stated that he found it inconceivable for such dramatic injuries to have occurred from such minor causes. He suggested a mechanism: "They have failed to recognize that most, if not all, of these babies suffered from the 'whiplash shake syndrome' and are victims of child abuse. While not totally pathognomonic of shaking, the constellation of SDH and retinal hemorrhage in the context of a historically trivial injury should be regarded as whiplash shake syndrome unless another etiology can be determined."[17]

Aoki and Masuzawa responded by stating that the incidence of child abuse in Japan is rare as compared to the United States, and that shaking was not used in their culture as a vehicle of abuse. They also believed that such injuries could be sustained by a fall to a soft Japanese mat, as the incidents were witnessed by the children's mothers and the "history presented by the mother was quite plausible in the situation."

1972, Cleveland

In his groundbreaking article "The Battering Child," Dr. Lester Adelson described five cases of fatal child abuse inflicted *by* children ranging from ages two to eight years.[18] Case 3 was a four-month-old girl who had originally been put to bed in her two-and-a-half-year-old boy cousin's room at her aunt's house. The aunt supposedly heard the baby crying and found the young male cousin running out of the room, saying, "Hit the baby, mommy. Baby bad girl." The aunt saw bruising on the infant and noted metal toys scattered about the room. She believed that the male cousin had hit the girl with a metal toy and then confessed to his actions.

The infant had stopped breathing at the scene, and the aunt's and police resuscitative efforts "were fruitless, and the child was pronounced dead on arrival at a nearby hospital." At autopsy, her injuries included cheek ecchymoses, multiple scapular hemorrhages, bilateral acute subdural hemorrhages, and subarachnoid hemorrhages over all lobes of the brain. Ocular findings were not described. The aunt offered that the male cousin was often "jealous of the baby."

While this baby may or may not have been shaken to death, the circumstances surrounding her death are suspect by today's standards. Creating such intracranial damage requires a good deal of strength and is commonly based on a rotational movement of the brain to cause the bridging veins to tear. A two-and-a-half-year-old does not have the strength to muster such force. It also seems that his "confession" could be viewed as an eyewitness account of something he saw his mother do.

1973, London, Ontario, Canada

Amacher and Li wrote about the presence of acute infantile subdural hematoma in a two-month-old girl as a result of "indirect" cranial trauma.[19] At the time of the incident, the girl had suffered a "coughing spell," leading to her being in respiratory distress and cyanotic. The young mother rushed across the hall of the apartment complex and sought help from a relative, who quickly suspended the infant upside down by her ankles. Three sharp blows were given to the midorsal region of the back, and the girl was immediately taken to the hospital. The incident was witnessed by several people. At the hospital, several hours later, the infant's anterior fontanelle bulged, she was irritable, and she had fresh retinal hemorrhages. Subdural taps produced fresh blood and continued to do so for the next twenty-one days. Eighteen months after the incident, the infant was "normal in all respects," with no recurrence of intracranial bleeding.

Both authors concluded that the back blows given to the infant were sufficient to cause "pendular motion of the head to establish differential inertial relationships between the skull-fixed dura and the brain"—thus producing the intracranial bleeding. They thought this action was a variant of the shaking mechanism that had been recently described by Guthkelch.[20] They warned against "deliberate or unintentional rough handling of infants." Their case report, however, is similar to reports of today in which perpetrators claim that cardiopulmonary resuscitation (CPR) is the cause for a shaken child's injuries. It appears likely from this early

1970s report that the girl's mother shook her to unconsciousness, leading to respiratory distress and cyanosis, causing the mother to panic and seek help from a nearby relative. Due to the paucity of information in those days about the mechanisms and forces needed to cause SBS, the girl's mother was not the target of investigation, and the girl's relative was most probably praised for "saving a life."

1973, Durham, North Carolina

Vitreous hemorrhaging in the presence of intracranial hemorrhage was the topic of an article by Shaw and Landers.[21] Of the eight cases that were presented, two were infants. One was a newborn who had suffered intrauterine complications and developed subarachnoid hemorrhage, along with subsequently diagnosed vitreous hemorrhage. The other was a four-month-old girl who was admitted to the hospital with generalized seizures and bulging fontanelle. Ocular examination found the girl's right eye showing "massive retinal hemorrhaging in the posterior pole and a large subhyaloid hemorrhage bulging into the vitreous cavity," and the left eye showing "diffuse retinal hemorrhaging involving the entire posterior pole and a subhyaloid hemorrhage surrounding the disk and extending into the vitreous cavity." LP revealed grossly bloody cerebrospinal fluid. When she improved several days later, she was discharged home "with a diagnosis of subarachnoid hemorrhage, etiology unknown." Two days later, she was readmitted with projectile vomiting, massive bilateral vitreous hemorrhages, and bilateral subdural hematoma. One year later, she still had remnants of vitreal blood, and her "development was retarded."

This is a case of SBS with what seems to be a diagnosis of traumatic retinoschisis in conjunction with her retinal hemorrhages. Though the concept of SBS had already been in the medical literature for several years, this was a tragic case that had been missed and led to further victimization and hospitalization.

1977, Newcastle, England

Bacon and associates presented the case of a two-month-old boy who was brought to their hospital supposedly after having been recently revived by his parents after an apneic episode.[22] The boy's father had been watching him in a carriage in the garden. The father found him not breathing and called the boy's mother, who held the infant over her shoulder while slapping his back repeatedly. Coughing and sputtering, the boy was revived temporarily, though blood stained his face and nostrils. At the hospital the boy was gravely ill; examination revealed fresh bilateral retinal hemorrhages. He was well nourished and had no external signs of trauma. Laboratory studies were normal, a skeletal survey was performed, and subdural taps were negative. He remained "irritable and hyperreflexive" the first three days of admission but soon responded to treatment (oxygen, IV fluids, and antibiotics). At discharge and the two-month follow-up, "he appeared entirely unscathed by the experience." The hemorrhages had resolved and his eyesight was normal. The boy's parents were both questioned extensively by the treating physician as well as the senior pediatrician and found to be innocent of any suspicion of child abuse: "Their answers throughout were frank, consistent, and entirely convincing, and the family doctor and health visitor attested to their excellent parenthood. Not a single feature emerged from the social background, the history, or the physical findings to support this suspicion."

Although the authors of this letter ascribed the infant's injuries to chest compression during the "life-saving measures" the boy's mother had performed, they fell victim to the myth of the "nice parents," when it seems more likely that the injuries were due to shaking by the boy's father. Studies on shaking and retinal hemorrhaging were not widespread in those days, and many parents got away with this type of abuse.

1980s, Chicago

In a classic paper on mistakenly diagnosing child abuse, Kirshner and Stein included a case that can now be interpreted as a missed case of SBS.[23] Ten postmortem cases were described that were initially believed to have been abuse cases but later were changed to such diagnoses as SIDS or meningitis. One case of a three-month-old, originally believed to have died from child abuse injuries, was changed to a diagnosis of SIDS at the postmortem examination. At the hospital, retinal hemorrhaging was found after failed resuscitation attempts at home by the infant's father. The authors attributed these hemorrhages to the "attempted vigorous resuscitation by chest compression"; in short, Purtscher retinopathy. What makes this a missed case of SBS is what is now known about the mechanism for abuse: CPR does not cause extensive retinal hemorrhages, and this history given by the infant's father is one that is often used by perpetrators of SBS.

1983, Buffalo

Springate reported on a case of clear misdiagnosis of a nine-month-old girl who was seen in the emergency room of Children's Hospital of Buffalo.[24] This was the last visit to three different hospitals over a two-week period. The story began when the girl was admitted to a hospital with a diagnosis of *H. influenzae* meningitis and placed on a ten-day course of IV ampicillin. Approximately one week later, the girl was seen at another hospital for fever, vomiting, and irritability and was "placed on clear fluids for presumed gastroenteritis." The next day, she was brought to Children's Hospital. Upon examination, she was found to be in the twenty-fifth percentile for height and weight, and had a slightly full fontanelle but otherwise normal physical and lab findings. Thirty minutes after the commencement of the examination, the girl's pulse was sixty-six and blood pressure was 115/75. Funduscopic exam revealed "unexpected" retinal hemorrhaging. A CT scan of the head revealed a linear skull fracture and subdural hematomas. "Appropriate investigation for possible child abuse was instituted, but remains inconclusive." The author concluded that accurate, early identification of abused children is vital for prompt medical treatment and would assist in averting future tragedy.

1986, Nottingham, England

McLellan and associates reported on a six-week-old girl with a brain aneurysm believed to be a misdiagnosed case of SBS.[25] Up front, the authors offered their opinion that the injuries initially appeared to be due to SBS. The girl had been fed by her twenty-one-year-old father early one morning, and four hours later the girl's sixteen-year-old mother noticed "a one minute episode of twitching of the left arm and hand." The twitching occurred throughout the day, and she "screamed uncontrollably during her evening bath, with a further left sided seizure." Later that night, the baby appeared "pale and sweaty." After calling the family doctor, the father returned to bed "but later accompanied her to [the] hospital and said that he had recently bounced the baby, sleeping in her pram, down the few steps to the garden." On arrival at the hospital, the girl had seizuring, irritability, a full fontanelle, and bilateral retinal hemorrhaging with a large right pre-retinal hemorrhage. A lumbar puncture showed blood-tinged cerebrospinal fluid. A head CT scan revealed a larger intracerebral hematoma, "incompatible with injury and to suggest spontaneous bleeding." A craniotomy removed the aneurysm, and the girl developed normally. The authors contended that even though the infant had retinal hemorrhaging combined with intracranial bleeding, other diagnoses needed to be ruled out, and this should not be seen as the hallmark of SBS. They called for "open mindedness to the interpretation of social factors in such cases." Aneurysms, though, do occur as a result of SBS.[6] A more thorough investigation might have led to a more conclusive diagnosis.

1988, Los Angeles

In their ground-breaking article, Rao and associates detailed the ocular findings in fourteen cases of fatal child abuse.[26] Yet one of the control cases, supposedly nonabused, was an eleven-month-old victim of a household fall reported to have hit his head on the leg of a table while playing with his father. Because of this innocuous injury, the boy sustained bilateral retinal hemorrhaging, subdural hemorrhage of the optic nerve, cerebral edema, and cerebral subdural hemorrhage. This now can be seen as an obvious case of missed SBS, once deemed as a "control" in analyzing cases of fatal child abuse.

1988, Detroit

Goetting and Sowa wrote an article in the April 1990 edition of the journal *Pediatrics*[27] describing a two-year-old developmentally delayed girl who suffered a "near-drowning" in her bathtub at home while being watched by a fourteen-year-old sister. The girl's circulation resumed after forty minutes of CPR, but she was comatose. "Funduscopic examination performed approximately 2 hours after immersion showed multiple large retinal hemorrhages bilaterally." The girl's coagulation and bleeding time were normal. She died four days later. "Skeletal survey, a complete forensic autopsy, and child protective services and police investigations all concluded that there was no preceding traumatic event."

This appears to be a shaking, drowning event by the girl's older sibling due to the history and retinal findings. The sister stated that from another room she heard nonrhythmic splashing for fifteen seconds, followed by silence. She found the victim one to two minutes later, submerged facedown. She removed the child from the bathtub and called paramedics, who arrived fifteen minutes later. As discussed in chapter 10, such large and numerous retinal hemorrhages are not caused by CPR. Also, the claim that a two-year-old, who could easily have righted herself, would drown in a bathtub is suspect in itself.

1990, Boulder, Colorado

In a letter to the editor of *Child Abuse & Neglect*, Mehl reported a case of a five-month-old infant boy who was admitted to a hospital with dehydration and initial glycosuria (abnormal amount of urine glucose).[28] He developed abdominal distention and vomiting with lethargy. On the third day of admission, the boy had seizures. After a normal neurological work-up, a head CT scan was done on the seventh day, showing bilateral subdural hematoma.

The boy's parents denied any abuse or shaking, though the mother did report that an "impact" episode may have happened in a borrowed car three days prior to admission. The woman was unfamiliar with the clutch shift of this car and forcefully lurched the vehicle forward several times. The infant was restrained in the backseat, "and in all likelihood his occiput struck against the car seat suddenly, but he did not appear to have suffered any harm at the time." It was suggested that this infant was not a victim of abuse due to the facts that the family was well known to the attending physician; the father was a graduate student; the mother came to every well-baby visit; the parents were viewed as loving; there were no other caretakers with whom the child was left; there was no retinal hemorrhaging during funduscopic examination; and the clutch incident happened in the presence of both parents and several neighbors.

The development of subdural hematoma occurs from traumatic events and seems questionable to have come from the proposed "clutch-release impact syndrome." It is also dangerous for any medical professional today to fail to consider SBS because of "nice parents." *Any* child can be a victim of physical abuse.

1993, Bombay, India

In the country's first report on SBS, two Indian pediatricians described a case they did not believe was intentional whiplash shaking.[29] Their report detailed a nine-month-old male who was admitted to the hospital with vomiting, lethargy, irritability, and seizures. He was found to have bilateral preretinal hemorrhages and bifrontal subdural hemorrhages. They suspected SBS but, upon questioning the boy's parents, found that the father "admitted to on and off throwing the baby up in the air and catching him as the child enjoyed this form of play." The baby had been left with a maid while the parents were working during the day and was supposedly well until the evening of admission.

The authors concluded incorrectly that this was not a case of intentional SBS, stating that "though child abuse was improbable in this child's home setting, affectionate playing by throwing the child up could have at an unguarded moment led to the injury."

1993, Baltimore

In one of the more difficult diagnostic cases on SBS ever documented, the authors of this particular case decided that coagulopathy was the culprit in an infant's demise, and not the infant's parents.[30] Wetzel and associates examined the case of a ten-week-old female who was brought to her pediatrician's office in respiratory distress and was subsequently transferred to a hospital. The physical work-up revealed hypothermia, a large bruise over her right buttock, thigh hematomas, and bilateral multiple retinal hemorrhages. Neurological examination "was consistent with brain death." A CT scan revealed severe cerebral edema (black brain), and subdural blood along the falx cerebri and tentorium. An abdominal CT scan "revealed an extensive gluteal intramuscular hematoma." Her laboratory work-up was normal except for prolonged prothrombin time (PT) and partial thromboplastin time (PTT). Because the girl was born at home, it was discovered that neither the midwife nor the infant's pediatrician gave a vitamin K prophylaxis. SBS was considered in this case, but when the vitamin K oversight was discovered, the diagnosis was changed to late hemorrhagic disease of the newborn. The parents' bleeding times were normal.

There are several key factors that make this a missed case of SBS. First, the gluteal hematoma is suspect, because this is an area that is typically the target of spanking in children. A few days before admission, the girl had rectal bleeding, which appears to be a result of the gluteal hematoma. Second, coagulopathy, or bleeding abnormalities, are common in traumatic brain-injury cases and can result from physical abuse, as proposed by Hymel and colleagues.[31] Next, the subdural hematoma the infant had lay between her cerebral hemispheres—a characteristic often unique to shaking injuries. The retinal hemorrhages the girl sustained are diffuse, multiple, and extend to the periphery of the retina—again a unique finding in SBS.[32] The cerebral edema was so extensive that the details of the convexities of the brain were obliterated on the CT scan. Finally, no other condition exactly mimics the collection of the injuries found in SBS.[33] This infant girl may or may not have had an underlying bleeding disorder, but the injuries she sustained demonstrate those of a shaken infant.

1994, Philadelphia

In a *reversed* case of SBS, Weissgold and colleagues described a circumstance of a six-week-old male infant being brought to the emergency room with irritability, vomiting, and hyperextension of the back.[34] Because of bulging fontanelle and a fixed downward gaze, the infant had a CT scan, which revealed intracerebral and subarachnoid hemorrhage with diffuse edema. The infant died several days later, following a ventriculostomy and intubation. The attending physician was suspicious, as the boy's parents "remained unusually stoic and uninvolved during the short hospitalization and at the baby's death." The parents also departed on a cruise after the funeral. Local prosecutors prepared to bring criminal charges against the parents for what the authors called "Battered/Shaken Baby Syndrome (BSBS)."

At autopsy, the infant was found to be without blunt trauma or fractures.

Along with the subarachnoid hemorrhage, there was blood present at the junction of the right optic nerve and eye globe. Microscopic investigation found "complex vascular malformation composed of variably-sized, generally thin-walled blood vessels." No retinal hemorrhages were present.

The authors concluded that these findings were natural malformations and were not indicative of abuse. They also concluded that the parents had their own way of emotionally dealing with their child's death, and any accusation of BSBS would have been a "tragic" mistake.

1998, Sheffield, England

This case described a nine-week-old Indopakistani boy who arrived at a local ER "floppy, slightly jaundiced and unconscious."[35] Rutty and associates noted that the boy had been given two injections of vitamin K, once at birth and once shortly afterward in the community. He also had been previously seen on several occasions for failure to thrive. For ten days prior to his final hospital presentation, he had suffered from diarrhea and vomiting. A CT scan showed a right-sided subdural hematoma, with midline shift and an infarction. The boy died twenty-four hours after admission. Autopsy showed bilateral retinal hemorrhages, and widespread perivascular and white matter hemorrhages. There was also a single external bruise in the midline of the chest. Several of the boy's blood-clotting factors and bleeding times were abnormal, and the diagnosis of "Late-form Hemorrhagic Disease of the Newborn" (LHDN) was made. The authors cautioned against medical providers rushing to a diagnosis of child abuse in light of intracranial and intraocular bleeding. This is sound advice, though in light of the vitamin K prophylaxis given (twice), the presence of retinal hemorrhages, the failure to seek care for the ill child, and the lack of social history presented with this case, it appears to be a case of SBS with a resultant metabolic imbalance.

1999, Dublin, Ireland

This case presented a six-month-old infant who was admitted to a hospital and treated for gastroenteritis.[36] Two days after discharge, the boy was returned to the hospital with "profound dehydration and in hypovolemic shock." Blood levels revealed hypernatremia with appropriately high levels of sodium, potassium, chloride, urea nitrogen, and creatinine. Other blood levels and bleeding times were normal. Funduscopic examination revealed massive bilateral retinal hemorrhaging, and a CT scan showed intraventricular subdural hematoma, diffuse subarachnoid hemorrhage, and diffuse cerebral edema. The boy soon died.

The authors claimed that because of the lack of evidence for trauma (a normal skeletal survey) and the high sodium levels in the boy's blood, he had succumbed to hypernatremia and not SBS. They quoted other studies that showed hypernatremic dehydration to be the cause of brain shrinkage and ultimate cerebral hemorrhage in infants and adults. "Elevated intracranial pressure leads to increased retinal venous pressure and results in retinal hemorrhages." Yet retinal hemorrhages are not typically found in hypernatremic infants. Nor does intracranial pressure promote intraocular bleeding. Instead, hypernatremia in this specific case was a result of misdiagnosed SBS. Abused infants can easily become dehydrated. This, along with intracranial pathology, such as subdural hematoma and edema, can lead to the state of hypernatremia, as confirmed by one recent study.[37]

2000, Nottingham, England

The case of an eleven-month-old male infant admitted to the hospital with fever, irritability, vomiting, and steady decline of consciousness was presented in a recent report.[38] The infant was found to have extensive retinal, intraventricular, and intracerebral hemorrhaging. Nonaccidental injury was considered, but because of the lack of external bruising and a normal skeletal survey, investigation was apparently not commenced. The boy died three days later.

Autopsy revealed "marked concentric hypertrophy of the left ventricle and fibrinoid necrosis of small cerebral arterioles, in keeping with severe antemortem hypertension. Extreme intimal proliferation was noted in the aorta, which was considered too severe to have arisen as a consequence of hypertension in the short period of this infant's life and indicated the presence of underlying fibromuscular dysplasia (FMD) of intimal type."

FMD is a disorder that affects the blood vessels and causes hypertension (high blood pressure). Chronic hypertension in a person with FMD can cause ischemic intracranial bleeding, often appearing like a "string of beads" or "stacked coins."

There are several problems with this case that was presented as a "natural," rather than nonaccidental, death. First, FMD is very rare in infants (approximately 1 percent, according to this report). It is also typically seen in young women, rather than infant males.[39] The subject of this report had intimal (inner vessel) type FMD, which is in itself rare (1 to 5 percent of FMD, according to this report). The authors assumed that because the intracranial bleeding was not what is typically seen in SBS (bilateral subdural hematomas), then it must not have been a shaking injury. They did not, however, identify the interhemispheric hemorrhage that is noted in the article photograph, a type very consistent with a shaking injury. There was also no appearance of the "string of beads" intracranial bleeding so common in FMD. Finally, the authors had nothing to offer as to what the presence of "extensive retinal hemorrhages" could be attributed to. Rather, it was again intimated that because there were no bilateral subdural hematomas, contusions, or other signs of violence, then the case could not be labeled as abusive, even though the signs of SBS were truly present.

✧   ✧   ✧

Mistakes occur, conditions are misdiagnosed, and learning to identify new syndromes takes time. Most of the cases described above were examples of children caught in abuse and perpetrators who got away with it. Jenny reported in her study of physician reports that they missed the diagnosis of abusive head trauma 30 percent of the time.[40,41] It is hoped that such a dramatic statistic will lead to better training of medical, law enforcement, and protective service personnel; social workers; and others who work with children. These individuals need to be sure to consider abuse and abusive head trauma when faced with an injured or deceased child.

Hospitals around the world have in their medical records cases of physical child abuse that have been missed.[42] Careful, comprehensive clinical assessment, which includes family history, past medical and social history, differential diagnoses, and complete physical examination, will aid in recognizing SBS.[43] Better education and training on SBS and physical child abuse injuries in medical schools, hospitals, and nursing programs are also vital in all communities. Only then will such cases not be missed.

NOTES

1. Staats OJ, Ceballos R, Miller RE. Brain Tissue Embolization Secondary to Cerebral Trauma. *Alabama J Med Sci* 1965; 2:394–396.

2. Staats OJ. Personal communication, January 2001.

3. Manschot WA, The Fundus Oculi in Subarachnoid Haemorrhage. *Acta Ophth* 1944; 33:281–299.

4. Levin AV. Retinal Hemorrhaging in Child Abuse. In: David TJ, ed. *Recent Advances in Pediatrics*. Vol. 18. London: Churchill Livingstone; 2000:151–219.

5. Jones RK, Shearburn EW. Intracranial Aneurysm in a Four-Week-Old Infant. *J Neurosurg* 1960; 17:122–124.

6. Lam CH, Montes J, Farmer J-P, et al. Traumatic Aneurysm from Shaken Baby Syndrome: Case Report. *Neurosurg* 1996; 39:1252–1255.

7. Holzel A, Smith PA, Tobin JO. A New Type of Meningo-Encephalitis Associated with a Rhinovirus. *Acta Paed Scandin* 1965; 54:168–174.

8. Russell PA. Subdural Hematoma in Infancy. *BMJ* 1965; 2:446–448.

9. Watts CC, Acosta C. Pertussis and Bilateral Subdural Hematomas. *Amer J Dis Child* 1969; 118:518–519.

10. Phelps CD. The Association of Pale-Centered Retinal Hemorrhages with Intracranial Bleeding in Infancy. *Am J Ophthal* 1971; 72:348–350.

11. Gutierrez FA, Raimondi AJ. Delayed Onset of Acute Post-traumatic Subdural Effusion. *Am J Dis Child* 1974; 128:327–331.

12. Schmitt B. Delayed Onset of Acute Post-traumatic Subdural Effusion—letter. *Am J Dis Child* 1975; 129:749.

13. Raimondi AJ. Delayed Onset of Acute Post-traumatic Subdural Effusion—reply. *Am J Dis Child* 1975; 129:749–750.

14. Sparacio RR, Khatib R, Cook AW. Acute Subdural Hematoma in Infancy. *NYS J Med* 1971; 71:212–213.

15. Curran JP, Wang JS. Fatal Intracranial Hemorrhage as the First Sign of Hemophilia B in an Infant. *Am J Dis Child* 1971; 122:63–65.

16. Aoki N, Masuzawa H. Infantile Acute Subdural Hematoma: Clinical Analysis of 26 Cases. *J Neurosurg* 1984; 61:273–280.

17. Rekate HL. Subdural Hematomas in Infants (letter). *J Neurosurg* 1985; 62:316.

18. Adelson, L. The Battering Child. *JAMA* 1972; 222:159–161.

19. Amacher AL, Li KT. Indirect Trauma as a Cause of Acute Infantile Subdural Hematomas. *Can Med Assoc J* 1973; 108:1530.

20. Guthkelch AN. Infantile Subdural Hematoma and its Relationship to Whiplash Injuries. *BMJ* 1971; 2:430.

21. Shaw HE, Landers MB. Vitreous Hemorrhage after Intracranial Hemorrhage. *Am J Ophthal* 1975; 80:207–213.

22. Bacon CJ, Sayer GC, Howe JW. Extensive Retinal Hemorrhages in Infancy—An Innocent Cause (letter). *BMJ* 1978; 1:28.

23. Kirshner RH, Stein RJ. The Mistaken Diagnosis of Child Abuse: A Form of Medical Abuse? *Am J Dis Child* 1985; 139:873–875.

24. Springate JE. Retinal Hemorrhaging in an Infant After Recovery from Meningitis. *NYS J Med* 1984; 84:61–62.

25. McLellan NJ, Prasad R, Punt J. Spontaneous Subhyaloid and Retinal Hemorrhages in an Infant. *Arch Dis Child* 1986; 61:1130–1132.

26. Rao N, Smith RE, Choi J, et al. Autopsy Findings in the Eyes of Fourteen Fatally Abused Children. *Foren Sci Inter* 1988; 39:293–299.

27. Goetting MG, Sowa B. Retinal Hemorrhage after Cardiopulmonary Resuscitation in Children: An Etiologic Reevaluation. *Pediatrics* 1990; 85:585–588.

28. Mehl AL. Shaken Impact Syndrome (letter). *Child Abuse & Neglect* 1990; 14:603–604.

29. Shivanand HB, Joshi MK. The Shaken Baby Syndrome. *Ind Peds* 1994; 31:715–718.

30. Wetzel RC, Slater AJ, Dover GJ. Fatal Intramuscular Bleeding Misdiagnosed as Suspected Nonaccidental Injury. *Pediatrics* 1995; 95:771–773.

31. Hymel KP, Abshire TC, Luckey DW, Jenny C. Coagulopathy in Pediatric Abusive Head Trauma. *Pediatrics* 99; 1997:371–375.

32. Levin AV. Understanding Retinal Hemorrhages: What Are They and What Do They Tell Us? Third National Conference on SBS. September 2000.

33. Alexander R. Junk Science in the Courtroom. Third National Conference on SBS. September 2000.

34. Weissgold DJ, Budenz DL, Hood I, Rorke LB. Ruptured Vascular Malformation Masquerading as Battered/Shaken Baby Syndrome: A Nearly Tragic Mistake. *Surv Ophthalmol* 1995; 39:509–512.

35. Rutty GN, Smith CM, Malia RG. Late-Form Hemorrhagic Disease of the Newborn: A Fatal Case Report with Illustration of Investigations That May Assist in Avoiding the Mistaken Diagnosis of Child Abuse. *Am J Foren Med Path* 1999; 20:48–51.

36. Fenton S, Murray D, Thorton P, et al. Bilateral Massive Retinal Hemorrhages in a 6-Month-Old Infant: A Diagnostic Dilemma. *Arch Ophthalmol* 1999; 117:1432–1434.

37. Handy TC, Hanzlick R, Shields LB, et al. Hypernatremia and Subdural Hematoma in the Pediatric Age Group: Is There a Causal Relationship? *J Foren Sci* 1999; 44:1114–1118.

38. Currie ADM, Bentley CR, Bloom PA. Retinal Haemorrhage and Fatal Stroke in an Infant with Fibromuscular Dysplasia. *Arch Dis Child* 2001; 84:263–264.

39. Mettinger K. Fibromuscular Dysplasia and the Brain. II. Current Concept of the Disease. *Stroke* 1982; 13:53–58.

40. Jenny C. Abusive Head Trauma: An Analysis of Missed Cases. Second National Conference on SBS. September 1998.

41. Jenny C, Hymel KP, Ritzen A, et al. Analysis of Missed Cases of Abusive Head Trauma. *JAMA* 1999; 281:621–626.

42. Jackson G. Child Abuse Syndrome: The Cases We Miss. *BMJ* 1972; 2:756–757.

43. Britton H. Shaken Infant Syndrome: The Basics. Second National Conference on SBS. September 1998.

✧   ✧   ✧

CHAPTER TWELVE

Procedures and Tests

THE TRAGEDY OF SBS BRINGS with it many clinical tests and procedures as part of an overall examination and treatment of injured children. Such processes can be very expensive and will typically expose a child to further pain and discomfort. Parents and other caregivers bear the emotional pain of seeing their child go through these procedures. Described in detail below are some of the aspects of diagnosis and follow-up treatment that a shaken child may need to experience.

DIAGNOSTIC IMAGING PROCEDURES

"Baby-Gram"

Once used regularly for the evaluation of child abuse injuries, the baby-gram is a process whereby an infant is placed on a diagnostic imaging area and a whole radiographic image is taken. It was considered a way to "cut costs" in the often expensive arena of diagnostic imaging. The problem with this test is that a diagnostician reading such an image will be faced with problems of underexposure, overexposure, image obscuration, and geometric distortion.[1] It is a process that is regarded as unreliable and inadequate, especially in evaluating child abuse injuries.

Computed Tomography (CT) Scan

Originally known as computed axial tomography (CAT), this scan combines the information from hundreds of tiny X-ray beams, collected and processed by a computer, to produce a cross-sectional final image of a body part. The technology of CT scanning has been greatly advanced in the diagnosis of traumatic head injury.

CT technology was finalized, marketed, and fully implemented in the 1970s. Images produced at that time were crude but gave medical professionals a new look at formerly hard-to-see areas of the body. Initially, it was proposed that CT be limited to use in cases of hydrocephalus, tumor, chronic subdural "effusions," and chronic seizures. Evaluation of head trauma was often limited to the condition and clinical course of the injured child.[2]

Today, CT scanning is one of the gold standards of thorough clinical work-ups of infants and children with head injuries or other neurological signs. The scanner appears as a large doughnut-shaped machine, through which a narrow stretcher can be moved. The device generates clicking and humming noises during scanning as images are being produced. There are a number of different settings on CT scanners, such as a "bone window" setting that shows the outer rim of a skull to highlight potential fractures. Another aspect of using CT is the angle at which the scans are produced; for example, a coronal CT facilitates diagnosis of subdural hematomas located in the midbrain. Changes may also need to be made to the child being scanned, such as "contrasting." Contrast is equivalent to a dye and is injected into the child's system. Initial sensations after injection of the contrast may be warmth or nausea, but they pass quickly. Contrast solution shows areas of high density within the brain (acute bleeding) more clearly. The addition of contrast can also help separate subacute from chronic injury. Sinal and Ball found, however, that most intracranial hemorrhages could be identified on CT scans without the need for contrast solutions.[3]

During CT scans, technicians often sedate and strap children in place, because they must remain still for reliable images to be produced. Parents or caregivers are usually allowed to be present to hold their children's hands, talk, or sing to them. Pregnant women and siblings, however, are not allowed in imaging rooms because of the exposure to X-radiation.

CT imaging is regarded as the method of choice for the initial evaluation of intracranial injury due to abuse.[4] It is readily accessible, less expensive than other imaging tools, and offers a quick view of intracranial injuries that may have occurred.[5–7] CT scans are also beneficial when used in combination with other imaging techniques, such as ultrasound.[8]

The findings on CT scans in the evaluation of shaken infants have been well documented over the years. Two groups of authors found that CT shows sub-arachnoid hemorrhage better than MRI scans.[9,10] Two other groups found serial (or follow-up) CT scans to be imperative in the tracking of intracranial injuries.[3,5] Sargent and associates delineated the types of bleeding seen on CT and warned of the misinterpretation of supposed diagnostic findings, such as "re-bleeding."[11] And finally, several other authors found, using a standard enhanced CT scan, that infants who develop a reversal sign, or "big black brain," will suffer grave consequences, such as death or irreversible brain damage.[12,13]

It is very beneficial to have pediatric radiologists read pediatric CT images. Such specialists may be able to more accurately interpret clinical findings, and thus have more complete evidence for a court of law.

Magnetic Resonance Imaging (MRI)

First available for general use in the 1980s, magnetic resonance imaging (MRI) offers a highly detailed view of specific body areas for diagnostic purposes. Though bulky and loud, MRI technology provides enhanced images that cannot be obtained through other means. The process uses electromagnetic radio waves, rather than ionizing radiation, to stimulate human atoms, which subsequently form a detailed image upon return to their state of rest. The process is one of the most expensive types of diagnostic imaging, at $800 to $1,400 per session.

MR imaging is usually done as a second-line procedure for diagnosing child abuse injuries, after abnormalities are initially found on CT. Children are usually medicated and asleep for an MRI, as there can be no movement if accurate images are to be produced. They are strapped to a platform and rolled into a large, cylindrical device. Family members are often allowed to stay in the imaging room and can wear earplugs during the MRI session. Many images are taken, and there is a very evident knocking during preparation and production of each image. MRI sessions may take up to an hour or more, depending on the images that are needed.

In most aspects of intracranial imaging, MRI is superior to CT due to its sensitivity and clarity of image.[14,15] MRI has become more and more versatile and useful in the diagnosis of SBS-related injuries. For example, this technique will show diffuse axonal injury lesions, cortical contusions, and small subdural hematomas more completely than CT scans.[16] Or, when a child has experienced several incidents of shaking prior to an acute condition seen when he or she is brought to the hospital, an MRI will differentiate older bleeding and show the intracranial breakdown of hemoglobin.[17] This aids professionals in determining the timing of shaking injuries.[18] Chabrol and associates suggested that MRI should be used several days after the child is initially seen in order to maximize the changes seen with hemoglobin breakdown.[19]

Further advances in diagnostic technology can aid in making MRI images clearer. Kleinman and Ragland recently reported on the use of the contrast solution gadopentetate dimeglumine for the enhancement of MRI images in cases of abuse.[20] They found that the contrast significantly aided the detection of small, hard-to-see subdural hematomas. Haseler and associates supplemented their use of MRI by way of proton magnetic resonance spectroscopy to determine what metabolic changes occurred in shaken children.[21]

More and more, the significance of clear imaging studies has become apparent. MRI brings such clarity to the forefront of clinical and legal cases. Children's lives can be saved through the proper interpretation and subsequent treatment of injuries found with the aid of this diagnostic tool. MRI done postmortem can be a useful complement to autopsy results and criminal investigation in suspected SBS cases.[22]

Nuclear Bone Scan

The nuclear bone scan, or nucleotide scan, enables detection of fractures missed by X-rays. Because of this, a nuclear scan is useful in the detection of physical child abuse injuries.[23–25] This type of scan requires the injection of a radioactive material (technetium 99m HDP) into the bloodstream. This substance will circulate through the body and will be taken up by the skeletal system by attaching itself to the bone. Resulting images will show up as "hot spots" in areas of rapid bone growth, such as recent fractures.

The process requires several hours before bone scan images can be made as isotopes gather in target areas. The dose of the material is very minute, and it is excreted within approximately twenty-four hours. Generally, sedation is not necessary for this procedure. During this scan, it is the radiation within the child that forms the image, whereas in other imaging studies, it is the X-ray that produces the radiation. There are no side effects from nuclear scans, and ample hydration is encouraged after the test. Nuclear scans have been found to be superior to X-rays in the diagnosis of skeletal trauma.[26]

Nucleotide scans cannot be performed after death for the purposes of criminal or medical examiner investigation. A more appropriate procedure would be to perform a postmortem skeletal survey. Nucleotide scans are expensive but work well in determining whether a child has any underlying fractures.

Skeletal Survey

When a fracture is found in an abused or shaken child, there may well be others. The skeletal survey is a series of X-rays used to evaluate every bone in the body. This should be a standard procedure when evidence of violence is found. Kleinman recommends the following for a thorough skeletal survey: anteroposterior (AP) and lateral chest, AP humeri, AP forearms, posteroanterior (PA) hands, AP pelvis, lateral lumbar spine, AP femora, AP tibiae, AP feet, AP and lateral skull.[4] Skeletal surveys should be repeated two weeks after the initial examination, as bones will be in the process of new growth around the site of any fractures.

Ultrasonography

This technology is being employed more frequently for the management of intracranial injuries. A device with a hand-held scanning wand produces ultrasonic waves, which are directed into an area of the body being evaluated. Different tissues in the body have different densities and elasticities. Ultrasonic waves bounce off organs and tissues, and then echo the shape of the part being examined.

In cases of SBS, ultrasonography is most useful in following the progress of a brain injury after acute diagnosis.[27] Ultrasonography allows for detailed images that may not be picked up by CT or MRI scans. When using ultrasonography in the evaluation of an infant, the wand is held against the fontanelle of the head and slowly moved in different directions to detect intracranial changes that may have occurred over time. This procedure is best used for infants six months or younger.[28] In older children, the cranial sutures will be closer together or completely closed, and ultrasonic waves do not transmit through bone.

A diagnostician looks for changes in intracranial bleeding, ventricle size and shape, and cerebral edema.[5,8] Any changes noted should be closely followed, allowing for more effective treatment.

X-ray

The X-ray, also known as radiograph, is the oldest of the diagnostic imaging techniques. The process of obtaining X-ray images is called roentgenography, named after the inventor, Roentgen. One of the main benefits of X-ray is the speed at which an image can be produced. The actual exposure time is only about one second. X-ray imaging gives off small doses of gamma radiation to the targeted area of the body. A lead apron usually blocks off the rest of the body. An X-ray beam goes through the body and into a cassette that contains unexposed photographic film, this being sensitive to X-rays as well as to visible light. The film is between two screens that contain crystals that give off light, thereby producing an image on the film. Bones are very dense and will appear as white. Fractures within the bones will appear as dark gray or black lines. Over time, fractures will heal and appear whitish, demonstrating new bone growth.

Infants and children need to remain still while X-ray images are being made. Often, a parent will wear a lead apron and hold his or her child in place for an image. An infant also may be placed in a special device in order to retain a stable position.

For skeletal trauma, the X-ray is the primary method of diagnostic imaging.[29] Skull, rib, and long-bone fractures are common in cases of physical child abuse and SBS. X-ray studies will show the extent of any such fractures and assist in the clinical management of these injuries. For example, skull fractures may widen within a short time, so follow-up X-rays are necessary.[30] Ribs fractures in infants are indicative of abuse.[6,31] Such fractures are also difficult to see when they are posterior. Because of that, Kleinman and associates suggest that a lower kilovoltage and an anteroposterior position be used in cases that are highly suggestive of abuse.[32] Long-bone injuries will show up clearly on radiographs, especially when new bone growth has begun. "Corner" or "bucket-handle" fractures, periosteal lesions, cortical thickening, and evident lines of fractures have all been seen in diagnostic evaluations using basic X-ray technology over many decades.[33]

Any medical provider suspecting, or even remotely considering, abuse as a differential diagnosis in an infant presenting to an emergency room or clinic should obtain basic X-ray studies. This can aid in the treatment of infants and children and in keeping them free from further harm while an investigation takes place. The prosecution of perpetrators of shaking crimes can sometimes be difficult; the use of highly detailed radiography in conjunction with autopsy images can provide irrefutable evidence in such cases.[1]

NONIMAGING TESTS AND PROCEDURES

Blood Studies

Coagulopathy, a disorder resulting from abusive head trauma, occurs when there is a problem with the clotting of blood. Prothrombin is a substance in the body that initiates the clotting mechanism. Obtaining a prothrombin time (PT) informs the medical provider as to the efficiency of a body's ability to clot blood. Hymel and associates have found that children with traumatic head injuries have a prolonged PT and activated coagulation.[34] If a family history of bleeding disorders, liver problems, or vitamin K deficiency is ruled out, such blood tests can aid in the diagnosis of abuse.

Brainstem Auditory-Evoked Response Testing

Evoked potential tests are electronic measurements of the brain's response to stimulus. Brainstem auditory-evoked response (BAER) testing measures the brain stem's auditory tract by the use of a series of auditory clicks in one ear. These clicks activate the eighth cranial nerve, as well as other parts of the auditory system. This type of testing will indicate brain stem damage as a result of SBS injuries.

Chemical Testing

Researchers have found high levels of glutamate, a neurotoxin, in persons who have sustained traumatic brain injury for days after the injury.[35] Tests are now being done on abused infants and children to look for high levels of glutamate in their blood. When a child receives a traumatic head injury, such as after a shaking incident, glutamate crosses the common limits of the brain and damages brain cells.

Quinolinic acid, another neurotoxin, has also been found in shaken children.[36] This toxin appears in higher concentrations in the cerebrospinal fluid of shaken children compared with children who have sustained accidental injuries. This finding may ultimately be used to determine the time of abuse.

High levels of both neurochemicals might also indicate prior injury. Sample sizes in initial studies have been small, so further investigation and testing need to occur before any definite conclusions are made.[37]

Craniotomy

The craniotomy is one way to surgically evacuate intracranial hematomas and stabilize other bleeding. It is the most invasive technique for the removal of such collections. Prior to performing surgery on an infant or child, a neurosurgeon will discuss the risks that are involved with parents or guardians. Infants and children who are shaken and have hematomas that require craniotomy may develop infection, have seizures, bleed further and possibly require repeat surgery, or die.

A craniotomy is often a lifesaving procedure. For children with high intracranial pressure (ICP), the procedure has been shown to reduce mortality and morbidity.[38]

The process is as follows: A child is given general anesthesia, and his or her scalp is shaved, prepped, and draped sterilely. A "horseshoe" skin flap is made with a surgical knife. It is elevated with a periosteal elevator, and a burr hole large craniotomy is performed with a pediatric perforator and craniotome. The resulting bone flap is then elevated and the dura is opened with a knife and scissors. Acute blood and clotted blood will be seen at this time and removed. Small bleeding veins can be cauterized to stop active bleeding. Bleeding from larger veins can be controlled with products such as Gelfoam powder or Surgicel. Cottonoids are placed to check for further bleeding. After five minutes of further inspection of the entire cranium using a brain retractor, the cottonoids are removed and often a subdural intracranial pressure monitor is implanted. The dura is then sewn together, and the craniotomy edges are lined with bone wax and Gelfoam powder. Prior to closing the skull, a Surgicel sheet is placed over the dura. The bone flap is sutured closed and a drain is set in place. The galea is closed with sutures, and the scalp is stapled.

Final checks include the adjustment of the ICP monitor, the suture of the monitor and the drain to the scalp, and the placement of foam tape around the entire head. A child can then be transferred to the pediatric intensive-care unit.

Electroencephalography

An electroencephalogram (EEG) helps medical providers evaluate the status of the electrical activity within the brain. A child will have electrodes pasted onto different locations of the scalp in order to accurately measure various sections of the brain. An electroencephalogram is the resultant recording.

The technology has become well advanced in recent years, with the standard use of computer-screen EEGs, rather than the version that formerly used moving needles on paper. EEGs are frequently "sleep-deprived," whereby the child is allowed only a minimal amount of sleep prior to the test. A sleep-deprived EEG is done to actively bring on a seizure in order to study and treat brain abnormalities. Strobe flashes from a device called a photic stimulator, or stroboscope, may also be used during an EEG while a child sleeps to bring on seizure activity. Technicians attempt to actively cause seizures in order to measure their intensity to ultimately provide treatment for the child that will best control the seizures. An EEG is an important technological component to determine cerebral function and behavior, prognosis following acute cerebral problems, and brain death.[39]

Electroretinography

This nonevasive process evaluates the functioning of various parts of the retina. It also has been found to be useful in determining the cause for persistent visual problems in shaken children.[40] An electroretinograph (ERG) will show whether the problem stems from a cortical or retinal deficiency.

Electrodes are pasted on a child's forehead and earlobes. Eyes are dilated with drops, and the child adapts to a darkened room for approximately thirty minutes. In sequence, a dim blue flash and standard white flash are presented, and the eyes' responses are recorded. After being allowed to adapt to a lighted room for ten minutes, the child's eyes receive a flicker stimulus, and the response is again recorded.

The ERG is usually not helpful immediately following a shaking incident. The procedure is most useful in detecting longitudinal problems of vision.

Hemosiderin Staining

Hemosiderin is a pigment that contains iron and is derived from hemoglobin in the disintegration of red blood cells. It is actually a way that the body stores iron until it is needed for later use in making hemoglobin. At autopsy, the testing of hemosiderin is performed to check for old hemorrhage in the eyes.[41] Medical providers and investigation personnel need to know this information for a more complete understanding of a child's injuries and for the purposes of court testimony.

Lumbar Puncture

Also known as a spinal tap, a lumbar puncture (LP) obtains cerebrospinal fluid (CSF) for diagnostic purposes or to reduce intracranial pressure. This process is standard in the evaluation of children who have been shaken or who may be experiencing underlying blood infection, such as meningitis.

The procedure for an LP is as follows: The infant or child is placed in a "C" position, with legs flexed to the chest and head lowered forward. The area between the fourth and fifth vertebrae is cleansed and may be isolated by a sterile paper towel. A fine-gauge, sterile needle is inserted into the subarachnoid space of the underlying spinal canal. The medical provider will feel a "pop." The stylet in the needle is removed, and CSF begins to flow. Two or three small tubes are collected for laboratory examination. A manometer may be placed after the stylet is removed to measure CSF pressure.[35] After the procedure is complete and the needle is removed, the tiny hole in the dura mater closes on itself and begins to heal.

Normal cerebrospinal fluid should be clear. Bloody or yellow-colored (xanthochromic) CSF indicates acute or old blood. Medical providers need to determine whether this blood is from a traumatic stick during the LP or from intracranial bleeding, such as a subarachnoid hemorrhage.[42,43] If the bloody appearance of the CSF diminishes after several tubes are collected, the trauma is from the process of giving the LP. The amount of red blood cells within the CSF can be counted microscopically.

Serious complications arising from an LP are rare. Occasionally, if the brain is under significant pressure, the brain stem can herniate, or become displaced downward, once the pressure is relieved through the opening at the LP site. This can cause intense headaches and sometimes arrest respiration. A similar, milder, and less dangerous headache may occur if CSF leaks into the spinal canal and transverses to the brain.

Shunts

The buildup of CSF in the cranium will cause hydrocephalus in an infant or child. Children also may have problems with chronic subdural hematomas. Because of this, there needs to be a way to divert fluids away from the brain to maximize normal functioning. A shunt is a method of diverting fluids into a body cavity that can absorb or excrete it.

There are several types of shunts that can be used in a child with hydrocephalus or poor drainage management. A ventriculoatrial (VA) shunt drains into the atrium of the heart; a ventriculopleural shunt drains into the chest cavity; the most common, the ventriculoperitoneal shunt (VP), drains into the abdominal cavity.

One end of the flexible shunt is surgically placed into the lateral ventricle of the brain, and the other end is tunneled under the skin to the abdomen, heart, or lung for drainage. These shunts are permanent. VP shunts have extra coils that are left in the abdominal cavity to allow for stretching as the child grows. Upon healing of the scalp, there will be a small, evident bulge showing the outline of the shunt. Most shunts have a reservoir for testing of the system.

Children with chronic subdural hematomas are placed with either subdural-pleural or subdural-peritoneal (SP) shunts.[35,44] These are nonvalve tubes that allow for drainage of fluid. Children with subdural collections from a complication with subarachnoid drainage have been successfully treated with temporary SP shunts.[45]

Complications can be numerous with the shunting process. Infection, if it occurs, will usually be present within days to weeks after surgical placement. VA and ventriculopleural shunts carry the risk of blood clots damaging the heart and lungs. Shunts may also malfunction because of kinking, overdrainage, or migration into the brain parenchyma.[46,47]

Shunts' complications are less common today because of technical advances. Play activities for children with shunts usually are not restricted.

Visual-Evoked Response Testing

A visual-evoked response involves using periodic flashing lights to measure brain activity. Electrodes are pasted to a child's scalp, and information is recorded from both occipital lobes to see if the "visual center" of the brain recognizes the flashed lights. Cortical visual impairment (CVI), common in SBS, represents damage to the visual cortex of the brain. Visual-evoked response testing can measure the gravity of CVI, as well as follow the development of the visual system over time.

NOTES

1. Kleinman PK, Blackborne ED, Marks SC, et al. Radiologic Contributions to the Investigation and Prosecution of Cases of Fatal Infant Abuse. *NEJM* 1989; 320:507–511.

2. Bachman DS, Hedges F, Freeman JM. Computerized Axial Tomography in Neurologic Disorders of Children. *Pediatrics* 1977; 59:352–363.

3. Sinal SH, Ball MR. Head Trauma Due to Child Abuse: Serial Computerized Tomography in Diagnosis and Management. *South Med J* 1987; 80:1505–1512.

4. Kleinman PK. Diagnostic Imaging in Infant Abuse. *AJR* 1990; 155:703–712.

5. Cohen RA, Kaufman RA, Myers PA, Towbin RE. Cranial Computed Tomography in the Abused Child with Head Injury. *AJR* 1986; 146:97–102.

6. Nimkin K, Kleinman PK. Imaging of Child Abuse. *Pediatric Clin N Amer* 1997; 44: 615–635.

7. Harwood-Nash DC. Head Injuries in Child Abuse. In: Poznanski AK, Kirkpatrick JA, eds. *Diagnostic Categorical Course in Pediatric Radiology*. Philadelphia: W.B. Saunders Co./Radiological Society of North America; 1989:47–55.

8. Zepp F, Bruhl K, Zimmer B, Schumacher R. Battered Child Syndrome: Cerebral Ultrasound and CT Findings after Vigorous Shaking. *Neuropediatrics* 1992; 23:188–191.

9. Feldman KW, Brewer DK, Shaw DW. Evolution of the Cranial Computed Tomography Scan in Child Abuse. *Child Abuse & Neglect* 1995; 19:307–314.

10. Merten DF, Carpenter BLM. Radiologic Imaging in Inflicted Injury in the Child Abuse Syndrome. *Ped Clin North Amer* 1990; 37:815–837.

11. Sargent S, Kennedy JG, Kaplan JA. Hyperacute Subdural Hematoma: CT Mimic of Recurrent Episodes of Bleeding in the Setting of Child Abuse. *J Foren Sci* 1996; 41:314–316.

12. Han BK, Towbin RB, Courten-Myers GD, et al. Reversal Sign on CT: Effect of Anoxic/Ischemic Cerbral Injury in Children. *AJR* 1990; 154:361–368.

13. Duhaime AC, Bilaniuk L, Zimmerman RA. The "Big Black Brain": Radiographic Changes after Severe Inflicted Head Injury in Infancy. *J Neurotrauma* 1993; 10 (suppl 1): S59.

14. Alexander RC, Schor D, Smith WL. Magnetic Resonance Imaging of Intracranial Injuries from Child Abuse. *J Peds* 1986; 109:975–979.

15. Ball WS Jr. Nonaccidental Craniocerebral Trauma (Child Abuse): MR Imaging. *Radiol* 1989; 173:609–610.

16. Sklar EML, Quencer RM, Bowen BC, et al. Magnetic Resonance Applications in Cerebral Injury. *Emerg Dept Radiol* 1992; 30:353–365.

17. Cox LA. The Shaken Baby Syndrome: Diagnosis Using CT and MRI. *Radiol Tech* 1996; 67:513–520.

18. Sato YS, Yuh WTC, Smith WL, et al. Head Injury in Child Abuse: Evaluation with MR Imaging. *Radiol* 1989; 173:653–657.

19. Chabrol B, DeCarie J-C, Fortin G. The Role of Cranial MRI in Identifying Patients Suffering from Child Abuse and Presenting with Unexplained Neurological Findings. *Child Abuse & Neglect* 1999; 23:217–228.

20. Kleinman PK, Ragland RL. Gadopentetate Dimeglumine-Enhanced MR Imaging of Subdural Hematoma in an Abused Infant. *AJR* 1996; 166:1456–1458.

21. Haseler LJ, Phil M, Arcinue E, et al. Evidence from Proton Magnetic Resonance Spectroscopy for a Metabolic Cascade of Neuronal Damage in Shaken Baby Syndrome. *Pediatrics* 1997; 99:4–14.

22. Hart BL, Dudley MH, Zumwalt RE. Postmortem Cranial MRI and Autopsy Correlation in Suspected Child Abuse. *Am J Forens Med Path* 1996; 17:217–224.

23. Haase GM, Ortiz VN, Sfakianakis GN, Morse TS. The Value of Radionuclide Bone Scanning in the Early Recognition of Deliberate Child Abuse. *J Trauma* 1980; 20:873–875.

24. Howard JL, Barron BJ, Smith GG. Bone Scintigraphy in the Evaluation of Extraskeletal Injuries from Child Abuse. *Radiographics* 1990; 10:67–81.

25. Sty JR, Starshak RJ. The Role of Bone Scintigraphy in the Evaluation of the Suspected Abused Child. *Radiol* 1983; 146:369–375.

26. Jaudes PK. Comparison of Radiography and Radionuclide Bone Scanning in the Detection of Child Abuse. *Pediatrics* 1984; 73:166–168.

27. Kleinman PK. Head Trauma. In: Kleinman PK, ed. *Diagnostic Imaging of Child Abuse*. Baltimore: Williams & Wilkins; 1987:159–199.

28. Walker C. Predicting Outcome after Cerebral Insult. *Headlines* Sept–Oct 1993:4–11.

29. Merten DF, Radkowski MA, Leonidas JC. The Abused Child: A Radiological Reappraisal. *Radiol* 1983; 146:377–381.

30. Meservy CJ, Towbin R, McLaurin RL, et al. Radiographic Characteristics of Skull Fractures Resulting from Child Abuse. *AJR* 1987; 149:173–175.

31. Hyden PW, Gallagher TA. Child Abuse Intervention in the Emergency Room. *Ped Clin N Amer* 1992; 39:1053–1081.

32. Kleinman PK, Marks SC, Adams VI, Blackbourne BD. Factors Affecting Visualization of Posterior Rib Fractures in Abused Infants. *AJR* 1988; 150:635–638.

33. Caffey J. *Pediatric X-Ray Diagnosis*. Vol. 2. Chicago: Year Book Medical Pub.; 1972.

34. Hymel K, Abshire T, Luckey D, Jenny C. Coagulopathy in Pediatric Abusive Head Trauma. *Pediatrics* 1997; 99:371–375.

35. Baker AJ, Moulton RJ, MacMillan VH, Shedden PM. Excitatory Amino Acids in Cerebrospinal Fluid Following Traumatic Brain Injury in Humans. *J Neurosurg* 1993; 79: 369–372.

36. Bell MJ, Kochanek PM, Heyes MP, et al. Quinolinic Acid in the Cerebrospinal Fluid of Children after Traumatic Brain Injury. *Crit Care Med* 1999; 27:493–497.

37. Hanley DF. Multiple Mechanisms of Excitotoxicity. *Crit Care Med* 1999; 27:451–452.

38. Cho DY, Wang YC, Chi CS. Decompressive Craniotomy for Acute Shaken/Impact Baby Syndrome. *Pediatr Neuosurg* 1995; 23:192–198.

39. Menkes JH. Introduction. In: Menkes JH, ed. *Textbook of Child Neurology*. 4th ed. Philadelphia: Lea & Febiger; 1990:1–27.

40. Fishman CD, Dasher WB, Lambert SR. Electroretinographic Findings in Infants with the Shaken Baby Syndrome. *J Ped Ophthalmol Strabismus* 1998; 35:22–26.

41. Elner SG, Elner VM, Amall M, Albert DM. Ocular and Associated Systemic Findings in Suspected Child Abuse: A Necropsy Study. *Arch Ophthalmol* 1990; 108;1094–1101.

42. Spear RM, Chadwick D, Peterson BM. Fatalities Associated with Misinterpretation of Bloody Cerebrospinal Fluid in the "Shaken Baby Syndrome." *Am J Dis Child* 1992; 146: 1415–1417.

43. Apolo JO. Bloody Cerebrospinal Fluid: Traumatic Tap or Child Abuse. *Pediatr Emer Care* 1987; 3:93–95.

44. Ransohoff J. Chronic Subdural Hematoma Treated by Subdural-Pleural Shunt. *Pediatrics* 1957; 71:561–564.

45. Tsubokawa T, Nakamura S, Satoh K. Effect of Temporary Subdural-Peritoneal Shunt on Subdural Effusion with Subarachnoid Effusion. *Child's Brain* 1984; 11:47–59.

46. Guertin SR. Cerebrospinal Fluid Shunts: Evaluation, Complications, and Crisis Management. *Ped Clin N Amer* 1987; 34:203–217.

47. Lawton KH, Meyers M, Donahue EM. Current Practices and Advances in Pediatric Neurosurgery. *Nurs Clin N Amer* 1997; 32:73–96.

CHAPTER THIRTEEN

✧   ✧   ✧

Survivors

F OR INFANTS AND CHILDREN WHO SURVIVE an incidence of shaking, life beyond the hospital walls can be harsh. For family members or others who carry the brunt of caregiving responsibilities, day-to-day processes can be onerous at best. This chapter focuses on the toll that SBS takes on a young recovering body, the challenges of therapies to regain and relearn simple functions, and the hope of current research that is being conducted worldwide.

ACTIVITIES OF DAILY LIVING (ADLs)

Children who are affected by brain injury have problems with nerve impulses and muscle responses, and experience problems when attempting basic activities. In these children, neurofiber messages of the brain become altered and have difficulty being transmitted. Specific areas of the brain control various functions; for example, the cerebellum coordinates the voluntary muscles, and the occipital lobe coordinates visual activity. Two types of nerves, motor and sensory, carry information from the brain to the muscles. Motor nerves allow for actual muscle movement; sensory nerves control the position of joints being moved and the tone of the muscle. Muscles have high- and low-tone properties. Low tone in muscles occurs when sensory nerves are abnormal or when there is injury to the brain or spinal cord. A low-tone muscle can become hypotonic or "floppy." Over time, the muscle will atrophy from not being used. High-tone muscles allow for proper movement, quick response, and so on. Following is an alphabetic list of ADLs and how they are affected by Shaken Baby Syndrome.

Bathing

Parents and caregivers can have a particularly difficult time bathing children who are disabled as a result of SBS. Just as there are bath seats for infants, there are also specialized devices for SBS survivors. Such special bath chairs, which help support the child's trunk, can be quite expensive, ranging in price from $250 to $300, and can be ordered from companies who carry special therapeutic equipment.

Parents and caregivers may also be able to get loaner chairs from social service agencies in their community, such as Early Childhood Intervention, United Cerebral Palsy, Easter Seals, Boys and Girls Club, ARC, or United Way, or from medical equipment closets through their churches.

Great care should always be used when bathing an infant or child so that he or she is not hurt by incorrect water temperature or slipping in the tub. Bath time can be a fun or even soothing time for children. It also becomes a therapeutic bonding time for the adult giving the bath.

Feeding

SBS survivors may have a difficult time when it comes to eating or being fed. This can lead to complications related to getting adequate nutrition.

Traumatic brain injury from a shaking incident may leave a child without the physiological capacity to suck, chew, or swallow. With the help of exercises given by speech therapists, children can master the basic elements of eating. For example, holding the sides of the child's jaws lightly can allow for basic tongue and lip control.[1]

Older children often experience difficulty with side-to-side or lateral movements to effectively chew "adult" foods. Speech or occupational therapists can offer suggestions for in-the-mouth exercises the child can do to strengthen the tongue muscles and coordinate lips to close correctly while eating.

Liquid or pureed foods may help other children with swallowing difficulties. Providing food that tastes good is also one of the most basic features to successful eating. Other children may thrust the tongue out of the mouth when eating. They can be assisted with the use of a small, soft brush (pacifier brush) and a special spoon, which parents and caregivers can use to gently manipulate where the tongue lies or to actually feed the child. Brushes work well in children who are sensitive to texture.

Children may be affected by gastroesophageal (acid) reflux and chronic vomiting. They might need a feeding or gastrostomy tube (G-tube) in order to get adequate nutrition. This tube is surgically attached to the stomach and is connected to a bag of liquid usually hung on an IV pole. Parents or caregivers are instructed in the use and care of the tube feeding device so that it can be used regularly in the home.

Mobility

Children affected by SBS may have significant mobility problems or loss of functioning in their limbs. Fortunately, there are exercises, activities, and equipment available to assist children as they grow toward mastering mobility. Many children, though, will be confined to wheelchairs for life.

Parents and other caregivers work in coordination with a professional therapist to exercise and strengthen a child's limbs and trunk if the child cannot move independently. A daily routine may include applying splints to a child's arms to keep hands straight, plastic casts to keep legs straight, or a body jacket to align the spine.

SBS children often need to be propped in a standing position to develop balance and leg strength, and to give them a sense of independence. Standers are devices whereby a child will stand for approximately twenty minutes at a time. A child will then work up to longer daily sessions in the stander. Standers are often equipped with trays where colorful objects and toys can be placed to keep children occupied during their time of "therapy."

Children affected by SBS often have musculature or orthopedic difficulties as a result of limb contracture or poor mobility. Weight-bearing exercises allow for limbs to build strength and receive proper development. Surgery may be required to correct musculature or orthopedic problems to allow for ease of movement, standing or walking. With orthopedic surgery, the hip joint can be altered for a better ball-and-socket fit. Physical devices, such as a knee immobilizer used at night, prevent a child from contracture and keep muscles flexible. In any post-hospital procedure, children will require physical therapy to aid in recovery.

Because children affected by SBS often have poor gross motor skills, walking can be a large final hurdle to independent mobility. Gait trainers, bouncers, exersaucers, and large infant walkers help toddlers with trunk control and support. When children are able to move in such devices on their own, they experience pride. It allows them the intrinsic sense of independence all children want and need.

Toileting

As a result of a shaking assault, and depending on the developmental milestones that had been attained prior to the shaking, children may never be able to independently toilet themselves. Guidance and reassurance by parents or caregivers can help them learn to accomplish this often-difficult act. Survivors of SBS often will depend on the steadiness of an adult hand or arm or a specialized potty seat. Children can also be trained through the habit of getting on the toilet seat soon after each meal.

✧   ✧   ✧

Children can become frustrated in their endeavors to become more independent in their ADLs. Calm encouragement serves to not only help a child, but also remind an adult caregiver or professional of the need for patience. Goals for the child should be set, as these keep everyone involved motivated in training efforts. High expectations will not help a child affected by SBS become more independent, however. Children go at their own pace.

THERAPIES

After discharge from a hospital, a parent or caregiver of a shaken child may be faced with many ongoing questions regarding their child's functionality and development. While hospitalized, an infant who has survived an incident of shaking should be evaluated to determine readiness for therapy. It is often hard to say what any shaken child will need due to severe impairment, because deficits develop over a long period of time. Any good rehabilitation program will tell families to treat infants sooner for better results. Because of this, health-care providers should order therapies after discharge. Any deficits immediately identified should be treated immediately.

Federally funded Early Childhood Intervention programs are available in every state for children from birth to age three. To be eligible for such a program, a child must have a disability or developmental delay, or be at risk of having one. Assessments are done to determine what services children and their families need. The family insurance company or child's Medicaid is billed for use of the program's services. No one is denied due to inability to pay. Older children are typically referred to school-related programs for ongoing therapies. Outpatient clinics may be connected with an inpatient hospital, or they may be independent agencies within a community. The more programs shaken children and their families can use, the more they will maximize potential for recovery.

Parent and caregivers should be wary of any program that takes a great deal of their personal time and money. Programs that are not covered by insurance should also be questioned. A child's pediatrician might be able to guide families on an adequate path of rehabilitation. Below are the descriptions of several fundamental therapies that make the lives of shaken children more endurable.

Occupational Therapy

This type of therapy maximizes a child's activities of daily living, which include everything from grasping objects to drinking from a cup. Occupational therapy considers a child's environment and guides parents or caregivers in what they can do to maximize the child's functioning. This allows for greater independence and positive feelings of success. The occupational therapist assesses not only a child's developmental abilities, but also a parent or caregiver's ability to work effectively with the child at home.

Therapists in hospitals, schools, and community-based agencies are in a unique position to identify cases of SBS and other types of abuse that may have been misdiagnosed.[2] Appropriate training of therapists on the nature of SBS injuries can make for a more thorough evaluation of affected children and their families.

Physical Therapy

Infants and children in physical therapy learn and develop normal movement patterns. This therapy works with a child's posture and movement and enhances the capabilities of the child. Range-of-motion exercises, tone response, and strength training are some of its basic features. Therapy sessions occur in both inpatient and outpatient settings, usually three to five times per week. Parents or caregivers need to be encouraged to practice the exercises and movements learned in physical therapy with the child at home.

Once an infant begins regular movements, these will be targeted to maximize muscular potential. As a child progresses, activities that emphasize the use of their gross motor skills, such as swimming and ball catching, can be fun and help build the child's self-esteem.

As children grow, they may need special devices to assist their long bones and muscles from becoming unstable. Arm splints and leg braces keep limbs rigid and in a correct position so as not to contract and lose functioning.

Physical therapists can support parents or caregivers emotionally simply by pointing out what their child with SBS *can* do, opposed to what he or she cannot do.[3]

Speech Therapy

The traumatic effects of shaking will often cause poor neuromuscular control, making it difficult for the child to form proper speech sounds. Speech therapy teaches children options in creating sounds and ultimately words. Children will often begin with a basic repetition of sounds to develop their potential for verbalization. If true deficits in speech production are present, therapists will work with children to find alternative ways to balance such problematic areas. Speech therapists also work with uncontrollable mouth movements of children. Facial muscles can be trained over time to function more properly. Parents and caregivers will also be encouraged to actively work with their children in the home to consistently provide feedback and training.

RESEARCH INITIATIVES

In recent years, scientific research has led to a better understanding of pathophysiology of SBS. Treatment advances have also taken steps toward helping surviving infants and their families lead better lives. Yet, with current technology, shaken infants fare no better than they did a decade ago. For example, management of the capricious nature of intracranial pressure is still imperfect. There is, however, hope that ongoing research initiatives will help guide medical professionals toward assuring a more rapid and complete recovery for injured children.

Intracranial Advances

Two recent articles have identified the benefits of using the drug tirilazad mesylate to combat the effects of cortical .OH (hydroxyl ion) levels and brain hemorrhaging in shaken, anesthetized male rats.[4,5] Cortical .OH is an alkali, free-radical oxygen compound that surfaces in the brain following traumatic brain injury. An excess of this compound indicates a disturbance of the brain cell and acts as a poison. This compound is thought to play a role in producing the hemorrhages that develop after brain injury and to increase the amount of damage already done by the initial violence as the compound extends.

Tirilazad is, basically, an antioxidant that significantly fights the effects of damaging cortical .OH. The drug has been found to reduce bleeding, help in the stabilization of brain membranes, and decrease the scavenging efforts of free radicals. Vitamin E levels (a natural antioxidant increased in the injured brain) were enhanced by the presence of tirilazad. The ultimate level of brain damage, however, as measured by the number of cells lost from the cerebral cortex, was not reduced by the use of the drug.

Yet a second article described the potentially positive effects of using tirilazad in combination with the drug riluzole to reduce progressive cortical degeneration. The researchers in this study believed that the neurotoxin glutamate, released in the brain during shaking, is key to the degenerative response of the brain after trauma. Riluzole is a glutamate inhibitor. In this study of shaken infants, tirilazad used alone reduced intracranial hemorrhaging, riluzole used alone did *not* reduce neural degeneration, and the combination of the two drugs significantly lengthened the time that brain neurons survived.

Another recent advance in intracranial research to accurately identify diffuse axonal injury (DAI) in shaken infants who have died is the process of beta-amyloid precursor protein (ß-APP) staining.[6] One study showed that the use of this particular staining process during autopsies could detect DAI when there was a question of the way an infant died. Another study used ß-APP staining within the cervical cord white matter of the spinal column and concluded that a positive stain supported a diagnosis of SBS.[7]

Intraocular Advances

Vitreoretinal surgery has been recently described as being a successful way to preserve the lens of the eye and help stimulate vision.[8] Such surgery was performed on nine infants, many of whom had been shaken. Eighty percent of the eyes after vitreoretinal surgery retained functional results. When blood does not clear from the vitreous of the eye, typically the eye's lens is removed. Researchers have reported a surgical way to spare the lens in order to optimize the function of the eyes. Vision improves and rehabilitation of the eye can begin.

Another way to clear intraocular hemorrhage and avoid vitrectomy without complications is by intravitreal injection with tissue plasminogen activator (tPA) and sulfur hexafluoride gas (SF_6).[9] Conway and associates found that weekly injections for several weeks can allow for fast resolution of intraocular hemorrhage with the potential for early recovery of vision.

In an important study, the use of ß-APP staining was found to be beneficial in the identification of axonal injury within the optic nerve in cases of fatal SBS.[10] The authors found that the majority of their cases of SBS had optic nerve axonal injury, determined by the use of ß-APP staining. Such findings supported their hypothesis that optic nerve axons, like intracranial axons, are susceptible to shear and stretch forces of whiplash trauma. The authors also found that ß-APP staining as a mechanism for identifying optic nerve axonal injury was clearly superior to conventional hematoxylin-eosin histology and NF immunostaining.

✧   ✧   ✧

As the mortality and the disabling effects of SBS have not changed in the last decade, society needs more and more research to help in the battle. In so many ways, a shaken child loses. The information described above is encouraging. Funding groups and the government should appropriately support research efforts to help scientists and medical professionals more thoroughly understand and treat injuries seen in SBS. There can only be hope that the next decade will lead in that direction.

NOTES

1. Batshaw ML, Perret YM. *Children with Handicaps: A Medical Primer*. Baltimore: Paul H. Brookes Pub.; 1986:134.

2. Davidson DA. Physical Abuse of Preschoolers: Identification and Intervention Through Occupational Therapy. *Amer J Occup Ther* 1995; 49:235–243.

3. Kang K, Paleg G. Therapists Can Help in National SBS Campaign. *Advance for Phys Therapists* January 5, 1998:33.

4. Smith SL, Andrus PK, Gleason DD, Hall ED. Infant Rat Model of the Shaken Baby Syndrome: Preliminary Characterization and Evidence for the Role of Free Radicals in Cortical Hemorrhaging and Progressive Neuronal Degeneration. *J Neurotrauma* 1998; 15:693–705.

5. Smith SL, Hall ED. Tirilazad Widens the Therapeutic Window for Riluzole-Induced Attenuation of Progressive Cortical Degeneration in an Infant Rat Model of the Shaken Baby Syndrome. *J Neurotrauma* 1998; 15:707–719.

6. Shannon P, Smith CR, Deck J, et al. Axonal Injury and the Neuropathology of Shaken Baby Syndrome. *Acta Neuropath* 1998; 95:625–631.

7. Gleckman AM, Bell MD, Evans RJ, Smith TW. Diffuse Axonal Injury in Infants with Nonaccidental Craniocerebral Trauma: Enhanced Detection by Beta-Amyloid Precursor Protein Immunohistochemical. *Arch Path Lab Med* 1999; 123:146–151.

8. Maguire AM, Trese MT. Visual Results of Lens-Sparing Vitreoretinal Surgery in Infants. *J Ped Ophthalmol Strabismus* 1993; 30:28–32.

9. Conway MD, Peyman GA, Recasens M. Intravitreal tPA and SF_6 Promote Clearing of Premacular Subhyaloid Hemorrhages in Shaken and Battered Baby Syndrome. *Ophth Surg Laser* 1999; 30:435–441.

10. Gleckman AM, Evans RJ, Bell MD, Smith TW. Optic Nerve Damage in Shaken Baby Syndrome: Detection by ß-Amyloid Precursor Protein Immunohistochemistry. *Arch Pathol Lab Med* 2000; 124:251–256.

Part Two

LEGAL ASPECTS OF
SHAKEN BABY SYNDROME

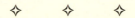

If your arguments be rational, offer them in as moving a manner as the nature of the subject will admit, but beware of letting the pathetic past swallow up the rational.

—Jonathan Swift

Children will still die unjustly even in a perfect society. Even by his greatest effort, man can only propose to diminish, arithmetically, the sufferings of the world.

—Albert Camus

CHAPTER FOURTEEN

Investigation of Shaken Baby Syndrome

E ACH YEAR, INFANTS AND CHILDREN are diagnosed as victims of SIDS, accidental falls, congenital disorders, and so on that are actually cases of murder by shaking. Autopsies are not performed, no one is prosecuted, and
homes are not investigated. As the pathophysiology of SBS becomes more widely
known, fewer such cases will be mismanaged. There will always be pockets of
ignorance and irresponsibility, but legislation regulations can change the way
professionals working with abused children do their jobs.

EXTERNAL INVESTIGATION

Deaths and injuries from SBS and other forms of physical child abuse are seriously underestimated.[1] When an infant is shaken and injured, there are several
issues on which to focus. The primary emphases should be the nature of the
injuries to the child, when the injuries were inflicted, and who committed the
shaking incident.[2]

The types of injuries found in SBS have been outlined thoroughly in this book
and in hundreds of other sources. Yet knowledge of these injuries and the way they
are produced is not common knowledge among law enforcement investigators,
pathologists, medical personnel, and social workers. Cases are missed and not
completely investigated. Harry Bonnell, a well-respected medical examiner in the
field of child abuse fatalities, carries the following philosophy: "You only find what
you look for, and you only look for what you know."[3] The more training oppor-

tunities there are for the professionals involved, the better they will be at identifying SBS injuries and fatalities. Only then can more cases be prosecuted.

Violent traumatic shaking leading to intraocular and intracranial bleeding and
rapidly progressing edema will be preceded by the onset of symptoms appearing
immediately or within minutes. Less severe shaking will produce less severe symptoms over a longer period of time.[4] Perpetrators of shaking incidents can be identified more readily if investigators and medical personnel are aware of this princi-
ple. A caretaker who offers an incomplete or skewed history of a symptomatic
infant's injury can invariably be identified as the perpetrator of the crime. It is
important that investigators review statements given to all medical personnel,
including emergency personnel, and other family members before an alleged perpetrator is questioned. These can support or negate the accuracy of injury details.

Investigations by law enforcement personnel are done to determine the
course of action appropriate to any criminal violation and to determine how victims can best be protected. All aspects of the family structure and quality of relationships should be documented. This includes the assessment of positive or negative interactions among family members, amount of time individuals spend at
home, and the type of emotional support that is received from extended family
members.[5]

Bass and associates found that further investigation into SIDS deaths led to
the finding that several of the infants were shaken to death.[6] They concluded that
information obtained during the death scene investigation should lead, when suspicious, to special examination of internal organs during autopsy.

An initial approach that scene investigators take is the observance of the child.
Breaking investigations down into steps allows for more thorough work. There is
usually only one chance to investigate a crime scene and few chances to investigate
a crime victim. So careful work must secure all necessary information at once.

There are a variety of questions to consider when investigating a shaken child:

- Is there external bruising, and if so, what type?
- Does the child appear well nourished?
- Did the child vomit?
- Is there any bleeding from the child?
- Are there any areas of swelling on the child's body?
- Are cutaneous marks present on the child's body?
- What was the position of the child when found?

The physical surroundings will be the next target in the investigation process.
This is very important, as careful observation and a detailed description are vital
in obtaining a case for the prosecutor. The whole room where a shaking incident
occurred must be properly examined. Findings can be compared with information given by an accused perpetrator; for example, a story given in the hospital of
an infant falling down a flight of stairs will be obviously conflicting if the investigator finds the home environment is a one-story dwelling.

The following should be noted:

- Condition of the living environment
- Discarding of infant clothing or other materials used in a "clean-up" process
- Height of infant sleeping area
- Condition of infant sleeping area
- Overt physical evidence (e.g., blood on a coffee table)
- Height of infant feeding chair
- Overt signs of alcohol or drug use (e.g., beer bottle, crack pipe).

Finally, investigators should thoroughly document interviews with all caretakers who were with the child within the last twenty-four hours. Much information can be garnered by simple observation on the part of the investigator or clinician.[7] How do family members interact? Is there appropriate eye contact? How do family members react to the findings that injuries to their child are abuse-related? Is there a willingness to cooperate? How do family members place themselves when sitting or standing? Specifically, investigators should note the following:

- Stories that do not match the gravity of the crime
- Excited utterances (e.g., "I didn't hurt that baby!")
- Differences in successive caretaker accounts of the same event
- When the child was last said to be well and acting normally
- Whether there are expectations of the child that are not age-appropriate
- When the incident occurred
- If the child was moved after the incident
- Accounts from other children present at the time of the incident
- The demeanor of the infant throughout the day
- Any recent psychosocial stressor affecting any of the infant's caretakers
- The condition of other siblings within the home.

Perpetrators of shaking crimes will offer stories that do not account for the severity of SBS injuries. An identified perpetrator for obviously inflicted injuries may give no explanation.[8] He or she may say, "The baby was fine one minute and was twitching and breathing funny the next." Though SBS is typically a crime of seclusion, there may be witnesses. Other children in the house, other caretakers, or other individuals who may have been present need to be interviewed completely away from the alleged perpetrator. Stories that do not match reveal answers for investigators.

Shaking incidents may arise from single moments of violence, wherein the caretaker lashed out in a rage at an infant. The perpetrator may or may not be a biological parent. No one can be absolved as a suspect until an investigation is complete and all persons connected with the crime have been interviewed. Shaking largely occurs within abusive homes. A pattern of abuse will emerge and be verified with a physical and diagnostic examination of the child. If there is a history of prior domestic violence or child abuse, investigators may not need to look too hard for potential suspects.

The process of interrogation is important to the process of the investigation. Proper interrogation will lead an investigator to the correct answers. In shaken infant deaths, investigators can interrogate at the crime scene or at the police station. The process is often aided by the interrogation being videotaped. The tape can be used in court at a later date and videotaping puts a potential perpetrator on edge emotionally. Richard Easter proposed that cardboard cutouts or dolls be used during the interrogation process to make the reconstruction of the crime more real.[9] Using such tactical methods can make excuses for injuries more ridiculous.

Investigators should question in the following way: "The child could not have been injured (or died) as you described. Help me understand by showing me just what happened." Or "I know you want to help me understand what happened to this child."[2] Phrases such as these may invite the accused into conversation with the investigator. The ego strength of such perpetrators is so immature in the first place that such a stance by the investigator will make the perpetrator believe he or she is really helping out. Building a rapport with the perpetrator can lead to a confession.

Videotaping the reconstruction with the perpetrator should occur prior to interrogation. The investigator and perpetrator can then look at the tape together and point toward any inconsistencies. Juries will also benefit from videotaped reconstruction, and they typically find such evidence persuasive. Once a confession is made, investigators should get the most out of the interview by asking the perpetrator about the number of shakes, the frequency of shaking incidents, and the severity of shakes. Having the perpetrator demonstrate on a doll, while being videotaped, can help a prosecuting attorney's case later in court.

Child Death Review

The majority of states have the structure for child death review teams in place, yet there are many counties without the funding and personnel for such programs. A child death review team is a task force of professionals, including physicians, pathologists, social workers, and attorneys, who meet regularly to review recent pediatric deaths. The team seeks to understand whether a death was potentially preventable, legal recommendations need to be pursued, and public or private agencies involved with the child functioned as intended.[10]

From such meetings, decisions can be made to determine future guidelines for child deaths. One significant study surrounding child fatality reviews found that there is frequently a practice of underreporting in many communities.[11] This may be due to lack of training in child abuse injuries, lack of tracking of cases, or poor investigation.

Active surveillance by child fatality review teams can minimize the practice of underreporting. Active surveillance means that there will be a requirement of thorough investigation and autopsy of all child abuse fatalities (or undetermined deaths), the collection of vital information, interagency collaboration, and policy adjustment.[12]

Review teams can work with community agencies, as well as county and state legislators, to ensure that children and their families do not slip through bureaucratic cracks of a faulty system. Monteleone suggests that review teams require consistent reporting, change custody laws, develop guidelines for child protective services (CPS) agencies to assess at-risk children, require that CPS abuse cases be kept open longer, perform computer checks on all babysitters and daycare workers where abuse is found, provide respite care, educate medical personnel, and establish better coordination between police and CPS.[10]

Once many of these things are in place, communities can have a better grasp on the needs of their children and families. In order for this to occur, states need to require statutes and provide financial support to assure follow-through on recommendations.

Coroners, medical examiners, prosecutors, CPS workers, and medical personnel need to be held accountable for their investigations into deaths from SBS and other methods of physical abuse. Death review panels should not be seen as adding to the growing list of responsibilities of investigating disciplines, but instead should be viewed as improving procedural efficiency.[13]

INTERNAL INVESTIGATION

Documenting an external investigation completely supports the finding of an internal investigation, that being an autopsy. By working with pathologists and medical examiners, investigators can secure information that will benefit a case for a prosecuting attorney. If a child's injuries are in question, both the investigator and the pathologist can ask whether there could have been intentional injuries that coexisted with other medical phenomena.[14]

The Autopsy

Individuals who are investigating the death of an infant or child suspected to have been shaken need to follow closely the protocol for child deaths.[15] Many states do not regularly investigate unexplained child fatalities, and when there is an investigation, even fewer require autopsy.[16] To secure a conviction of a perpetrator in a shaking death, autopsies need to be performed. To distinguish SBS from SIDS deaths, questionable infant deaths need to be thoroughly examined.

For families of deceased children, autopsies can be particularly difficult, as the process may seem to add a form of insult to an already devastating injury. But autopsies can also be important for families, as they may find definitive answers as to the exact nature of what happened.[17] Autopsies of abused children can also be an emotional challenge for pathologists, who see the totality of injuries that caused death. The importance of a thorough autopsy can not be underemphasized. Adhering to strict protocol not only can detail the cause of death in an abused child, but also can lead to a successful conviction of an accused perpetrator. Autopsy results are the only way an infant can communicate the abusive incidents he or she endured. Richard Easter called this "listening to the child's body and what it tells you."[9] A thorough autopsy is one way of being an advocate for the life of an abused, shaken child.

Autopsy of a shaken child should include the following:[18–20]

- Skeletal survey
- Comparison of body height, weight, and head circumference to norm
- Documentation of external bruises (estimate ages), internal injuries, and skin lesions
- Stripping dura mater from brain and examination of skull for fractures or hematomas
- Examination of whole brain for hematomas, lesions, tissue damage, or other injuries
- Estimation of age of intracranial abnormalities
- Microscopic examination of brain (e.g., determination of diffuse axonal injury)
- Examination of total spinal cord and vertebrae
- Enuclation of eyes and microscopic exam for hemorrhage or other ocular injuries
- Estimation of age of intraocular abnormalities
- Microscopic examination of fractures to determine aging
- Examination of all viscera and microscopic inspection of all lesions
- Examination and swabbing of all orifices, and analyses of findings
- Analyses of blood, tissue, vitreous fluid, urine for microbiological and toxicological studies
- Photographing findings
- Sketching and labeling findings
- Consulting with other specialists
- Reporting findings to proper authorities.

Investigators should be present at a shaken child's autopsy to take photographs and interview the pathologist. Photographs can be used during interrogation and in courtroom presentations. Many investigators alternate between autopsy pictures and normal or studio pictures of the infant when interrogating a perpetrator. This can frequently bring a self-recriminating statement and ultimate confession. The investigator should also interview the pathologist during the autopsy, as knowledge of specific injuries and causes can aid in knowing how to question during interrogation.[11] Investigators need to communicate their findings to the pathologist in return. Such teamwork among disciplines will allow for more accurate results.

Autopsy conclusions should include all pathological findings, historical information, consultant opinions, and final diagnoses and recommendations.[21]

The pathology results, though critical to the prosecution or defense of perpetrators, need to be reported accurately without an attempt to conform to police or counsel theories.[2]

Keeping abreast of the latest research on SBS and other child abuse fatalities is vital to the work of a pathologist.[22] Such knowledge can make all the difference in courtroom proceedings. The more standardized testimony provided to juries, the less often perpetrators of shaking crimes will go unpunished.

Autopsy results are an ironic legacy a shaken infant leaves behind. In life, an infant is unable to speak for his or her own protection. In death, an infant's body speaks volumes about what happened.

CASE HIGHLIGHT

Justice after Twenty-One Years

In May 1978, five-month-old Ryan Wanta died after being in the care of Linda Sobish, who ran a daycare from her home. Ryan had been rushed to the hospital when he stopped breathing after supposedly choking on strained peaches. Sobish had tried cardiopulmonary resuscitation, yet the boy did not respond. At the hospital, his heart was restarted, but a ventilator was needed to sustain his breathing. Ryan died several days later. Injuries found in the hospital and at autopsy included severe bilateral retinal hemorrhaging and intracranial bleeding. Investigations were made by both police and child protection officials, though no action was taken against Sobish. Ryan's autopsy was ruled as "undetermined."

In 1996, Sobish was investigated because of complaints that she was tying children to their beds while they napped at her daycare. In 1997, Sobish pleaded no contest to running her daycare without a license. Ryan's mother, Arlene, heard about these allegations against Sobish and contacted the Portage County prosecuting attorneys in Steven's Point, Wisconsin. She pressed them to investigate the circumstances around Ryan's 1978 death. In August 1998, Sobish was arrested on a charge of second-degree murder after an investigation led officials to believe Ryan died from Shaken Baby Syndrome.

At Sobish's trial, many doctors testified that what is known today about Shaken Baby Syndrome is far and above what was known in 1978, just six years after it was first named. More details of what happened to Ryan came out at the trial: Nothing had been found to be blocking his airway; there were no signs of choking or vomiting in Sobish's home; bruises were found on the back of Ryan's head; and there was no finding of aneurysm or intracranial malformation in Ryan's brain. The defense argued that the boy had suffered from dehydration and anemia.

The eleven-day trial ended on October 21, 1999, with the jury finding Linda Sobish guilty of second-degree murder in the death of Ryan Wanta. It took them less than three hours. Sobish was sentenced to ten to twenty years in prison. Justice for Ryan was finally found.

NOTES

1. Lundstrom M, Sharpe R. Getting Away with Murder. *Pub Welfare* 1991; 49:18–27.

2. Parrish R. *Battered Child Syndrome: Investigating Physical Abuse and Homicide.* NCJ 161406. U.S. Dept. of Justice. Office of Justice Programs; July 1997.

3. American Public Welfare Association. Tiny Victims Leave Tiny Clues. *Pub Welfare* 1991; 49:22–23.

4. Kirschner RH, Wilson HL. Fatal Child Abuse: The Pathologist's Perspective. In: Reece RM, ed. *Child Abuse: Medical Diagnosis and Management.* Philadelphia: Lea & Febiger; 1994:325–357.

5. Weston JT. The Pathology of Child Abuse and Neglect. In: Kempe CH, Helfer RE, ed. *The Battered Child.* Chicago: University of Chicago Press; 1968:240–271.

6. Bass M, Kravath RE, Glass L. Death-Scene Investigation in Sudden Infant Death. *NEJM* 1986; 315:100–105.

7. Wissow C. Talking to Parents and Families. In: Wissow LS, ed. *Child Advocacy for the Clinician: An Approach to Child Abuse and Neglect.* Baltimore: Williams & Wilkins; 1989: 40–48.

8. Showers J, Apolo J, Thomas J, Beavers S. Fatal Child Abuse: A Two-Decade Review. *Pediatric Emer Care* 1985; 1:66–70.

9. Easter R. Scene Investigation in Shaken Baby Syndrome Investigations. Second National Conference on SBS. September, 1998.

10. Monteleone JA. Review Process. In: Monteleone JA, Brodeur AE, eds. *Child Maltreatment: A Clinical Guide and Reference.* St. Louis: G.W. Medical Pub.; 1994:309–325.

11. Ewigman B, Kivlahan C, Land G. The Missouri Child Fatality Study: Underreporting of Maltreatment Fatalities among Children Younger Than Five Years of Age, 1983 Through 1986. *Pediatrics* 1993; 91:330–337.

12. Schloesser P, Pierpoint J, Poertner J. Active Surveillance of Child Abuse Fatalities. *Child Abuse and Neglect* 1992; 16:3–10.

13. Stangler GJ, Kivlahan C, Knipp MJ. How Can We Tell When a Child Dies from Abuse? *Pub Welfare* 1991; 49:4–12.

14. Wissow C. Fatal Maltreatment. In: Wissow LS, ed. *Child Advocacy for the Clinician: An Approach to Child Abuse and Neglect.* Baltimore: Williams & Wilkins; 1989: 172–184.

15. Illinois Dept. of Children and Family Services. Autopsy Protocol for Child Deaths. In: Ludwig S, Kornberg AE, eds. *Child Abuse: A Medical Reference.* 2nd ed. New York: Churchill Livingstone; 1992:497–508.

16. Advisory Board on Child Abuse and Neglect. Current Issues: Training Weaknesses. In: *A Nation's Shame: Fatal Child Abuse and Neglect in the United States.* U.S. Dept. of Health and Human Services; 1996.

17. Beckwith JB. The Value of the Pediatric Postmortem Examination. *Ped Clin N Amer* 1989; 36:29–36.

18. Norman MG, Newman DE, Smialek JE, Horembala EJ. The Postmortem Examination on the Abused Child. *Perspec Ped Path* 1984; 8:313–343.

19. Pearl GS. Traumatic Neuropathology. *Clin Lab Med* 1998; 18:39–64.

20. Graham M. The Role of the Medical Examiner in Fatal Child Abuse. In: Monteleone JA, Brodeur AE, eds. *Child Maltreatment: A Clinical Guide and Reference.* St. Louis: G.W. Medical Pub.; 1994:431–458.

21. Goode R. Forensic Investigation of Pediatric Deaths. In: Ludwig S, Kornberg AE, eds. *Child Abuse: A Medical Reference.* 2nd ed. New York: Churchill Livingstone; 1992: 383–402.

22. Dorandeu A, Perle G, Jouan H, et al. Histological Demonstration of Haemosiderin Deposits in Lungs and Liver from Victims of Chronic Physical Child Abuse. *Int J Legal Med* 1999; 112:280–286.

CHAPTER FIFTEEN

SIDS versus SBS

UNDREDS OF CASES OF Sudden Infant Death Syndrome (SIDS), also known as "crib death" or "cot death," have been described in the medical literature. Many of these were probably cases of shaken infants before SBS was identified or commonly recognized. Physicians did not recognize the signs of SBS and therefore did not question parents or other care providers about statements such as "I just found her that way."

SIDS is a condition that affects infants for unknown reasons. The syndrome seems to affect infants up to eight months of age, but becomes much less frequent after age six months.[1]

In 1992, the American Academy of Pediatrics recommended putting infants down to sleep in a supine position (on their backs). A baby sleeping prone (face down) has approximately three times the risk for SIDS as when sleeping supine, and supine positioning is better than side positioning.[2] Since this advice was published and prevention efforts put in place, the practice of placing infants on their backs to sleep reduced the worldwide incidence of SIDS by 30 percent. Breast feeding has also been found to significantly reduce SIDS.[3]

On the other hand, premature or low-birth-weight infants have an increased risk for SIDS. Other risk factors include smoking during pregnancy; exposure to household smoking; excessive sleep clothing; sleeping on a nonfirm mattress, such as a waterbed; and being surrounded by excess crib materials, such as stuffed animals, bumper pads, comforters, and so on.[4]

It seems that every so often, new culprits are being named as causes of SIDS, the listing of which has been lengthy. One recent study from a group in Wichita found persistent levels of a blood chemical called hemoglobin-F (HgF) in victims of SIDS in the weeks or months after birth, well after those levels should have declined. Research continues in the anomaly known as SIDS, but one cause that can be missed is SBS. Shaking can, in fact, lead to parents, caregivers, and investigators finding infants dead in their beds. Autopsies may not be performed, or untrained investigators may accept it as fact that such infants were found as victims of SIDS. SIDS deaths need to be thoroughly investigated, including autopsies and death reviews.

At the same time, it must be recognized that parents who have innocently experienced the trauma of SIDS may find the investigation process a breach of their privacy and their grief. Wendy Valerie Harman frankly divulged such personal feelings in her commentary, "Death of My Baby," in 1981.[5] She realized quickly that she would never forget or accept the SIDS death of her ten-week-old son, Charles. Besides the loss of her baby and the grief that came with it, she and her husband also experienced distasteful interchanges with police investigators and even the media. Parents who lose a child to SBS may have a similar experience with such personnel. Investigations should be done with tact and respect for all family members affected by such a loss. What parents and others often do not realize is that the sole purpose of all the investigations is to seek to know the truth of what happened. And this will usually mean interviews and autopsies. Only after these are completed can officials rule out SIDS or child abuse.[6]

There are medically valid reasons for caution before a diagnosis of SIDS is made. One study looked carefully at twenty-six cases presented as SIDS deaths.[7] The authors found that 69 percent of the deaths appeared to have been from various causes other than SIDS, including two cases of SBS. They also called for thorough death scene investigation to be done prior to autopsy. The results of such information would then be forwarded to the medical examiner's office and lead to "special examinations of the brain, spinal cord, eyes, and skeleton."

Other factors that should give rise to suspicion when an infant is found dead include unlikely or inconclusive stories by the infant's caretakers, a history of previous death of one or more siblings from alleged SIDS, the presence of bruising or malnutrition, prior protective service involvement, or the infant being described as hard to care for or discipline.[1] Emergency medical technicians (EMTs), along with police or other investigators, should note the living conditions of the infant, as well as the emotional conditions of the household, as part of the larger picture of determining how an infant died.

When autopsies are performed on SIDS infants, there should be limited abnormal findings. SIDS does not cause subdural hematoma, external bruising, fractures, retinal hemorrhaging, or brain edema.[8] Betz and colleagues have concluded that the simultaneous appearance of conjunctival or eyelid petechiae and acute pulmonary emphysema at autopsy in "SIDS" deaths are instead highly suggestive of death by asphyxiation.[9]

In 1972, Richards and McIntosh studied 226 consecutive infant deaths and found that investigators, more often than not, relied on unverified parental or caretaker accounts when confronted with an infant death.[10] Three cases, which they presented from the early 1970s, are highly suspicious of child abuse deaths, though formally listed as SIDS:

SIDS at Three Weeks

When the father had not arrived home by 7:30 P.M., the baby's mother went to her mother-in-law's house, taking with her the baby and her other child, a toddler. The father arrived later, drunk, and they all set off for home at 9:45 P.M. When they arrived outside their house, the mother, fearing there was going to be a row, left the baby with her husband while she and the toddler went back to spend the night at his mother's. On waking in the morning, he found the child to be dead.

SIDS at Eight Months

The baby was illegitimate and spent the first four months of its life in a children's home. The father, who was unemployed, said they had abandoned their three children one week after his wife had come out of the maternity hospital because "the state refused to give us clothing and so they can . . . get on and look after them." The home was very dirty. The baby, who had appeared well on the previous day, was found dead in her cot at 10 A.M., having last been seen at 10 P.M. the previous night.

SIDS at Four Months

The parents had separated, the twenty-year-old mother having left her three children with her husband. Because of financial difficulties, the electricity supply was cut off, and the father asked a woman (whose identity is not known) to look after the baby while he and the older children went to stay with his mother. The baby is reported to have been well but one morning was discovered dead in its cot.

Cases such as these still today may or may not be questioned or even thoroughly investigated. Many medical practitioners feel that SIDS deaths are over-investigated. Former Iowa medical examiner Thomas Bennett has been blamed in several cases of infant deaths of erroneous diagnosis. Critics have stated that Bennett has ruled that an infant died of SBS when the child had actually been a victim of SIDS. They blame Bennett by stating that he sometimes based conclusions of abuse on microscopic injuries that could have been caused in other ways. One judge, in a case where Bennett determined that an infant had been shaken to death, ruled that the baby's parents were wrongly accused and released them after they had served nine months in prison. A reversal in another SBS case of which Bennett had been a part helped lead to the reversal in this particular case. After this ruling, defense attorneys stated that several other Iowa parents had also been falsely accused of killing their children. Bennett has defended his findings, as he makes such determinations when he finds signs of SBS, such as intracranial bleeding and retinal hemorrhages, that are not found in SIDS deaths.

This controversy serves to emphasize the necessity of full and accurate observation and record keeping on the part of medical, law enforcement, and legal personnel. Children do not need to suffer, nor should parents and other caretakers escape culpability for violent actions. SIDS can be an all-inclusive term for deaths for which inexperienced professionals can not find a cause. Meadow states that the term SIDS should be used in a much more limited fashion than at present, adding that it has a history of being "used at times as a pathological diagnosis to evade awkward truths."[11]

In 1993, 1999, and 2001, the AAP Committee on Child Abuse and Neglect and the Committee on Community Health Services proposed the following recommendations for medical professionals when confronted with an unexplained infant death:

- There should be accurate history taking by emergency responders and other medical personnel around and at the time of death. This should be made available to the coroner or medical examiner.
- Intentional asphyxiation should be considered in cases of unexpected infant deaths.
- Pediatricians and other medical professionals should maintain a supportive approach to parents during the cause-of-death process, with prompt informing sessions once the cause is determined.
- Pediatricians should advocate for proper death certification.
- Pediatricians should support legislation requiring autopsies of all children whose deaths resulted from trauma, are unexpected, or are unexplained.
- Pediatricians should support legislation that establishes comprehensive and prompt death scene investigation.
- Pediatricians should be involved in the training of death scene investigators regarding SIDS, child abuse, and pediatric disease to determine the cause of death.
- Pediatricians should be involved in the death review process.
- Initiatives that relate to the prevention of childhood death should be supported.[12–14]

People smother their children for reasons similar to why they shake them: to quiet them, because they do not want them, or because they are abusive individuals. Because SBS injuries are mostly internal, a diagnosis of SIDS can frequently be given. Children who survive SBS injuries may also be given a spurious diagnosis of "near-miss" SIDS—that is, of having almost succumbed to SIDS death. Giving complete physical examinations and carefully obtaining information in such cases can avoid errors of diagnosis.[15,16]

NOTES

1. Reece RM. Fatal Child Abuse and Sudden Infant Death Syndrome. In: Reece RM, ed. *Child Abuse: Medical Diagnosis and Management*. Philadelphia: Lea & Febiger; 1994:107–137.

2. Oyen N, Markestad T, Skjærven R, et al. Combined Effects of Sleeping Position and Prenatal Risk Factors in Sudden Infant Death Syndrome: The Nordic Epidemiological SIDS Study. *Pediatrics* 1997; 100:613–621.

3. Valdes-Dapena MA. Sudden and Unexpected Death in Infancy: A Review of the World Literature 1954–1966. *Pediatrics* 1967; 39:123–138.

4. American Academy of Pediatrics. Does Bed Sharing Affect the Risk of SIDS? *Pediatrics* 1997; 100:272.

5. Harman WV. Death of My Baby. *BMJ* 1981; 282:35–37.

6. Emery JL. Child Abuse, Sudden Infant Death Syndrome, and Unexpected Infant Death. *Am J Dis Child* 1993 147:1097–1100.

7. Bass M, Kravath RE, Glass L. Death-Scene Investigation in Sudden Infant Death. *NEJM* 1986; 315:100–105.

8. Gilliland MGF, Luckenbach MW, Chenier TC. Systemic and Ocular Findings in 169 Prospectively Studied Child Deaths: Retinal Hemorrhages Usually Mean Child Abuse. *For Sci Inter* 1994; 68:117–132.

9. Betz P, Hausmann R, Eisenmenger W. A Contribution to a Possible Differentiation Between SIDS and Asphyxiation. *Foren Sci Inter* 1998; 91:147–152.

10. Richards IDG, McIntosh HT. Confidential Inquiry into 226 Consecutive Infant Deaths. *Arch Dis Child* 1972; 47:697–706.

11. Meadow R. Unnatural Sudden Infant Death. *Arch Dis Child* 1999; 80:7–14.

12. American Academy of Pediatrics, Committee on Child Abuse and Neglect. Investigation and Review of Unexpected Infant and Child Deaths. *Pediatrics* 1993; 92:734–735.

13. American Academy of Pediatrics, Committee on Child Abuse and Neglect. Investigation and Review of Unexpected Infant and Child Deaths. *Pediatrics* 1999; 104:1158–1160.

14. American Academy of Pediatrics, Committee on Child Abuse and Neglect. Distinguishing Sudden Infant Death Syndrome from Child Abuse Fatalities. *Pediatrics* 2001; 107:437–441.

15. Berger D. Child Abuse Simulating "Near-Miss" Sudden Infant Death Syndrome. *J Peds* 1979; 95:554–556.

16. Altman R. The Shaken Baby Syndrome (letter). *NEJM* 1998; 339:1329–1330.

✦   ✦   ✦

CHAPTER SIXTEEN

Pretrial and Trial Aspects

O F THE MANY DIFFICULTIES that SBS presents in the courtroom, the most basic is understanding what is necessary to cause the syndrome. Juries, judges, and attorneys all need to be educated. Elementary instruction on biomechanics, physiology, neurology, and ophthalmology are all components that may need to be offered in this type of court case. For the attorneys, there is the burden of proving that the alleged perpetrator was the shaker, as there may have been multiple individuals who had access to the infant.

This chapter deals with the legal aspects of an SBS-related case from the time of the determination of what criminal charges will be brought against an alleged perpetrator to the moment of sentencing. All jurisdictions are not the same, so this chapter should be used only as a guide. The chapter finishes with a detailed account of the most influential court case to date: the Eappen-Woodward trial.

PRETRIAL ASPECTS

Law enforcement personnel can assist in cases against perpetrators of shaking crimes long before a trial date by coordinating thorough investigations. The last caretaker with the injured child may not always be the perpetrator. Investigators need to determine who had an opportunity to be alone with the child, the condition of the child prior to injury, and the dynamics of the home situation, so that the correct person will be charged for the crime. Medical personnel can also do their part through accurate diagnoses, accurate charting, accurate history taking, and being available to assist in interpreting clinical information.

Prosecuting attorneys should be actively involved in SBS cases early in the legal process. Being involved means that the prosecutor has discussions with medical personnel about the descriptions of injuries related to SBS and how they relate to their specific case. Being involved also means that meetings are held with family members to learn the dynamics of the home environment. If death occurs, being involved will mean meeting with the pathologist who performed the autopsy. Finally, being involved means solid case preparation. This involves speaking with child abuse experts about physical findings and biomechanics, as well as researching completely the variances of SBS.

Penalties and Charges

Depending upon the state, various kinds of penalties and charges are brought against perpetrators of shaking and other physical child abuse crimes. District attorneys and prosecutors differ from region to region as to what criminal charges will be pursued. Some prosecutors are more aggressive, seeking first-degree murder charges in most child fatality cases; others are prepared to plea bargain for substantially lower charges.

When children die from shaking injuries, their perpetrators could be charged with first- or second-degree murder, based on intent; reckless (reckless action causing death) or negligent (negligent action causing death); homicide, or manslaughter. The definition of first-degree murder is that the act was one of deliberate premeditation. In many states, there is another definition: extreme atrocity or cruelty. Second-degree murder charges encompass this label. In 1997, the commonwealth of Massachusetts prosecuted Louise Woodward under this particular definition. The idea is that if a person commits an intentional act that would cause a reasonable likelihood of death—such as the violent shaking and impact of Matty Eappen's head—that is extremely atrocious or cruel, second-degree murder will be charged. Involuntary manslaughter is used for an unintentional action that a person commits when he or she should have known that there would be endangerment of life. Voluntary manslaughter, on the other hand, is used for an act of intention done in the "heat of the moment."

If an infant dies as a result of SBS injuries, this will not always result in a charge of intentional murder. Prosecutors may charge the perpetrator with a lesser felony charge if they feel that a case is not clear-cut and the facts better support a conviction at that level. SBS is a crime of isolation, where there are typically no witnesses. This is a source of frustration among many child abuse prevention advocates, who feel that the death or injury of a child should automatically result in a murder or attempted murder charge. Prosecutors who support felony murder charges against a perpetrator of SBS are stating that this individual intentionally shook to inflict harm upon a child. If death results, then it was a certain result of their conduct.

For children who survive shaking incidents, charges may include felony assault of a child, reckless endangerment, felony child abuse, battery, or child endangerment. Many of these are felony charges, which means that the perpetrator not only faces substantial prison time, but is guaranteed the right of a trial by jury. Prosecuting attorneys balance the facts that emerge from the investigations in cases of SBS to decide what charges will be made, taking also into account the possible disabling consequences of the injuries.

Prosecutors need to realize that shaking and other abusive crimes against children should not be tolerated. Delivering strict charges and sentencing will send the message about our societal tolerance of abuse.

There is little uniformity among states in the charging of physical child abuse and child homicide. Most states support a felony charge of murder, child abuse, or child endangerment, based upon the fate of the child.[1] In Nevada, state statutes 200.010, 200.030, and 200.508 have been implemented to deal with any nonaccidental physical injury of a child under age eighteen. Such an injury is considered child abuse. When there is resultant substantial bodily harm, the perpetrator faces a charge of felony child abuse, with a sentence of two to twenty years. When death results because of abuse, the perpetrator faces a charge of first-degree murder, regardless of intent to kill. Such statutes greatly assist prosecutors in their job to convict perpetrators of child abuse crimes. *Labastida v. State of Nevada* (112 Nev. 11, 1996) set in motion the responsibility of persons who witness child abuse crimes, establishing that a witness could be charged with first-degree murder by child abuse if that person did nothing to prevent the abuse from occurring. This statute also makes a clear statement about tolerance of physical child abuse.

Statute of Limitations

The statute of limitations defines the amount of time that may pass between the crime and the filing of criminal charges, beyond which the alleged perpetrator cannot be prosecuted for that crime. There are different statutes of limitations for felony crimes and for misdemeanor crimes.

Most states have no statute of limitations for murder or manslaughter; all other felony crimes, such as aggravated assault, carry statutes of limitations anywhere from three to seven years, depending on the state. This issue is frequently an issue for parents and caregivers of shaken children, especially if they have experienced poor law enforcement investigation or hesitancy on the part of a district attorney to prosecute. Families need to press for expeditious investigation and follow-up prosecution before the statute of limitations can be invoked.

After the Arrest

Arraignment of a crime usually occurs within twenty-four to forty-eight hours after an arrest is made. It is an accused individual's first appearance before a judge. The charges are read to assure that the accused knows what they are, and the accused is asked to plead guilty or not guilty. On charges of murder, and in some states on all charges involving felonies, there is an automatic "not guilty" plea. Often the accused person's attorney does the actual speaking for him or her. The presiding judge then decides if the charges are appropriate and sets a bail amount and a court date for further proceedings.

A person who is arrested and placed in jail has the right to a preliminary hearing. States differ on the timing of this hearing, but it is generally held for a detained defendant within ten days.[2] An individual released on bond is entitled to a preliminary hearing within thirty days. At this hearing, the accused is informed of the charges and penalties. A prosecutor will present evidence and/or witnesses, along with probable cause, to attempt to show that a crime has been committed by the accused. The accused and his or her attorney may question witnesses and evidence, and the presiding judge will then make a determination.

At the preliminary hearing is also the time when a judge sets the amount of bond that the accused must pay in order to be released rather than remain in jail while he or she goes through the judicial process. A judge hears both prosecution and defense statements before setting bond for a perpetrator. In many jurisdictions, a person accused of a crime will need to pay only 10 percent of the bond, in cash, before being freed to wait for an upcoming trial or plea agreement, but there are no state or county rules that apply to setting bond. Judges use their own discretion and base their decisions on the egregiousness of a crime, past criminal record, the charge made, and whether an accused is likely to flee from justice. Advocates of child abuse prevention are frequently dismayed when judges impose a low bond, but the court system follows the tenet that a person is innocent until proven guilty. Hence, judges must weigh all facts when considering bond. Clearly, as with charging, enormous discrepancies occur within the scope of bonding perpetrators of shaking crimes.

If probable cause is evident, the case will next go to a grand jury; if not, the judge will dismiss the charge, but the prosecutor still can present evidence of probable cause to a grand jury. A grand jury usually consists of twelve to twenty-three people, who hear accusations and evidence of a crime, and then determine if there is enough to support a charge that has been made and therefore the accused shall be required to stand trial. A grand jury does not try cases, nor does it determine guilt or innocence. But a grand jury may request expert or material witnesses to testify under oath to help it decide whether a defendant should be indicted (a "true bill") or excused ("no true bill"). The accused may have no input into the process.

Plea Bargains

Plea bargains are agreements between prosecutors and defendants for a reduced sentence or charge in exchange for a plea of guilty. This practice often leads families of shaken infants to believe that true justice was not served. There are known cases of SBS where the perpetrator has plea-bargained from a charge of murder to reckless homicide and was sentenced only to probation. Such cases will continue to occur as long as child abuse laws are left in their current state.

Plea bargains may be entered into for several reasons. The prosecutor may think the case is weak due to lack of evidence and/or witnesses, or may believe that a jury would acquit the defendant or dismiss the more serious charges. Sometimes the prosecutor will reduce the charges or agree to a fixed sentence to ensure that the the accused does some time in prison so as to "mark" him or her as having been convicted on some crime, so that others will be warned. Or the prosecutor may wish to save taxpayer money on a lengthy trial with a potentially poor outcome.

Families of shaken children may need to encourage prosecutors not to plea-bargain cases, but they must also realize there is a risk in not doing so. Families often will see this as a crevice in the judicial system. Judges are not bound by plea bargains, although such pleas are always heavily considered in the courtroom.

Pretrial Motions

Pretrial motions encompass such things as when the prosecution and the defense ask the court to accept or reject evidence into admission for the upcoming trial. Such evidence may not be tangible evidence; for example, the prosecution may raise the question of admissibility of prior physical abuse by the accused, or the "doctrine of chance" or opportunity the accused had when alone with the victim, or the intent to harm the child with the finding of Battered Child Syndrome or Shaken Baby Syndrome.[3]

Scientific evidence may also be introduced as potentially admissible. This was a significant aspect in the pretrial motions for the Woodward case. The prosecution may even submit evidence that the accused had a history of malice toward the victim or had a history of shaking the victim in order to discipline him or her. Judges may or may not accept into admission any evidence that is submitted by the prosecution or defense. Prior acts by the accused can greatly aid the prosecution's case. Other pretrial motions may include modifications of jury instructions, exclusion of expert witness testimony, intent to introduce graphic elements, and admission of hearsay.[4,5]

TRIAL BY JURY

Shaken baby cases are heard in three types of courts: criminal, family (or juvenile), and civil. Families of shaken infants may become involved in any or all of the three courts. This often depends on the outcome of a criminal proceeding.

Criminal offenses against a minor are prosecuted in criminal court. This is where perpetrators of shaking crimes may or may not be convicted. Criminal court is also the only place where punishment is by incarceration.

When a minor commits a shaking crime against another minor, as when a young babysitter shakes an infant, the defendant is generally prosecuted in juvenile court, though states do allow young persons to be prosecuted as adults in criminal court, especially in cases of murder or manslaughter.[1]

Family, or juvenile, court focuses on the issues of protection and placement of a child and siblings in an abusive family, pending the identification of the perpetrator of the crime. This is often frustrating for innocent families of shaken children. For example, a babysitter or daycare worker may have abused a young infant of a very loving, responsible family, but until this situation is clarified, the infant is placed in foster care. When a child protection worker removes a child from his or her home, or places a child under temporary guardianship, the worker has a very short time to petition a family court justice for an order of protection. Issues regarding child placement and protection cases tend to require less need for proving that abuse is beyond a reasonable doubt than do criminal cases. There are no fines levied or prison term sentences imposed in family court. The only issues considered are adjudication, whether the child does or does not become a ward of the court, and disposition, where the child should be placed.[6]

Although a jury may acquit the accused on criminal charges, he or she could still be found guilty in a civil case. A civil suit is a financial suit. Families of victims may sue for various reasons, including loss of potential income, hardship, outstanding medical and/or burial bills, or attorney fees. They may sue the perpetrator; the perpetrator's insurance company, if there is coverage, as in childcare facilities; or the perpetrator's employer, such as an au pair agency). In few situations are civil attorneys the same prosecutors as in a family's criminal trial.[2] When families are seeking legal representation for a civil case, they should interview a variety of attorneys on possible courses of action that might be pursued and their expectations of the case. The attorneys will need to secure medical witnesses who are expert in the field of child abuse or other professionals who are used to testifying in such cases.

Subpoenas

Subpoenas are one of the first details in the coordination of a trial. These are court-ordered documents that require the appearance of named individuals scheduled to testify. Records such as hospital charts and doctor's notes can be subpoenaed as well, though most medical institutions have a confidentiality clause protecting privileged communication.

On a subpoena, an individual will be directed when, where, and at what time he or she should appear to testify. Persons who ignore subpoenas may be charged with contempt of court and arrested.

Juries

All individuals charged with crimes are constitutionally entitled to trial by jury. A jury has the responsibility of weighing the facts of a case to determine whether an accused individual is guilty or not guilty of the crime or crimes of which he or she has been charged.

Juries are typically composed of twelve members of the community, although some states use six-person juries for lower-level felonies.[2] The role of the prosecution is to prove the guilt of the accused beyond a reasonable doubt. In a civil action, the burden of proof is only that there is a "greater probability of truth" or "50% plus 1."[7] Prosecutors and defendants can agree to waive the right to a trial jury.

In most states, a guilty verdict must be by unanimous vote once all the facts are presented. Some states allow an eleven to one or even a ten to two vote by jurors.[2] In unanimous verdict states, even if one juror remains steadfast in an opinion contrary to that of the rest of the jury, the trial ends in a mistrial or "hung jury." Prosecutors may retry the charges with a new jury, or the charges may be dismissed. Civil cases seldom use twelve jurors, and some states do not require a unanimous verdict.

Before a criminal trial begins, a jury is selected. Prosecutors and defense attorneys interview prospective jurors to ensure that they are appropriate for the upcoming task. Several factors can automatically rule out a potential juror, such as case bias, knowing the victim's family or the perpetrator, past experience with SBS issues, or in-depth knowledge of the current case.

The Trial

Once the jury is selected, the trial begins. Jurors sit and listen to testimony over a period of days, weeks, or months, depending on the complexity of the case. In most states, they are not allowed to speak or ask questions of witnesses; however, there is a growing trend to allow jurors to submit written questions to witnesses. All communication goes through the court bailiff.

Jurors come from various walks of life and can be swayed by such things as negativity, complexity, or poor testimony. It is the job of the attorneys to make complex information related to the case as easy to understand as possible for the benefit of the jurors and judge. Jurors seem to invariably find it difficult to believe that an infant can be shaken so violently as to cause death or serious injury, so the defendant has an advantage from the start of courtroom proceedings. Judges, too, can have difficulty in believing there was criminal intent in an SBS case. In recent years, a Missouri man pleaded guilty to second-degree murder for the shaking death of his infant. The judge in the case sentenced the individual to probation, as the judge thought the mandatory sentence of ten years was too harsh for a father who had made a "mistake." If there was more education on SBS and child abuse to the greater community, potential jurors and judges would not find it so hard to believe that such a crime is possible.

One mother of a shaken infant suggests that an interesting scenario would be a trial by a jury of the *victim's* peers. "Imagine the group reaction of a panel of one- to two-year-old jurors hearing, 'Members of the jury, this child, your peer, was egregiously injured by this adult. This is what happened to your peer.' (Demonstration of shaking.) We hear the harrowing cries of an injured baby, and as it will be, the jury of the victim's peers follows suit, and all begin wailing. The court convicts the perpetrator of a most deplorable crime against children and is immediately sentenced to life in prison. And only when they see the perpetrator being dragged off in chains do the jurors' wails begin to subside."

In the end, jurors bring with them common sense and their own experience, which can benefit the prosecution. Most people know that an infant requires the utmost caregiving by someone who acts responsibly. This includes regular feedings, diaper changing, holding lovingly and carefully, and so on. When jurors are presented with a fatal case of shaking or a child who was seriously debilitated by shaking, their common sense will tell them that the act of violence that caused this was wrong, and that an infant debilitated by severe shaking will not return immediately, or ever, back to a normal state of well-being. A good prosecutor will instruct the jurors to see through the complex medical testimony to the essence of a case.

Legal Representation

Parents and caregivers need legal representation to look after their interests, which ultimately allows families to be available for their children. Families often think that since they were not the perpetrator, they do not need a lawyer, then realize too late that they should have obtained legal counsel in light of their child's assault. Such families are often too overwhelmed with their child's clinical condition to even consider hiring an attorney. Families also believe that law enforcement, protective services, and other investigation teams will follow a logical path of "going after the perpetrator." Too often this is not so, however, and they themselves are investigated and their rights to their child are temporarily or permanently taken away.

County agencies may potentially staff poorly qualified personnel. Because of this, child protection services (CPS) can become a bureaucracy that makes decisions for families and the future of the injured child solely by the book. Without legal representation, parents and other caregivers have no advocacy or protection. Parents might lose their rights to their child, justly or unjustly; cases may be mismanaged or be managed by multiple personnel; legal paperwork may not be fully explained; medical information may not be shared; authorization for medical procedures may not be allowed.

Each party in an SBS case needs an attorney to help protect him or her against losing important civil or legal rights. Even when CPS has excellent legal representation, the result may be to pursue actions that minimize or block the ability of parents or caregivers to do what *they* think best for the child. Proper legal representation will support and guide all family members. A guardian ad litem (meaning guardian for that lawsuit) is a person who is appointed to protect the interests of a child in a legal action. This guardian is a third party acting as an officer of the court and whose role is one of advocacy.[4] Such persons generally do not serve as legal counsel, trustee, or caregiver. Guardians ad litem can be attorneys, but most typically these are social workers or caseworkers. Guardians ad litem use their best judgment for the best interests of their client and may present evidence, question witnesses, and offer placement recommendations to the court.[5]

Always in the minds of CPS representatives is the concern that an abused child will return to the care of the alleged perpetrator. If a crime against a child is not substantiated, but only alleged, the child may very well return to his or her home. Follow-up home visits may be few and far between, so the officials of CPS tend to take the view that the best interest of a child is *not* to be returned to the former place of care.

Defense and Prosecution

Both sides of the legal system want one result in a courtroom case—a successful outcome. Both the defense and the prosecution may use dramatic measures to influence a jury in their behalf. Attorneys have the duty of presenting their client's case in the most favorable light possible. They may not make statements that they know to be untrue, as by misquoting a document from which they are reading, but defense attorneys, in particular, are under no obligation to be objective. For example, they must, when necessary, continue to assert their clients' total innocence even if they have just urged them to plead guilty. Protection of the rights of the defendant in our criminal law system is built around the idea that it is better that many guilty persons should go free than that one innocent person should suffer unjust punishment.[8] Prosecutors are bound by an ethics standpoint to seek justice. This may mean that some cases are dismissed when evidence absolves a defendant of criminal culpability.[2] Culpability states that an individual who shakes an infant and causes serious injury or death is responsible for this outcome, regardless of his or her motivation. With shaking crimes, there are two possible motivations. There may be deliberate intent, whereby a person wanted to violently control an infant for whatever reason, such as transference of past negative feelings onto the child. And there are those who shook but did not mean cause harm or death. These are the perpetrators who claim the "out-of-control" defense and may be sincerely regretful for their actions.

SBS is a complex syndrome at one level, but very easy to prosecute at another. Medically and biomechanically, it is just now being understood by medical and forensic personnel. This tends to complicate the legal aspects of the syndrome, as made evident in the Eappen-Woodward trial. On the other hand, SBS is a consequence of blatant child abuse, and medical providers know the forces required to cause the dramatic injuries that accompany the syndrome. So in this sense, perpetrators should be easily prosecuted for their crimes.

The problem arises in the fact that the general population is not versed in the clinical aspects of the syndrome, and the attorneys on both sides know this fact. When juries consider the evidence and testimony in child abuse and shaking cases, they are often emotionally unable to accept that such things could be done to young infants. Juries want to believe that the injuries to the victim were caused by an accident. Prosecutors are therefore left with considerable work to prove their cases and will benefit from the inclusion of pediatric specialists who have worked with victims or survivors of SBS. These professionals will bring greater expertise to the witness stand than some other medical personnel. Prosecutors can also strengthen their cases by trying to corroborate the medical information presented by their side when cross-examining defense medical specialists. This occurred throughout the Woodward case, so that the prosecution was able to whittle away the claims of the defense experts, backing them into a testimonial corner.

DEFENSE. Defense attorneys use many different tactics in order to win their cases. The "sympathetic" defense is one where there is a shift of focus toward blaming an innocent party, such as the partner of the perpetrator or the victim's parents or other caregiver. Defense attorneys could pose to the jury that their client:

- is a new parent and had never been instructed on how to care for his or her child
- didn't know that shaking was a bad thing, and just wanted the baby to be quiet
- had been going through some emotionally rough times lately
- sought medical care, therefore was a good care provider
- tried to resuscitate his or her child unsuccessfully
- was abused as a child

- was under the influence of drugs or alcohol
- kept the baby away from the hospital because it appeared to be okay
- witnessed the baby fall but saw no signs of injuries.

Such defenses are simply excuses, but unfortunately, many times juries accept them and acquit the accused. Jurors understand that it is very stressful to care for a baby, especially one who continually cries. There are also perpetrators who admit their crime but express remorse and grief. An attorney might use this to gain the jury's or court's sympathy. Such individuals tend to be biological fathers. Female babysitters or licensed or unlicensed child-care providers are the least likely to confess or express remorse.[9] Some perpetrators have true remorse and feelings of guilt, but by law they must still answer for their crimes. Others express remorse only in order to obtain the sympathy of the jury and escape or minimize punishment.

Another strategy perpetrators and defense teams like to use is to point a finger of blame in an alternative direction. An abuser will often rely on the fact that he or she took the child to the pediatrician on numerous occasions, with multiple issues, such as falls, sibling injuries, or apnea spells. When SBS is diagnosed later, the abuser places blame on the doctor for the original misdiagnosis so as to generate an atmosphere of reasonable doubt to persuade the jury not to convict. Defense teams are also aware that most people find it hard to believe that fellow members of their community would intentionally injure a defenseless infant.

Another defense strategy is to dwell upon how many people had access to the infant on the day that the shaking allegedly took place. Because there are multiple caregivers in today's society, this broadens the complexity of such cases.

Finally, defense attorneys know that juries are typically uninformed about the clinical and biomechanical aspects of SBS. Because of this, defense teams may attempt to use misconceptions to their advantage, such as the idea that "rough play" or "mild shaking" may cause shaking-related permanent brain damage or death.

PROSECUTION. To win a case against a perpetrator of a shaking crime, the prosecutors need to be fully knowledgeable about SBS. They must put into clear focus the responsibility of the accused from the very beginning of the trial—for example, by insisting that frustration with a crying infant is *not* a reason to shake it and is *not* a valid defense. SBS is caused by violent actions by violent individuals and must be presented to the jury in this way.

A simple strategy that prosecutors can use is to direct the jury on the basics of caretaking and handling of infants. Infants' heads and bodies need support and care during holding. By contrast, perpetrators of shaking crimes handle infants in such an extreme fashion that any reasonable person—including the perpetrator—would interpret it as involving a substantial risk of serious injury or death to the child. This is also the consensus of the American Academy of Pediatrics.[10] Such a statement can be supported with another: that shaking a child in such an extreme way is worse than striking a child.

The prosecution successfully used another technique in the Woodward trial in Boston. Perpetrators can frequently be backed into the situation of having to make up an explanation for their behavior. Individuals who do not readily admit to shaking crimes typically do not want to be viewed as inept caretakers, either. They may answer no to such questions as "Did you leave the child unattended?" or "Did you cause the child to fall?" If so, the perpetrator will place himself or herself in a corner by admitting he or she was with the child throughout a specified time. If the accused was the only person with the child, and if there was no other way the child was injured, then that individual must take responsibility for what happened.

Timing of injuries can often be based on knowing the state of the child when he or she was left with the accused. It would be helpful to have witnesses who can testify that the child was happy and healthy prior to being with the accused.

Infants with multiple injuries, such as healing fractures, bruises, and/or burns, who are also shaken tend to provide a more conclusive case for the prosecution. Such injuries reveal the pattern of abuse the infant experienced as part of a violent home environment.

Good medical experts can be very important for the prosecution, because of their unique knowledge of shaking injuries and biomechanics. However, there also can be a conflict of evidence when the defense team presents its "expert" witnesses who disagree on the effects of violent shaking or what was found on clinical exam or in diagnostic images. There may even be conflicting testimony as to possible differential diagnoses that may appear like SBS. This is one reason why sound medical examination and documentation are imperative in these cases. They could mean the difference between conviction and acquittal.

Judges

Some judges have no tolerance for crimes against children. Others, unfortunately, see children as unequal members of society and punish perpetrators of shaking crimes less severely than they would a similar crime against an adult. Judges are human, and as with juries, they too can form opinions early in a criminal cases.

In cases where judges allow perpetrators of shaking crimes to go free, it may be difficult for the partners to obtain custody. In one case, a judge felt that because a child's mother had been regularly taking the child to pediatrician appointments, the child could not have been abused. The girl was shaken, the mother was found not guilty (though she had, in fact, done what she was charged with), and the father had to go to family court to try to obtain custody.

Judges are not medical professionals and must rely on the information on physiology, diagnostics, and so on that is presented by legal counsel and witnesses. Often, they are too easily persuaded to go along with defense theories as to what really happened to a shaken infant. A judge may also get pulled into the sympathy strategy of the accused, as happened to Judge Zobel in the Louise Woodward case.

Findings, Documentation, and Evidence

A solid case against a defendant will have solid investigative findings, documentation, and evidence. These are all vital to the successful prosecution of such cases. Investigative findings include pictures of rooms, sleeping areas, bottles consumed, diapers changed, food jars, toys played with, and so on. They give a picture of how well an infant fared prior to his or her injuries. Investigative interviewing will include well-guided questioning, which is transcribed or videotaped.

Thorough documentation across disciplines not only is sound professional practice, but will aid in the prosecution of an offender as well. Documentation includes such things as emergency medical technician (EMT) notes, medical record notes, social work progress notes, and nursing observations and findings.

Evidence can be demonstrative, direct, circumstantial, or testimonial.[6] *Demonstrative evidence* displays the substance of clinical findings, such as X-rays, CT or MRI scans, surgical findings, or ophthalmological findings. *Direct evidence* refers to a witnessed account of a shaking incident or the testimony of the accused. *Circumstantial evidence* means that the court or jury is asked to infer that abuse has taken place based on demonstrative evidence and testimony of expert witnesses in SBS and abuse. Expert witnesses with special qualifications, who testify whether or not abuse occurred on the basis of the facts presented in court, give *testimonial evidence*. Unlike other witnesses, they may give opinions or facts on events that they did not personally observe.

Attorneys and expert witnesses will use such things as slides, graphic representations, charts, autopsy photographs, videos, and/or demonstrations with dolls to support or deny the allegations of shaking. These demonstrations can be very influential for juries, as visual examples are much more significant than mere description. Such evidence is either based on factual clinical findings or on supposition by witnesses' experience and/or research. The American Prosecutors Research Institute maintains graphic resources that can be loaned to prosecutors in child abuse cases if none are available.

Behavior

Any case involving a child is likely to be very emotional, and often families are concerned about showing emotion in the courtroom, believing that if they cry or express anger, that this will negatively influence the jury. In the Woodward trial, the press picked up on the demeanor of Debbie Eappen, mother of the deceased, and implied that she was the abuser, because she did *not* shed tears on the witness stand.

Most attorneys tell their clients to act natural in court. Rob Parrish, a prosecuting attorney and expert in SBS legal cases, proposes the following for parents and other caregivers: "Be yourself and don't do anything that is contrived or 'staged,' no matter what."[11] He also states that it is typically the defendants in SBS cases whose behavior comes across as contrived, since they have often been coached by their attorneys before they testify.

Witnesses

In trials, both the defense and prosecution call witnesses, who testify under oath. Prosecutors can benefit from medical providers who testify in the simplest of terms so that their findings can be understood by a jury. Defense attorneys will seek out medical experts to discredit the evidence posed by the medical witnesses of the prosecution.

There are primarily four types of witnesses used in a criminal court trial: expert witnesses, defense experts, character witnesses, and eyewitnesses. *Expert witnesses* are persons with specialized education, experience, and training. They can be used in any part of the legal process: serving as behind-the-scenes attorney consultants, supporting certain elements of the case, or testifying in the trial. Experts educate not only the judge and juries, but also the counsel, on complex medical evidence and facts. They may be physicians, nurses, social workers, medical examiners, scientists, physicists, law enforcement officials, or special investigators. They are usually paid for their time and preparation, and their fees may sometimes be exorbitant. They can be asked under oath what fees they are charging, and an unreasonably high figure makes a bad impression on most juries. Expert witnesses help explain both clinical findings and processes, and will testify about differential diagnoses or questionable findings. They can be asked the likelihood of a certain event happening, which is also known as opinion testimony.[12]

It is important for expert witnesses to prepare for their testimony. This is done through meetings with the counsel who called them and by reviewing pertinent evidential materials, such as medical records, taking notes to highlight certain important clinical aspects.[13]

Torrey and Ludwig describe three aspects to the expert witness appearing in court: qualification, direct examination, and cross-examination.[14] During the phase of qualification, the attorney who called the witness will qualify him or her by establishing the witness's credentials. During direct examination, the witness presents and comments on material relevant to a case. Cross-examination allows the opposing counsel to challenge aspects of the expert witness's testimony. More latitude is given to attorneys in cross-examination than when each side questions its own witnesses. For example, in cross-examination, asking leading questions is allowed. Cross-examination can be stressful for witnesses, as they are open to all types of rigorous questioning. Thomas Bennett, a pathologist well versed in the art of medical testimony, says that witnesses should remain calm under cross-examination, "Some lawyers like to be confrontational. Be cool, not cold or hot. Think of them as a best friend who is a little slow at times. You would show patience to a friend."[15]

Expert witnesses often use "demonstrative evidence" to help demonstrate or explain their claims. In the Matthew Eappen murder trial, Dr. Eli Newberger, a well-known expert in child abuse, demonstrated the shaking and slamming simply by using his hands to explain the forces needed for such a shaken impact injury as the young boy sustained. Courts may also allow dolls to be used for purposes of demonstration. Other expert witnesses may use devices to show the more scientific aspects of SBS, such as using a transillumination (backlighting) box to highlight images of retinal hemorrhaging in the victim.[16] Johnson wrote an indispensable guide on the use of charts and models to supplement physician testimony in court in SBS and physical abuse cases.[17]

Expert witnesses should possess several characteristics to appropriately influence those in the courtroom: They must be likeable, well educated, articulate, trustworthy, knowledgeable about the case, licensed, and willing to serve as a witness. They should have credentials and practical experience, and have written relevant papers, books, or reviews. They should avoid converting reasonable, clear medical facts into complicated theories and probabilities. If they do this, they may face intensive defense cross-examination and can confuse jurors.[18] Expert witnesses should not be too absolute in their opinions and should be ready to answer, "I don't know." "From what studies have shown (or what I have seen), this finding is not typical in Shaken Baby Syndrome" is an honest opinion that gives jurors options to help make final conclusions.

Defense experts help their side defend a case. In a 1997 SBS case tried solely by a judge, the defense obtained three well-known expert witnesses to testify that an infant could fall twenty-three inches, as claimed by the mother, and sustain retinal hemorrhages, subdural hematoma, and edema—injuries characteristic of SBS. This unfortunately led to a "not guilty" verdict.

There are instances where physicians, medical examiners, and other medical professionals have testified irresponsibly for the defense in order to disprove that an abusive event occurred, going beyond their medical expertise. Medical professionals should limit their professional testimony to their area of medical expertise. Many times defense expert witnesses do not follow such a tenet and use statements such as "without a doubt" or "my conclusive findings" to confirm that what they are testifying is true. Families or prosecutors concerned about such irresponsible statements or dubious practices during court cases have recourse. Letters of complaint can be written to medical societies and medical licensing boards in the state where testimony occurred or in which the expert resides. Although there is no enforcement in cases of questionable ethical testimony, the American Medical Association, in its code of ethics, encourages medical professionals to provide assistance in securing patients' legal rights objectively, without being partial to either side during testimony, and to maintain their professionalism at all times. The American Academy of Forensic Sciences and the National Association of Medical Examiners have ethics committees as well.

Character witnesses testify in court about the personality characteristics of the accused. Such witnesses may be in support of the accused ("He isn't capable of hurting anyone") or testify against the accused ("She has a temper that often flares").

Eyewitnesses are individuals who have actually witnessed the shaking incident. Such testimony is very valuable, but rare in shaking crimes. Eyewitnesses can describe not only the character of the accused, but also the nature of the assault, such as whether there was an impact at the end of the assault. Eyewitnesses are invariably more believable than expert witnesses who propose scientific and biomechanical postulates to explain away what clearly happened.

SENTENCING

Depending on the county, state, and judge, a perpetrator may receive substantial prison time or none at all if convicted. First-degree murder can carry sentences that include the death penalty, life imprisonment without parole, or a term of a minimum of twenty years. Second-degree murder carries approximately fifteen years' to life imprisonment (though some states do not have this type of sentence). A manslaughter conviction carries up to twenty years' imprisonment or even the possibility of immediate parole.

There is a term known as the "prosecutor's paradox," which states that "the worse the case is for the victim, the better the case is for the prosecution."[5] In terms of sentencing, under the guidance of an able attorney, this statement is an accurate one. Prosecutors need to treat the sentencing portion of an SBS trial as the ultimate appeal for justice. Recommendations should reflect the seriousness of a crime.

Families of the victim and of the accused can both make impact statements at the time of sentencing. Impact statements can influence judges either way in sentencing; they can also influence juries in civil court, who put a dollar figure on damage awards. Such statements focus on all aspects of the hardship that the victim's or accused's family has been put through—emotional, financial, physical, and psychological. They include messages of grief and loss, related to the death of the child, loss of the child's potential, and/or how the tragedy has affected the lives of family members.

APPEALS

A person convicted of a crime has the right to appeal the court case. Appeals are only rarely heard in cases where the defendant has pleaded guilty or no contest. An appeals court reviews the original trial of the convicted individual and considers arguments by both the prosecution and defense to decide whether to reverse the conviction or to reduce the original sentence. During the appeals process, a person may be released from detention, but arguments will be heard if there is thought to be a risk of the convicted person absconding or repeating the offense.

CASE HIGHLIGHT

The Life, Death, and Legacy of Matthew Eappen

On February 4, 1997, eight-month-old Matthew Spellman Eappen was shaken and slammed on a hard, flat surface in his home by his caretaker Louise Woodward, an au pair from Elton, England. On February 9, 1997, he died. The entire world watched as the case, trial, and sentencing unfolded. Why did this particular case draw such attention and controversy, and why did it become the groundbreaking one among the thousands of Shaken Baby Syndrome cases that have occurred over history?

The circumstances behind this tragedy are what proved controversial in the end. There was the eighteen-year-old au pair from a different country residing with a couple, both physicians, and their two young children—Brendan, two years old, and Matthew, an infant. Both boys were happy, playful, and well nourished.

Sunny and Debbie Eappen sought an au pair to care for Matty, as they called him, when Debbie returned to her medical practice. Their home in Newton, Massachusetts, was not glamorous, and the Eappens had loans to pay from medical school. Louise Woodward was seeking an au pair position to experience the thrill of life in the United States. Before the Eappens hired Woodward in November, they had briefly used two other au pairs for Matty. Woodward had been transferred to their home from another au pair placement. With this new family, Woodward was given regular instructions on caregiving expectations.

After some time, Woodward became increasingly challenging for the Eappens, with countless trips into Boston, late nights out, long telephone conversations with friends, and so on. Her priority as au pair soon diminished. At one time, Sunny Eappen came home from work early and found his two boys alone in the family room, as Woodward spent the next fifteen minutes down in the basement.

Sunny and Debbie both spoke with Woodward on January 30 about how to improve in her role as caretaker, suggesting that she could leave if she was not happy with this particular appointment. She apologized and vowed to change, but her ways did not improve. The Eappens put Woodward on a curfew so that she might stay focused on her caregiving responsibilities each morning. Little did the Eappens know that their au pair's pent-up anger and frustrations would soon change their lives forever.

THE TRAGEDY

"I was a little rough with him."
—Louise Woodward

The following sequence of events was never substantiated and is based only on reports Louise Woodward gave to investigators. Before she gave Matty his final bath, Woodward said, he had been fussy and crying most of the morning. She dropped the boy onto a bed in the morning. In the early afternoon, after bathing Matty, she lightly shook him, as she was frustrated with his crying, and dropped him to the bathroom floor after placing a towel down, where he banged his head. She changed his diaper, placed him in his crib, and rested a musical toy on his chest. She soon returned to find Matty in distress: His eyes were rolled back in his head, he had shallow breathing, and he was unresponsive. She wiped vomit out of his mouth, breathed into his mouth several times, and then called 911. (The fact that he had vomited was never substantiated.) After hearing the details of his condition, the dispatcher who took the call instructed her several times to place the boy on his stomach.

The first police officer responding telephoned the home en route and found the phone line busy. Upon arrival, he found that not only was the door to the house closed, but Woodward was on the phone. He asked the location of the injured boy. Woodward continued talking on the phone. She was asked again where Matty was. It was then that the officer saw his feet in the living room, just as the emergency medical response team arrived. Matty was found on his *back, not on his stomach as instructed, and he was in the first-floor living room, not in the second-floor bathroom. Woodward was still on the phone. Another officer removed the phone and escorted her into the living room to have her tell what had happened to Matty. The boy was rushed to Children's Hospital in Boston in critical condition.*

Police were called to the scene and interviewed Woodward. Debbie Eappen called Woodward from the hospital and asked for more details of the afternoon's incident, as doctors needed such information for the treatment of Matty. It was soon afterward that Woodward was detained and questioned more thoroughly by police. The next day, February 5, 1997, the au pair was formally charged with assault.

THE HOSPITAL
"We were holding Matthew and we prayed."
—Debbie Eappen

Matty Eappen never regained consciousness, and his clinical status declined steadily after he was admitted to the hospital. He was found to have a subdural hematoma, progressive cerebral edema, and retinal hemorrhaging. A two-and-a-half-inch occipital skull fracture was later confirmed at autopsy. These features, in combination, were all consistent with Shaken Impact Syndrome. A wrist fracture, several weeks old, was also found, showing previous abuse by Woodward. Matty clung to life for five days, his family staying at his bedside constantly.

On February 9, 1997, the Eappens prayed, received communion, lit a candle belonging to Debbie's grandmother, and held the child as he died—a tender, loving moment to a tragic ending of an innocent boy's life. The assault charge against Louise Woodward became a charge of murder.

THE CASE AND TRIAL
"It [Matty's injury] was equivalent to having been thrown from
a second-story window onto concrete."
—Dr. Eli Newberger

"But, I didn't do anything. I didn't hurt Matty."
—Louise Woodward

Lynn Rooney, assistant district attorney, was assigned to the Woodward-Eappen case and quickly requested that no bail be set for the au pair. Woodward pleaded not guilty to first-degree murder in Middlesex Superior Court on March 7, 1997. Debbie Eappen wore a button with a photograph of Matty's face pinned to her lapel. When bail was denied, the international controversy began. Supporters of Woodward contended that she was unaware of the U.S. court system and should not have been kept in a correctional facility with other women who were "more dangerous." Members of a local clergy association had written a letter of support for Woodward's bail, and the Newton mayor had even signed it. This was a theme that would play continually throughout the trial and afterward: the poor, young foreigner being accused of a tragic crime by an upper-middle-class couple of doctors.

Medical examiners and child abuse professionals from the Children's Hospital stated that Matty's injuries were equivalent to that of a long fall. Andrew Good, Woodward's attorney, wanted to suppress statements she had made—one to the responding officer after she called 911, and a second to detectives, who read her rights before interviewing her.

Hiller Zobel was assigned as the judge in the case and originally set a July trial date. Woodward's team recruited Barry Scheck, a forensic attorney featured on the O.J. Simpson defense team, to help with their arguments. One of the first challenges for the defense was to try to gain the admissibility of a polygraph test that Woodward had taken, with guided questions such as "Did you ever hit or strike Matthew on the head?" Judge Zobel ruled that it was inadmissible, as independent evidence could not corroborate that polygraph tests were accepted within the scientific arena.

The defense created its own delays with the trial date and planned its strategy by working its way through all the medical evidence, positing several clinical explanations for the injuries Matty sustained. First, the defense asked that DNA testing be performed to see if the boy had an underlying medical condition that could have affected his bone strength and caused intracranial bleeding. This was to delay the trial by three months and was structured to coincide with the pregnancy due date of prosecutor Lynn Rooney. Judge Zobel would not extend the trial another three months, as Rooney requested to take maternity leave, so she was replaced by Gerry Leone.

Next, the defense focused its attention on two-year-old Brendan, Matty's brother, as the perpetrator, as he was the only one in the house besides Woodward the day of the incident. The prosecution replied that no two-year-old could have inflicted such damage on an infant. Then the defense proposed that the cause of Matty's retinal hemorrhaging was by a sudden increase in intracranial pressure induced by the rebleeding of a prior head injury, not by violent shaking.

In late September, the defense team asked to have the case dismissed after medical experts testified that sections of dura mater (brain lining) taken during Matty's autopsy were missing. The defense contended that these sections would have showed prior injury. Dr. Umberto De Girolami, the head of neuropathology for Brigham and Women's Hospital, had previously examined the dura mater in question, and it revealed no dark spots indicating a previous injury, which corroborated with the findings of Dr. Gerald Feigin, the medical examiner who had performed Matty's autopsy. Zobel denied the defense motion, saying that the dura sections could have been lost during Matty's surgery to remove his subdural hematoma soon after hospitalization, and questioned why this was brought up two weeks short of the newly scheduled trial date.

When the trial finally began on October 6, 1997, both legal groups gave medical evidence as support for their side. And the medical experts did offer their testimony. The neurosurgeon who had performed the operation to remove the subdural hematoma also said there was no evidence that the hematoma was an old one that had begun to bleed again. The ophthalmologist offered key *testimony on the retinal hemorrhages found in Matty, something the defense team could not counter. And Feigin, who had performed the autopsy, testified that he had seen no evidence of a prior head injury or bleeding within Matty's skull. He stated that the skull fracture was recent in appearance, and the boy died from head trauma and subsequent brain swelling.*

Police detective William Byrne, who was on the scene after EMTs were called for Matty, testified that he had interviewed Woodward and thought her story sounded feasible. It was not until he spoke with medical personnel at the hospital that he arrested the au pair the following day. His report details the description of what Woodward told him had happened on February 4, 1997.

When Woodward took the stand in her own defense, she reacted to her defense attorney's questioning by grinning after she was asked, "Did you slam Matthew Eappen? Did you do anything to hurt Matthew Eappen?" Woodward also denied that she ever told Newton police that she had "tossed" the baby on the bed before a bath and later "dropped" him onto the bathroom floor.

Three weeks later, when all testimony was finished and closing arguments given, the judge ruled that Woodward's jury could consider only two charges: first- or second-degree murder. Her defense team had requested that a lesser charge of manslaughter be excluded from the jury's consideration, as they hoped for an acquittal. The prosecution protested Zobel's ruling and appealed to the state's Supreme Judicial Court, but the appeal was denied without a hearing.

The jury deliberated for several days, and on October 30, 1997, nine women and three men found the British au pair guilty of murder in the second degree in the death of eight-month-old Matthew Eappen.

Woodward collapsed into the arms of her defense attorneys and screamed out, "Why did they do that to me? Why did they do that to me? I'm only nineteen. I didn't do anything. I didn't hurt Matty."

THE JUDGE'S REVERSAL

"It is, in my judgment, time to bring the judicial part of this
extraordinary matter to a compassionate conclusion."
—Judge Hiller Zobel

On November 10, 1997, Superior Court Judge Hiller B. Zobel reduced Woodward's second-degree murder conviction to manslaughter. The second-degree murder conviction carried a life sentence with the possibility of parole in fifteen years. Normally, judges do not exercise their judgment on jury verdicts, yet Zobel felt that the au pair was confused and frustrated with Matty, and did hurt him in her care. Even more dramatically, Zobel sentenced Woodward to time served (279 days since the original arrest). Zobel had cited a state law known as Rule 25 when he lowered the verdict to manslaughter. The judge was to initially post this decision on the Internet, but computer problems altered that plan.

Supporters of Woodward in the United States and Britain cheered as the decision was announced. Cameras directed on citizens in Elton, England, cap-

tured champagne bottles being popped with the news of Zobel's decision. Supporters of the Eappens, on the other hand, were left shocked and befuddled by this breach of justice.

Woodward left the courtroom and went to a presidential suite at a Boston hotel with her parents. Prosecutor Gerry Leone did not anticipate the reduction of the sentence to manslaughter and was completely surprised by announcement of "time served." Sunny and Debbie Eappen returned home with their three-year-old son, Brendan, and a constant tragic memory of another son they once had.

THE AFTERMATH AND BEYOND

"I think the challenge for us today—the community at large, the medical community, the legal community, all of those who work on the child abuse unit— is to meet the challenge of 'Never again.'"
—Former Middlesex Assistant District Attorney Martha Coakley, who prosecuted Woodward

"Matthew should be here today. This day is as painful as it is beautiful. It gives us a lot of comfort that he won't be forgotten. We're all going to be his voice, and that's the job we have now."
—Deborah Eappen at the opening of the Matthew Eappen playroom
at New England Medical Center

"How was heaven today, Matthew?"
—three-year-old Brendan Eappen

One of the initial legacies that Matthew Eappen provided was his heart. During his testimony, pathologist Gerald Feigin said that two of Matty's heart valves had been removed when he was taken off life support on February 9 and donated to another child. This was an act typical of the giving nature of the Eappens.

The battle of the appeal process began soon after Judge Zobel's decision. The prosecution hoped an appeal would return the manslaughter verdict to murder. The defense, on the other hand, hoped for an outright acquittal.

Supreme Judicial Court Justice Ruth Abrams heard the arguments in December, and she chose not to return Woodward to prison while awaiting the actual appellate hearing. The hearing was scheduled for March, wherein seven justices would hear brief summarization and arguments from both sides. The decision would come in mid-June.

In the meantime, several changes began to occur throughout the United States and Britain in terms of child-care practices. In Britain, parents became hesitant about sending their daughters into an au pair program, fearful of another Woodward case. For some au pair agencies, the number of British women applying had fallen by half. Other aspects of the child-care system in the United States began to be more closely scrutinized. For example, in-home video monitoring sales skyrocketed after the Eappen-Woodward case broke. Some colleges offered nanny-training courses. And local and state legislation launched efforts to prevent tragedies such as Matty's from ever happening again.

One Massachusetts bill proposal put au pair agencies under the jurisdiction of the state's Office of Child-Care Services, which regulates daycare centers. The bill was presented to improve the training that au pairs receive before and after going into homes. It also required that criminal and other background checks be performed.

In February 1998, one year following Matty Eappen's death, a children's playroom was dedicated in his name at the New England Eye Center's pediatric ophthalmology/ear, nose, and throat clinic. This center is a part of the larger New England Medical Center. The playroom offers games, toys, and puzzles for pediatric patients, and a plaque is in place in Matty's honor.

On May 25, 1998, Deborah Eappen gave birth to son Kevin, who weighed seven pounds, eight ounces. He was born one day after Matty would have turned two. Kevin brought renewed happiness to the lives of Sunny and Debbie, who had endured great emotional pain for many months. Kevin's birth was another indication that the Eappens were moving forward with their lives.

Shortly before the Supreme Judicial Court's decision was announced in June, the Eappens announced the formation of The Matty Eappen Foundation, based in Chicago. The thrust of the foundation is to educate the public about child abuse, specifically Shaken Baby Syndrome, provide support to families of child abuse victims, and to honor Matty's life.

On June 16, 1998, the Massachusetts Supreme Judicial Court upheld Judge Hiller Zobel's decision to reduce Louise Woodward's second-degree murder conviction to manslaughter. Three members of the court contended that Zobel had misused his authority and voted to keep the second-degree murder conviction, yet four claimed that Zobel's decision was within his legal power, though not necessarily right. Hence the verdict stood, with a four-to-three vote, and Woodward was allowed to return to England. The ruling showed that the judges supported the idea that Woodward was responsible for the death of Matty, but it undercut juries, as it upheld the court's ability to overrule verdicts.

That afternoon, the Eappens filed a civil suit in federal court, for several reasons. First, Debbie and Sunny wanted to prohibit Woodward from receiving any financial gain from this tragedy. The couple was seeking compensatory and punitive damages for Matty's pain and suffering before his death and the hospital and funeral expenses they had paid.

On June 28, a federal judge made permanent an injunction that prevented Woodward from using any financial reward she might receive regarding the case until the civil lawsuit was settled.

In July, Woodward failed to respond in court in the United States to the civil suit, and hence merely defaulted. She claimed not to have the money to hire attorneys. The actual amount that Woodward had to pay would not be decided on until January 1999. Woodward signed an agreement in the court settlement not to profit from her story. If she ever attempted to make money on the tragedy, she would donate any profits received to a charitable organization (UNICEF).

In September 1998, Debbie and Sunny Eappen joined 850 other professionals, parents, and caregivers at the second National Conference on Shaken Baby

Syndrome in Salt Lake City, Utah. Both Eappens talked about their emotions from the ordeal and gave inspiration to all attendees through their drive to fight child abuse. Three-month-old Kevin accompanied the couple on this trip, which appeared to be a catharsis of sorts, as they interacted with other parents who had similarly suffered. Their presence also brought about a feeling of completeness for hundreds of professionals who worked with child abuse daily and had followed the case so closely.

This chapter ends with an ironic note. People *magazine in December 1998 wrote an update on the life of Louise Woodward since she had returned to England. She had enrolled in law school and claimed she wanted to help others so they wouldn't experience a fate similar to what she had endured, giving a blackened version of what a loving couple was doing in their son's memory an ocean away.*

The Matty Eappen Foundation has since helped make SBS training mandatory for all au pairs employed by EF Au Pair, the company that had hired Woodward. The foundation also is advocating for background criminal checks on child-care personnel, as well as providing general SBS information to parents and professionals.

NOTES

1. Parrish R. Personal communication, December 1998.

2. Gensel B. Personal communication, March 2000.

3. Holmgren BK. Charging, Plea Negotiation and Sentencing Strategies in Shaken Baby Syndrome Cases: How Medical Science Should Inform Legal Practice. Second National Conference on SBS. September 1998.

4. National Center on Child Abuse and Neglect. Representation for the Abused and Neglected Child: The Guardian Ad Litem and Legal Counsel. U.S. Dept of Health and Human Services. Children's Bureau; August 1980.

5. Goldner JA, Dolgin CK, Manske SH. Legal Issues. In: Monteleone JA, Brodeur AE, eds. *Child Maltreatment: A Clinical Guide and Reference*. St. Louis: G.W. Medical Pub.; 1994:387–430.

6. Munro JU. The Nurse and the Legal System: Dealing with the Abused Child. In: Campbell J, Humphreys J, eds. *Nursing Care of Survivors of Family Violence*. St. Louis: Mosby; 1993:343–358.

7. Araujo JJ. *The Law and Your Legal Rights: A Bilingual Guide to Everyday Legal Issues*. New York: Fireside Pub.; 1998.

8. Guthkelch AN. Personal communication, January 2000.

9. Showers J. Personal communication, May 1998.

10. American Academy of Pediatrics. Shaken Baby Syndrome: Inflicted Cerebral Trauma. *Pediatrics* 1993; 92:872–875.

11. Parrish R. Personal communication, July 1998.

12. Meyers JEB. Medicolegal Aspects of Child Abuse. In: Reece RM, ed. *Child Abuse: Medical Diagnosis and Management*. Philadelphia: Lea & Febiger; 1994:430–446.

13. Leake HC, Smith DJ. Preparing for and Testifying in a Child Abuse Hearing. *Clin Peds* 1977; 16:1057–1063.

14. Torrey SB, Ludwig S. The Emergency Physician in the Courtroom: Serving as an Expert Witness in Child Abuse Cases. *Ped Emerg Care* 1987; 3:50–52.

15. Bennett T. To be Believed or Not Believed. *Iowa Medicine* March 1997; 112–113.

16. Nolte KB. Transillumination Enhances Photographs of Retinal Hemorrhages. *J Foren Sci* 1997; 42:935–936.

17. Johnson CF. The Use of Charts and Models to Facilitate a Physician's Testimony in Court. *Child Maltreatment* 1999; 4:228–241.

18. Bonnell H, MD. Personal communication, August 1998.

CHAPTER SEVENTEEN

Post-Trial Aspects

T HERE ARE MANY LEGAL ASPECTS of SBS that occur outside the courtroom walls that are important to the lives of children everywhere. Some of these issues need to be mandatory, such as professionals reporting to proper authorities that physical abuse has occurred or is suspected. Other issues occur more rarely, such as formal adoption of a child survivor of SBS. These and other legal procedures are discussed below.

OTHER LEGAL PROCEDURES

Mandatory Reporting

Soon after Kempe's groundbreaking article describing the battered child was published (1962), the Children's Bureau, what was then the Department of Health, Education, and Welfare, proposed legislation on reporting. Five basic features were listed: reporting by physicians or institutions suspecting child abuse; procedures for reporting; immunity from liability; disallowance of physician-patient and husband-wife privileged communication in cases of abuse; and penalties for failing to report.[1] These first child abuse laws were passed in the mid-1960s and served as a model for other countries as well. In 1974, Congress passed the federal Child Abuse Prevention and Treatment Act (CAPTA). By this year, all fifty states now required professionals who worked with children to report cases of suspected abuse or neglect to child protection agencies. Failure to report could result in a felony charge against the professional, a loss of license, or a malpractice suit.

Today, in SBS and all other cases of abuse or neglect, parents or caregivers of injured children should be informed that the medical professionals are required by law to make a report to proper authorities in light of their findings. This creates an open, honest environment so that no one will be taken aback when child protective services (CPS) and law enforcement personnel become involved. This is especially important for the medical professional, as the identity of the perpetrator may not be known, and keeping a neutral ground will avoid misguided accusations.

Mandatory reporting consists of completing a child-at-risk form, making a telephone call to CPS and law enforcement officials within twenty-four hours after initial contact with the child, and submitting a follow-up written report within forty-eight hours after phoning in the incident. When a report is made, CPS and police will investigate. The process is usually an immediate one in order to establish the safety of the child, determine the identity of the perpetrator, interview key medical personnel, inspect the crime scene, and so forth. Once abuse is substantiated, CPS and law enforcement personnel will plan how to deal with the particular case.

Approximately 60 percent of all cases of child maltreatment are substantiated, but too frequently, child abuse cases go unreported. There are several reasons for this. A medical provider may believe that he or she does not have the proof necessary to support a report. However, individuals who report need only suspect that something happened to a child. There might even be a case where a nurse or social worker suspects that a child has been shaken, but the attending physician disagrees. If so, a report should be made in order that an investigation may be carried out. CPS workers will then be made aware of a potential perpetrator, and if abuse is ever substantiated, there will be confirmatory evidence of a pattern of abuse. Health-care facilities should have in place a policy of support for staff who report objectively, even if other staff members disagreed. Medical providers also may not report certain cases if they feel they are finding an individual guilty before being proven innocent. Yet the focus and purpose of mandatory reporting systems should be the protection of the child.[2] Also, medical providers are not exempted from filing a report under the heading of provider-patient privileged communication.

Making reports frees medical and other professionals from liability so long as they are using clinical judgment and reporting in good faith.[3,4] Professionals have an obligation to their clients or patients by protecting those who cannot care for or protect themselves. Most states allow a physician to keep a child in custody without parental consent or court order if placing the child back into his or her living environment presents an imminent danger to the child's health or life.

Interdisciplinary and interagency cooperation in cases of SBS and other forms of child abuse is vital, sending a message that there is teamwork on a united front and ensuring seamless care of the injured child and his or her family.

Order of Protection, or Restraining Order

Family members can receive an order of protection, also known as a restraining order, if a perpetrator of a shaking crime is released on bail, has completed serving a sentence, or was not prosecuted for the crime. Orders of protection can be granted in an individual's county of residence. An individual who is seeking an order of protection will have to appear in court to obtain one. These proceedings may or may not be closed to the public, though individuals seeking orders of protection can asked that it be closed for reasons of safety.

Orders of protection typically are created for the child and the rest of the family. This is frequently the only time that there is a specific focus on child protection, as the usual legal processes tend to be focused on determining whether a crime has been committed.[5]

A judge will set a standard limited distance that a perpetrator needs to respect or face incarceration. If the perpetrator violates the order, police may be called, and the individual may be arrested. Most restraining orders provide for up to one or two years of incarceration per violation. The local civil clerk can provide information and assistance on such orders.

Parental Rights

If a mother or father of a shaken infant is convicted as the perpetrator of the crime, the spouse may begin legal proceedings to terminate the abuser's parental rights. Custodial parents may also wish to terminate visitation rights from a perpetrator's parents. Often, however, the best the custodial parents can hope for is supervised home visitation. If the custodial parent remarries, a designated surrender is needed in many states, with the knowledge and intention of an adoption by a new spouse.

Central Registry

State child protection offices maintain a computerized registry of all reported cases of abuse and/or neglect that have been substantiated. This is to keep a record of multiple reports in families and to assure that children are protected by comprehensive follow-up services.

Perpetrators of abuse often hospital-shop to avoid attention and possible questioning. Investigators receiving reports from medical providers and other personnel can regularly compare suspect names with those in the state's central registry. This should not supplant the practice of reporting questionable cases; it merely shows investigators if there is a history and a pattern of reported abuse.

Foster Care

There were approximately 500,000 children in foster care placement in 1995, an increase of 70 percent from 1982.[6] The decision to remove a child and place him or her in a foster home should be based on a complete evaluation. Historically, this has been the exception, rather than the rule. There is such a great variability in placement decisions that there are often no set criteria in the determination that a child should be taken from his or her home.[7] When injuries are found to have been caused by SBS or other blatant physical abuse, CPS workers usually can assure that the living environment of the child is safe and loving if he or she is placed in foster care.

Foster placement can be short-term or permanent. An example of short-term placement is when an older sibling of a shaken infant is removed from the home during an investigation of crime. Shaken children who survive will also be placed in short-term foster care. Visitation by a child's parents, if allowed by the court, will tend to be limited initially. Arndt suggests that brief visitation, depending on the parent who is visiting, can be beneficial for all parties involved.[8] Children will reap emotional benefits from seeing and interacting with their biological parents, unless one of them is the perpetrator. If the child has been raised in a hostile environment by both parents, foster parents can offer helpful suggestions to the biological parents about quality parent–child relationships. And parents can observe proper parenting through the positive interactions between their child and foster parent.

The purpose of foster care is to provide a safe, loving environment to children in need of services. Most foster care homes do give children these basic provisions. However, there are also foster homes that are highly dysfunctional and even abusive. Foster parents are paid monthly to provide for placed children. Unfortunately, some providers are motivated by the pay they receive, while inadequately caring for their foster children. CPS officials oversee the foster care process, though due to the inordinate amount of casework such workers typically have, they may not regularly be in direct contact with the foster parents. CPS workers may not be able to monitor whether there is appropriate visitation, clinical follow-up appointments, new clothing, and so on.

In 1997, the Safe Adoptions and Family Environments (SAFE) Act (S.511), introduced by Senators John H. Chafee and John D. Rockefeller IV, was passed. This was one of the first steps toward necessary improvements in the foster care and adoption programs. The bill allows federal dollars to be used both for reunification services for families and for the care of a child with a parent in a residential substance abuse treatment program. The bill also requires states to develop and implement accredited guidelines for the care of children residing in out-of-home settings, assist public and private provider agencies in meeting the guidelines, and judge compliance with the guidelines by measuring improvement in child and family outcomes. The bill also emphasized that federal funds be used for staff retention and cross-agency training within child welfare agencies. This is very important, because child protection agencies typically have a high turnover and poor training.

Adoption

To lower the number of children in foster care in 1980, Congress passed Public Law 96-272, the Adoption Assistance and Child Welfare Act. This law imposed on states the requirement to make reasonable efforts to prevent placement of children, reunify families as soon as possible if placement occurs, and require a judicial determination of whether reasonable efforts have been made to prevent placement.[9] If these requirements are not met, states will not obtain financial assistance in providing for a particular child. In cases of SBS and other physical child abuse, this requirement will be withheld, if necessary, to protect the child from further harm.

Next-of-kin frequently become the legal guardians and ultimate adopters of SBS children. This puts the child in a least-restrictive environment and one with which the child may already be familiar. It also provides some reunification of the family, though there may be strict limitations on visitation by anyone who may be a risk to the child.

Life-Care Planning

A life-care plan uses input from medical professionals to plan for specific needs and costs for a disabled individual, such as medical, surgical, and therapeutic requirements; equipment; transportation; and education.

Certified professional life-care planners assist parents and caregivers in developing an appropriate long-range plan and assist attorneys in civil suit cases or with settlement and negotiations. For example, a child may be able to take care of himself, or there may be a need to hire people to provide care when he becomes an adult. Medications alone can be a significant out-of-pocket expense and must be highlighted in a life-care plan.

Good life-care planners are knowledgeable of a variety of disabilities, including traumatic brain injury. They also can determine the needs of children in custodial care, what costs will be like when the primary caregiver dies, and what their needs will be during the various developmental growth stages. Ultimately, life-care planning is based on a child's current physical state, medical complexities, and living situation.

Parole

Though persons convicted in shaking crimes may be sentenced to a term of months or years in prison, they rarely end up serving this allotted time. They may go before the parole board for good behavior, they may be given a provision for a minimum amount of time served prior to seeing the parole board, and so on.

The parole board is made up of state officials who job it is to review a person's crime and sentence and make a decision as to the safety of the community if this person is released. Often, parole board officials are under pressure to weed out certain low-risk criminals and provide early release because of overcrowded conditions in prisons and the expense of caring for large numbers of prisoners.

Families of shaken children are typically anxious and fearful when it comes to the time of parole hearings for perpetrators of their cases. Impact statements given by family members can be made to the parole board in order to maximize the length of the perpetrator's sentence. Letters to parole board members can be written by community advocates, government officials, and friends of the child's family. These supportive efforts may be enough to persuade the parole board to reject the plea for parole. One woman collected all the hate mail she received from her boyfriend while he was in prison and mailed them to his parole board. He was denied parole based on the threats of further injury to the family.

CASE HIGHLIGHT

The Shirron Lewis Case

In May 1999, in Media, Pennsylvania, a judge refused a petition to end life support for a twenty-month-old boy who was left blind, deaf, and insensitive to pain after being shaken by his father. Judge Joseph Battle signed an order denying a county petition to terminate life support for Shirron Lewis, who had been kept alive by a mechanical respirator since March 1998, when he first arrived at the hospital at the age of five months. His doctors said he would not recover.

The boy's father, forty-two-year-old Ronald Lewis, was being held in jail on a charge of attempted murder, which carries a maximum penalty of twenty years in prison. He faced a first-degree murder charge and the death penalty if the boy was taken off life support and died. Yet Delaware County case workers believed it would be in the boy's best interests to remove him from life-support systems, and a child advocate asked for custody of the toddler. The boy's parents, from Chester, Pennsylvania, wanted him kept alive on religious grounds.

On January 3, 2000, Shirron died after showing signs of distress while comatose. At this writing, the boy's father is pending trial.

NOTES

1. Isaacs JL. The Law and the Abused and Neglected Child. *Pediatrics* 1973; 51:783–792.

2. Silver LB, Barton W, Dublin CC. Child Abuse Laws—Are They Enough? *JAMA* 1967; 199:101–104.

3. Johnson CF. Abuse and Neglect of Children. In: Nelson WE, Behrman RE, Kliegman RM, Arvin AM, eds. *Nelson Textbook of Pediatrics*. 15th ed. Philadelphia: W.B. Saunders Co.; 1995:112–116.

4. Wissow CA. Reporting Suspected Child Maltreatment. In: Wissow LS, ed. *Child Advocacy for the Clinician: An Approach to Child Abuse and Neglect*. Baltimore: Williams & Wilkins; 1989:201–208.

5. Halverson KC, Elliott BA, Rubin MS, Chadwick DL. Legal Considerations in Cases of Child Abuse. *Primary Care* 1993; 20:407–416.

6. Simms MD. Foster Care. In: Nelson WE, Behrman RE, Kliegman RM, Jenson HB, eds. *Nelson Textbook of Pediatrics*. 16th ed. Philadelphia: W.B. Saunders Co.; 2000:105–106.

7. Runyan DK, Gould CL, Trost DC, Loda FA. Determinants of Foster Care Placement for the Maltreated Child. *Am J Pub Health* 1981; 71:706–710.

8. Arndt HCM. Quality Foster Care: A Service to Children and Their Parents. In: Lauderdale ML, Anderson RN, Cramer SE, eds. *Child Abuse and Neglect: Issues on Innovation and Implementation*. Proceedings of the Second Annual National Conference on Child Abuse and Neglect. April 1977; 101–106.

9. Goldner JA, Dolgin CK, Manske SH. Legal Issues. In: Monteleone JA, Brodeur AE, eds. *Child Maltreatment: A Clinical Guide and Reference*. St. Louis: G.W. Medical Pub.; 1994:387–430.

Part Three

SOCIAL ASPECTS OF
SHAKEN BABY SYNDROME

✧   ✧   ✧

Grown men can learn from very little children for the hearts of little children are pure. Therefore, the Great Spirit may show to them many things which older people miss.

—Black Elk

So long as little children are allowed to suffer, there is no true love in this world.

—Isadora Duncan

✧ ✧ ✧

CHAPTER EIGHTEEN

Perpetrators

A PERPETRATOR OF A CRIME is the person who performs the crime. Perpetrators of SBS can be *anyone*. Grandmothers, uncles, babysitters, siblings, and daycare workers all have fallen into the category of perpetrator. New parents can be dangerously naive about those who care for their infant son or daughter, believing that no one would ever bring harm to their baby. They might even think that abused and shaken infants are only extreme cases one reads about in the newspaper and sees on television. The idea that anyone can be a perpetrator of SBS needs to reinforced with new parents or caregivers.

Most individuals who shake infants do not fall into a specific category, yet research has shown that certain characteristics make a person more at risk at being a perpetrator of SBS. These characteristics are listed here, as well as some red flags that indicate that a person is likely a perpetrator.

CHARACTERISTICS OF PERPETRATORS

Abused as a Child

This can be a common defense within a courtroom setting, and juries have been known to accept this excuse as justifying a person's actions. Yet abuse of another human is always wrong, especially abuse of a child without any sort of defense capabilities. Effective prosecutors will respond to such defense claims with an acknowledgment of the abuse history of the accused and a statement such as "Well, then, you knew what you were doing was wrong because of your own experience."

When individuals who were truly abused as children grow up, they tend not to have appropriate skills for dealing with anger and will have a need to control their environment. Such people believe that corporal punishment is justified, because this has been their way of living for many years, and that a crying child needs to be controlled. Shaking may be a mode that seems acceptable to a formerly abused adult.

Some perpetrators create an environment of negativity, which pervades every aspect of their lives. These individuals like commanding loved ones, enjoy the power of harsh words and threatening behavior, and use others as targets of their wrath. Such perpetrators bring with them a history of violent behavior, which more often than not stems from a childhood of physical, emotional, or sexual abuse.

When children are born into a controlling, negative environment with abusive individuals, they become easy prey. Other children may be innocently introduced into such an environment when their mothers or fathers choose new partners.

In a perpetrator's mind, young children are a way to get back at people from the perpetrator's own negative past. This vicious cycle perpetuates violent behavior. There are losses all around. No one is able to win unless the violence comes to a halt. Typically, prevention programs are unable to break through such a strong wall of abuse.

Alcohol or Substance Abuse

Alcohol and substance use often typifies domestic violence. When infants are involved in a tense home environment, they often become innocent participants in a web of violence. Tragedy also can occur when children are left alone with those who regularly abuse substances. Rational thinking is not possible for an individual abusing substances, and no one will effectively care for a child while under the influence.

When a caretaker of an injured infant come to a hospital emergency room and appears intoxicated or under the influence of substances, police should do a thorough investigation. Breathalyzer tests and urine drug screens should be performed on suspected perpetrators.

Anger Control Issues

Defense attorneys and perpetrators often use the "nice person who snapped" assertion to substantiate why a shaking incident occurred. As loving parents and caregivers know, this is not an adequate defense. A competent caregiver will seek assistance when frustrated by a crying or fussy baby. He or she will try other strategies to soothe a baby, such as putting the baby down somewhere out of harm's way, drawing the baby in close to his or her chest, or allowing the baby to cry. Those with anger control problems will, instead, violently shake or strike out in response to an infant's demands.

Delay in Seeking Medical Treatment

P. D. Scott, in his early review of fatal cases of child abuse, listed "unnecessary delay in seeking help" as the main characteristic of fathers who battered their children.[1]

Description of a Situation Not Matching the Infant's Injuries

Stories or explanations that accompany a shaken infant to an emergency room are frequently erroneous. A common excuse used is that an infant fell from a couch or bed.[2] Articles from the past two decades have assured the lack of serious injury of infants in falls from one to four feet.[3-5] Even falls down flights of stairs or from several stories rarely produce life-threatening consequences. Police investigation will compare a story of injury given at a hospital with the actual scene where the injury took place to determine the hardness of the landing surface, if there was a crushing injury with the fall, and so forth. Medical providers should address inconsistent stories with professionalism, stating something like "Your daughter's injuries are very serious. We do not see this in falls (out of arms, off a bed). To treat her the best we can, could you tell us if anything else might have happened?"

Reviving infants from episodes of sleep apnea is another common excuse given by perpetrators, who may even seek praise for acts of heroism. In truth, infants can easily become apneic after an episode of shaking.[6,7] This often complicates the medical diagnosis, as medical providers might not consider abusive trauma in an initial work-up. In past decades, parents and other caregivers were actually instructed to gently shake infants or children who were not breathing in order to revive them. This has since been discontinued in the instructions at cardiopulmonary resuscitation (CPR) and other classes.[8]

Another "heroic measure" that has been disproved as a viable explanation for injuries seen in SBS is the use of CPR.[9-11] This is a typical defense strategy. The fact that an infant has retinal hemorrhaging does not mean this was received during an episode of CPR. Hemorrhages are underlying and appear beyond any efforts of resuscitation.

Finally, light shaking, blows to an infant's back, or tossing games in the air will not produce SBS.[12,13] Innocuous activities such as these were thought to be damaging and played a significant role in the diagnosis of SBS when it was initially described and for many years afterward. But studies and witnessed events have proved otherwise. For SBS to occur, there needs to be substantial violence while shaking an infant.

Emotionally Unattached

Loving parents who have an established bond with their infants will not shake them. Individuals who shake do so out of rage or because of their own inadequacies and do not have such an established bond. When an adult caretaker does not have an emotional bond with an infant, a blockade is established.

Frequently, perpetrators are not biological parents. They may be relatives, babysitters, daycare workers, or siblings.[14] Perpetrators who are emotionally unattached may abuse because they do not like children or because of a psychological motive. They may be jealous of a baby who is breast-feeding or demands a great deal of attention from their mother. Perpetrators may be jealous that a baby is not their own or that a baby cries in their arms and not in other people's.

Altemeier found that unwanted pregnancies heralded overt rejection by one or both parents after a child was born.[15] This will set the stage for disdain from the start of an infant's life, as well as physical and other types of abuse.

Focus on Discipline

This is a red flag to any clinician who works in an environment that deals with injured infants and their caretakers. When an adult focuses the discussion on his or her need to discipline the child, it is typically a statement of guilt. What the individual is trying to do is to express his or her reasons for causing injury to the child in masked terms.

Such statements can be subtle and thus missed by clinicians. For example, when a person states, "It was important for me to do something about that crying—she needs to learn that she can't have everything," this is a line of thinking that needs to be further questioned. Statements like "I didn't do anything wrong" are psychologically tempting words subconsciously put out to others by perpetrators. When such words are challenged, lives can be saved.

Insensitive to the Needs of an Infant

The cry of an infant is an important communication tool, and the only one the infant can use to have its needs met. A perpetrator of SBS often believes that an infant is "out to get" him or her when it is crying.[16] He or she does not readily consider the physical or emotional needs of the infant and the many factors that can cause an infant to cry or be irritable. Instead, the infant's needs are ignored, which can give rise to further crying.

A quick way for an abusive caretaker to control a crying infant is by shaking it. Rendering the infant unconscious will take care of the crying. Further crying will lead to further, more violent, shaking and more physical damage.

Limited Parenting Skills

Incorporating soothing strategies when caring for a crying infant is an important skill for new parents and other caregivers. Dealing with infants and their, at times, constant demands can be frustrating and taxing, even for the most competent caregiver. Many individuals are not able to provide the love, care, and support that infants need and should never be left on their own with that responsibility.

Perpetrators quickly exhaust any soothing and caring strategies they may possess and will focus on disciplining and controlling an infant. They do not consider giving up their caretaking role to call someone for help in a desperate situation. These are the moments when tragedy strikes, as they attempt to control infants in their own ways.

An effective strategy that competent caregivers use when alone and exasperated by a crying infant is to place the child in a crib or bassinet in a safe room, close the door, and walk away. This is viewed as an adult "time-out." The caregiver will then call someone for help and support. This is a way to successfully use positive parenting skills.

Male

Approximately 60 to 70 percent of perpetrators of SBS are male.[17,18] There are several reasons for this. Studies have shown that men often respond negatively to the stimulus of infant cries, simply through physiological reactions.[19] Heart rate increases, subtle sweating begins, respiration increases, and so on.

On a social level, men do not have the amount of caregiving exposure as do women, hence they tend to have fewer options from which to choose in caring for and soothing infants. Men also might become more frustrated in the chores of caregiving, not wanting to perform certain duties, such as diaper changing.

Men are more likely to choose control and containment as ways of dealing with stressful situations, such as fussy or crying infants. They may not be emotionally flexible. Shaking may be a way they try to control a seemingly unmanageable situation.

Starling and Holden's 2000 study found that men, as the most common perpetrators of abusive head trauma, did not differ when comparing two geographic U.S. populations.[20] Of a group of twenty-seven children who were shaken, impacted, or a combination of both, fathers were perpetrators 45 percent of the time and mothers' boyfriends 25 percent of the time. (Female babysitters were found to be the third-highest group of perpetrators.)

Multiple Life Stressors

When individuals are faced with multiple issues, such as job loss, relationship problems, and financial stressors, there can be substantial tension. The feeling of chronic stress, coupled with the demands of an infant or toddler, can be a strong indicator for an abusive situation. Some people find it difficult to separate stressful life issues from positive child rearing, whereby the child assumes the brunt of the person's negativity.

Anyone can carry his or her personal life stressors with him or her while caring for a young child. This is dangerous, as such individuals will typically put up a front of positive regard when with the parents, and then impart harm toward the child after the parents are not present. Parents and others need to be instructed not to leave their children with caretakers who are known to be experiencing substantial life stressors. They may be compounding a caretaker's problems. If the parents have no other choice, they should instruct the caretaker on ways to appropriately care for their child, and tell him or her to contact a parent if problems arise. Although this will not ensure a safe environment for the child, the caretaker will be left with positive options.

Rarely Confess to Shaking

Few perpetrators will quickly and honestly step up to the claim "I violently shook the life out of this child." Most individuals who have shaken a child use excuses (an infant fell from a bed) or minimize their actions (tossed an infant in the air). Often there is a face-saving element to lying or minimizing one's actions, as people want to be seen in a good light by the significant people in their lives. Most perpetrators of crimes will seek the path of least resistance—it is a part of human nature and stems from a childhood fear of "getting caught." Perpetrators of shaking crimes will also lie to avoid prosecution and punishment.[21] The legal implications of shaking an infant can be great, so that for perpetrators, it often seems better to skirt responsibility than to face a potentially life-altering judgment in court.

Shake When No One Is Present

The American Academy of Pediatrics consensus statement on Shaken Baby Syndrome was published in 1993 and 2001.[22,23] In the 1993 statement, they wrote, "While caretakers may be unaware of the specific injuries they may cause by shaking, the act of shaking/slamming is so violent that competent individuals observing the shaking would recognize it as dangerous." This was reiterated in its 2001 statement. Perpetrators know that they are inflicting harm on infants by violently shaking them, which is why they do not usually do it in the presence of others.

Most caregivers will hand an infant to another person in the house or at a place of employment when they become frustrated. This is called tag-team parenting or caregiving. When another person is present to hand a crying infant to, the infant usually will not be shaken. Yet for some individuals, outward expressions of violence are normative, and they will shake regardless of who is present.

Unrealistic Expectations for the Infant

Many parents and caretakers expect their children to perform outside their level of development, such as having a two-month-old stand, a six-month-old crawl or self-feed, or an eleven-month-old toilet-trained. When a performance by an infant does not match what a caretaker expects, this can be a "trigger event" to an episode of shaking.[24]

Among training programs in childbirth education, postnatal parenting classes, and support groups, there needs to be instruction on the developmental aspects of infants and children. Well-child visits to pediatricians should always include a review of what a child has been doing and what parents and caregivers should soon be expecting.

Young

Persons who shake infants are typically in their teens or early twenties. Such individuals do not have significant experience caring for an infant. Young parents often do not have the maturity or mental resources to cope with a crying child and will be quicker to react than to pause to consider appropriate caregiving alternatives.

Overpeck and associates found a strong correlation between childbearing at an early age and infant homicide.[25] They felt that prevention programs related to child abuse should be targeted more actively among the adolescent population.

This recommendation is on track with other prevention initiatives that call for early training of young, less-experienced caregivers.

✦   ✦   ✦

Perpetrators of shaking crimes often are not aware of other options. They make snap decisions, target the very innocent, and then plea for leniency in their cases. Smart defense attorneys play on the hearts of juries and can get dismissals and light sentences for their clients. But ultimately, what any crime against a child comes down to is that it is sorely a breach of trust and responsibility. Individuals need to be culpable for their crimes. Training and prevention programs are just a start to lead the way toward better caregiving for today's children.

CASE HIGHLIGHT

The Strange Case of Virginia Jaspers (1948–1956)

On August 27, 1956, a thirty-three-year-old pediatric nurse, Virginia Jaspers, was brought to the detective bureau in New Haven, Connecticut, to be questioned about the death of an eleven-day-old infant. During five hours of questioning, police officials were astounded when she admitted to causing not one, but three deaths, as well as inflicting injuries on two other babies. This confession ended an eight-year spree of physical child abuse at the hands of a qualified, seemingly competent caretaker.

In 1942, Jaspers, the daughter of a state senator and recent high school graduate, took an eighteen-month course in child care at St. Agnes Home in West Hartford, Connecticut. She then began home nursing in New Haven and the surrounding area. Over her career, she served as an infant caretaker within hundreds of homes. One mother described her personality as "immature." Jaspers had a childish delight in eating, especially ice cream and soda, and regularly took pictures of the babies in her care. She was also known to talk and laugh constantly.

Jaspers, though, was anything but gleeful with her victims. She stood six feet tall and weighed 220 pounds—a physical nature that proved to be lethal, along with an emotional disposition as deadly as a ticking bomb. At her arrest in 1956, she explained that her temper frequently became uncontrollable, and she would sometimes go into "moods" wherein she would weep without apparent reason.

The initial infant death occurred in 1948. A twelve-day-old girl named Cynthia Hubbard was originally thought to have died of natural causes (SIDS before it was so named). Yet a local pediatrician, Robert Salinger, suspected otherwise when he was called in for consultation on her death. He stated: "The case was discussed widely at the time. We did not know whether it could be blamed on intent, awkwardness or just chance. But an autopsy was performed and we did feel that the baby had been dropped or thrown." He would be key in Jaspers's arrest eight years later.

Even after Cynthia's death, Mrs. Hubbard hired Jaspers for her second child. She once recalled: "I have to admit that at the time she handled the baby well. True, she was heavy-handed. When she burped the baby, she seemed a little strong. I remember we kidded her about it a few times but thought nothing serious about it."

The next death occurred in 1951: three-month-old Jennifer Malkan, the adopted daughter of Willard Malkan and Joan Brainerd. Her death was attributed to aspiration of vomitus, and no autopsy was done. Jaspers was very distraught about this infant's death. According to Brainerd: "Afterward, she frequently sat across the street and stared at our house. She seemed very lonely and I never trusted her." Brainerd even swayed several other parents from hiring her. "I didn't know at the time if she had anything to do with Jennifer's death or not."

In 1955, Jaspers fractured the leg of a three-week-old boy in her care, Bruce Schaeffer. His leg was treated in the hospital and splinted with a tongue depressor. The doctor who treated him was Dr. Salinger, who was now too familiar with Jaspers's pattern of abuse. Yet a state police report on this injury showed no indication that the youngster's leg was deliberately broken. The Schaeffer case was the only complaint about Jaspers referred to the police for investigation. The district attorney's office became involved at the insistence of Bruce's father, Marvin. It was then that the DA became aware that Jaspers was the pediatric nurse in two infant deaths; still, nothing was pursued.

When Virginia Jaspers fatally shook Abbe Kapsinow on the evening of August 24, 1956, it was because the eleven-day-old girl would not take her formula and go to sleep. Abbe's young mother was recently hospitalized with complications from giving birth. She and her husband hired Jaspers from a list of home nurses provided to them at the hospital.

After Abbe was found unconscious by her mother and brought to the hospital, it was thought that she might be suffering from intracranial bleeding. In the hours before she died, two spinal taps revealed bloody spinal fluid, a clue that she was a victim of violence. There were also peculiar marks on her head.

Several doctors were called in that night, one of them Dr. Salinger and the other Dr. Lawrence Michel, a young resident in pediatrics. After discussion about the case and discovering that Jaspers was the caretaker, Dr. Michel urged Abbe's mother to authorize an autopsy.

An emergency postmortem was ordered and X-rays completed, showing subarachnoid bleeding. It was determined that the child had died of physical abuse. Police were immediately contacted and an investigation commenced.

Questioning gave detectives a complex picture of Jaspers as a woman who appeared one way with her clients and another way while alone with their children. She described the nature of her crimes by saying that she would place two thumbs on an infant's chest and extend the tips of her fingers around a baby's sides and back. She confessed that she would then squeeze and vigorously shake the youngsters to stop them from crying. As an explanation for the deaths,

Jaspers only said, "It was all uncontrollable. I didn't know why I did it. Children sometimes get on my nerves."

In November 1956, she pleaded guilty to manslaughter and was sentenced to ten to twenty-two years for the Malkan and Kapsinow deaths (the Hubbard death was not included because of a statute of limitations). She served less than one year, because a judge, within reach of her father's influential power of his former state senate office, reduced her term.

She remains living at the age of seventy-eight. The Malkan and Kapsinow families have been pulled apart, and the Jaspers case has been virtually forgotten, until now.

NOTES

1. Scott PD. Fatal Battered Baby Cases. *Med Sci Law* 1973; 13:197–206.

2. Chadwick DL, Chin S, Salerno C, et al. Deaths from Falls in Children: How Far Is Fatal? *J Trauma* 1991; 10:1353–1355.

3. Helfer RE, Slovis TL, Black M. Injuries Resulting when Small Children Fall Out of Bed. *Pediatrics* 1977; 60:533–535.

4. Nimityongskul P, Anderson LD. The Likelihood of Injuries when Children Fall Out of Bed. *J Ped Orthopedics* 1987; 7:184–186.

5. Williams RA. Injuries to Infants and Small Children Resulting from Witnessed and Corroborated Free Falls. *J Trauma* 1991; 31:1350–1352.

6. Johnson DL, Beal D, Baule R. Role of Apnea in Nonaccidental Head Injury. *Ped Neurosurg* 1995; 23:305–310.

7. Rosen CL, Frost JD, Glaze DG. Child Abuse and Recurrent Infant Apnea. *J Ped* 1986; 109:1065–1067.

8. Chadwick D. Stop Shaking for Treatment of Apnea (commentary). *Amer Acad Peds News* 1988; 6.

9. Gilliland MGF, Luckenbach MW. Are Retinal Hemorrhages Found after Resuscitation Attempts?: A Study of the Eyes of 169 Children. *Am J Med Path* 1993; 14:187–192.

10. Goetting MG, Sowa B. Retinal Hemorrhage after Cardiopulmonary Resuscitation in Children: An Etiologic Reevaluation. *Pediatrics* 1990; 85:585–588.

11. Kanter RK. Retinal Hemorrhage after Cardiopulmonary Resuscitation or Child Abuse. *J Ped* 1986; 109:430–432.

12. Spaide RF, Swengel RM, Scharre DW. Shaken Baby Syndrome. *Amer Fam Prac* 1990; 41:1145–1152.

13. Lancon JA, Haines DE, Parent AD. Anatomy of the Shaken Baby Syndrome. *New Anatomist* 1998; 253:13–18.

14. Dix J. Homicide and the Babysitter. *Amer J Foren Sci & Path* 1998; 19:321–323.

15. Altemeier WA, O'Connor S, Vietze PM, et al. Antecedents of Child Abuse. *J Ped* 1982; 100:823–829.

16. Lazoritz S, Hudlett JMM, Weathers L, Brooks W. True Confessions: Perpetrator Admissions and Clinical Correlations. Second National Conference on SBS. September 1998.

17. Lazoritz S, Baldwin S, Kini N. The Whiplash Shaken Infant Syndrome: Has Caffey's Syndrome Changed or Have We Changed his Syndrome? *Child Abuse & Neglect* 1997; 21:1009–1014.

18. Butler GL. Shaken Baby Syndrome. *J Psychsocial Nurs* 1995; 33:47–50.

19. Brewster AL, Nelson JP, McCanne TR, et al. Gender Differences in Physiological Reactivity to Infant Cries and Smiles in Military Families. *Child Abuse & Neglect* 1998; 22: 775–788.

20. Starling SP, Holden JR. Perpetrators of Abusive Head Trauma: a Comparison of Two Geographic Populations. *South Med J* 2000; 93:463–465.

21. Showers J, Apolo J. Criminal Disposition of Persons Involved in 72 Cases of Fatal Child Abuse. *Med Sci Law* 1986; 26:243–247.

22. American Academy of Pediatrics. Shaken Baby Syndrome: Inflicted Cerebral Trauma. *Pediatrics* 1993; 92:872–875.

23. American Academy of Pediatrics. Shaken Baby Syndrome: Rotational Cranial Injuries—Technical Report. *Pediatrics* 2001; 108:206–210.

24. Hyden PW, Gallagher TA. Child Abuse Interventions in the Emergency Room. *Ped Clin N Amer* 1992; 39:1053–1081.

25. Overpeck MD, Brenner RA, Trumble AC, et al. Risk Factors for Infant Homicide in the United States. *NEJM* 1998; 339:1211–1216.

CHAPTER NINETEEN

✧ ✧ ✧

Families of
SBS Victims

A LTHOUGH FOR VICTIMS OF SBS the outcome in physical terms varies all the way from complete recovery through permanent disability to death, their families have much in common. They share not only the emotional costs—which are lifelong—but also, in many cases, disruption of their lives and substantial financial costs as well. All these are the results of a few minutes of senseless violence.

One mother, writing to other parents and professionals on an Internet mailing list, effectively highlighted the experience of families of SBS:

> We share the special memories we had with our children. We share the tremendous anger we had toward all the perpetrators who killed or hurt our innocent children. We share the sadness of "how could we let our kids go." We share the joys of every "milestone" our kids make. We discuss the strategies to get justice, and also we talk about how to protect our wounded families. We share many, many things here together. Those things [are] not so easily understood by co-workers, best friends, and defense attorneys.

Listed below are several key issues that are everyday reminders in the hearts of families remembering or caring for these special children.

KEY ISSUES OF FAMILIES

Mandated Parenting

Many individuals believe that legal mandates should be placed on persons who are about to become new parents. Some think that courses should be required for first-time parents. To help young people be prepared for parenting, many schools throughout the country are offering caregiving courses as electives. The "Baby Think It Over" program in most states offers an opportunity for middle and high school children to carry a baby over an entire weekend. This lifelike model cries sporadically during the day and night and can be soothed with proper positioning and handling. If all else fails, there is a special key that turns off the crying. This is an appropriate solution for a teenage student, but live infants do not come with keys; they are born with basic needs that are frequently not met by their caretakers.

Defense arguments in SBS court cases frequently come down to one of ignorance: "I didn't know that shaking was bad." Jurors may or may not be swayed by such an argument. If basic parenting courses were required prior to being able to care for an infant, then such tragedies like SBS would occur less frequently and not be tolerated. Knowledge about the dangers of shaking infants needs to be an integral part of our society. Such knowledge can be shared among friends, with neighbors, at places of worship, and at places of commerce.

One legal professional who supports this concept states, "I would love to see the day when 'never shake a baby' is such household knowledge that only hermits who have had no exposure to anyone for five or ten years could fail to be aware of the dangers of shaking a young child or infant."

New parents and caregivers who have no previous experience of providing for an infant can easily become frustrated. They receive advice from many sources, including their own families. Such advice typically will *not* include "Let the baby cry, and take an adult time-out." New parents and caregivers have an internal desire to fix the issue of a crying baby, and many seem to feel that they will be failures if they cannot do this. Validating that such feelings are common should be a part of parenting and childbirth education classes.

In a hospital obstetrics unit, education about caregiving and soothing infants should be given to both parents. SBS prevention brochures for after discharge should be handed out, and follow-up in-home visits scheduled. The visits would be an opportunity to assess a family's needs and offer guidance. These often seem like expensive proposals to hospitals and insurance companies, but the cost is trivial compared with saving the lives of children.

More Children

Having more children is a sensitive issue for many parents of shaken infants. They may have a child who died or who was severely disabled. First-time parents who never previously experienced the joys of parenting might want to have more children to regain a semblance of normalcy. Couples who have children with SBS injuries may want more children in an effort to replace the "loss" they have experienced.

Other families may want to avoid having more children for a multitude of reasons. They may be so distraught by the memory of the first child that they want to protect any future children from similar suffering. Or because the care-giving needs of a child with SBS injuries are so overwhelming, they are not phys-ically or emotionally able to handle other children.

Couples affected by SBS need to communicate openly about having further children. The partners may or may not agree. Counseling can help couples dis-cuss feelings, be more objective, and come to an ultimate resolution.

Needs of Families

Too frequently, spouses or other family members attempt to jump back into a life of normalcy without taking time to grieve and feel the pain of loss—of the life of an infant or the infant's potential. More often than not, parents and other family members are never the same after such loss and experience deep emotional pain. Different people have different needs and react in their own individual ways to such a tragic event. A tragedy such as SBS can bring a couple together, yet intense emotions can also pull them away from each other, leading to separation or divorce.

Parents of shaken children may feel shame or other emotions that cause feel-ings of separation from others in society. Friends, family, and professionals can best support parents of shaken children by listening to them and letting them know that help is available through kind words and actions. Validating their emo-tions can allow healing in the midst of pain.

The comfort of other families of shaken children can help fill the need for comparable sharing. These families need to hear strategies for caregiving, work-ing through grief, and getting resource assistance.[1] Families new to this tragedy depend upon others who have had similar experiences.

Respite or Visiting Programs

As new parents return home from the hospital with a newborn, there are typ-ically follow-up home visits by a visiting nurse, who checks on how the mother, father, and baby are adjusting and discusses important issues such as breast-feed-ing. For "at-risk" parents, a case manager may be available from the birthing hos-pital to make follow-up calls or visits. For infants who have been shaken and their families, there is usually no in-home program after discharge.

Hospitals and community agencies that do have respite programs available for families of shaken infants offer an important service. Some insurance plans may even allow for a nurse or social worker to visit a family to provide hands-on caregiving to an infant while the parent is given a well-deserved break. Many health-care professionals have even developed their own respite businesses.

Families should discuss options with visiting nurse organizations and ask about implementing such services if none exist. Ideally, respite should be a free community service. Family and friends can always aid in respite, but professionals should also be available, as technical or level of functioning questions may arise.

Schooling

As children who survived shaking become older, they may have not only unique care needs, but unique educational needs as well. The amount of services that will be needed within the classroom setting will depend on a child's level of potential.

The Americans with Disabilities Act of 1992 requires that children be placed in the "least restrictive environment," allowing for children disabled as a result of being shaken to be mainstreamed into a standard classroom. Such a mainstreamed child will need to receive an individualized educational plan (IEP) to maximize his or her learning abilities.

Having a special-needs child in a mainstreamed environment can be a challenge for a teacher. One child may have difficulty with attention deficits, whereas others may have problems with mobility, sight, or cognition. Most teachers and special-needs instructors have limited experience in the ways of teaching a child with a traumatic brain injury. A parent can become the teacher's teacher by giving him or her special tips and sharing resources on different strategies that may work for the child. At home, parents can help their child educationally by practicing skills learned at school, such as block or cursive writing.

Parents often worry about how their child will do socially with other children within a mainstreamed environment. Classmates may tease a child survivor of SBS, or they may welcome the child gladly into their social network. Parents may find that children in a lower grade provide a better setting for their disabled child to function socially, because of the younger age of the students. If the child is ambulatory and can function independently, organized sports in school are an important social skill that can boost a child's esteem.

If parents and caregivers of shaken children become advocates for change in their community, they will most likely become advocates within their child's school setting too. One issue that may be addressed is the physical accommodations for the child. Another issue may be educating school staff on the many aspects of SBS. Supporting others along their child's educational path is often the best thing parents can do.

Spirituality

Keeping faith in one's spiritual beliefs may be an effort for parents and other family members of shaken children. They have questions like "Why did this happen?" or "If God is all-loving, how could He allow my child to experience this tragedy?" These are questions that cannot be readily answered, yet people often find that they somehow need some kind of answers during emotionally wrenching times.

Other individuals may deeply rely on their faith to see them through their pain. Many scholars have written that humans are not supposed to be aware of God's plan, but instead are put on the earth to deal with the polarity of our human composition. Good and bad people have been described as having the potential for loving-kindness or for evil. Human beings have the right to choose their path. Many believe that because of this, God does not intervene in what we do, rather, God is there to support humans that are in need.

Spiritual moments can guide parents, families, and caregivers. Such moments may not be clearly evident. They may come in the form of a chaplain at a hospital bedside, a neighbor providing meals and words of support, a visit to a gravesite of a shaken child who has died, or a walk through the woods. Such moments can revitalize people and spur them to do something positive in the darkness of a tragedy.

Allowing spiritual moments in our lives on a daily basis can often be a struggle. Both professionals and family involved in the life of a shaken child need only to look around themselves for spiritual moments. The world can be a very good place, even when it seems that each moment is too painful to proceed forward. By doing so, we as humans become more aware of our true spiritual nature.

Stares and Questions

After the initial impact of SBS has passed, parents and caregivers attempt to regain a semblance of normalcy in their lives. The pain of the shaking event may be revisited again and again by feelings that arise and through conversations with others.

The sting of these powerful emotions can also be brought forth through others' words of ignorance. A question posed about one's children to a parent whose only child has just died is an example of ignorance. The parent may realize that the person inquiring was truly unaware of his or her loss, but the pain of the question remains.

People can also be ignorant through their actions. Parents and caregivers frequently face stares when they are out with their disabled child who has survived shaking. Children can be unintentionally hurtful with questions like "Why does he look that way?" or "How come she doesn't talk?" Parents and caregivers can use these opportunities to educate. Though the pain of repeated stares and questions can be overwhelming, the feelings raised by such encounters may temper with time.

It typically requires concentrated effort to get past critical, awkward moments and carry on. One mother states: "I think the pain will always be there, when my son won't be able to do the things his peers are doing, whenever his blindness is discovered, whenever someone's thoughtless comments are heard. I try to ignore what needs to be ignored and deal with each of the others as best I can cope at that time. Some times are easier than others."

Suffering

One issue that plagues many parents and caregivers is the question of suffering an infant may have experienced during the violence of shaking. They wonder how long a child may have been in extreme pain, confusion, and fear.

This can be answered in several ways. If a child is very young (less than three months old), he or she is unable to formulate in his or her mind such an advanced concept as confusion. Usually there will be yelling, throwing, and possibly hitting prior to an act that renders a child unconscious. These negative stimuli will cause the child to cry more, as he or she will most likely have the innate ability to experience fear. Once shaking commences, all cognitive processes stop. Thoughts of "Where is my mommy and daddy?" and "Why is this happening?" will not be present.

Children who experience repeated incidents of abuse will feel fear and confusion more readily, as they live with such negative emotions on a daily basis. Such children will cry at the sight of their abuser or when being held by him or her. As young children are unable to vocalize their fears, nonabusing parents and other caregivers may assume that such crying is due to separation.

The most important thing for parents and caregivers to realize is that they must give the responsibility of the shaking incident solely to the perpetrator. Too many families blame themselves for shaking tragedies and for any suffering endured by the child. In our society, we all carry a certain amount of trust in order to be able to live our lives. We trust that when we leave our son or daughter in the care of another person, he or she will be a responsible caregiver. When we leave our son or daughter in the care of a husband, wife, or significant other, we expect that he or she will lovingly provide care and seek help if needed. Yet individuals will let us down in the most extreme ways. We, as parents and caregivers, need to understand this, accept this, and move forward with the comfort that we have been the best we could have been to our children.

TEN THINGS PARENTS OF CHILDREN WITH SBS WANT YOU TO KNOW

The following is a reprint of an address that was made at the first National Conference on Shaken Baby Syndrome in 1996.[2] The author of the work and presenter is the mother of an SBS survivor. It was a call to the professionals in the audience to take heed to the needs of families directly affected by the tragedy of SBS. That call is ever-present today.

As Bettelheim says, "What cannot be talked about can also not be put to rest; and if it is not the wounds continue to fester from generation to generation.

1. "Be an empathic listener. Develop a willingness to hear anything, including rage, sorrow, and horror. Allow us to tell our stories over and over, and as they unfold over time.

2. "Role play, rehearse, and prepare us as completely as you can for court, and any legal processes. Think about providing our family with an advocate for criminal and civil trials. Educate us about the process, all of it. We will be less traumatized by this experience if we can prepare ourselves for what could happen. Involve us in decision-making. Debrief the experience afterwards.

3. "Recognize the importance of social support for us. Ask us directly about our support systems. Realize these can disappear or change over time. Our extended family, and other support systems in our community, may become overwhelmed by support for the long-term. Think to include grandparents in support efforts for they are doubly victimized, having a grandchild who is a victim and their own child (the parent) who is a victim of SBS.

4. "My child and I may experience blame, disbelief, moral judgments, skepticism, negative comments and evaluations, distancing, curiosity, or rejection from others just by being in the world. Please don't let us experience these from you or your organization, too.

5. "Believe us when we say that the 'conspiracy of silence' about SBS is very real and very damaging to all of us. For you to silence us too, even in the service of justice within the criminal justice system, may traumatize us further. Recognize that our own family members may also wish us to keep silent.

6. "The treatment of a child with Shaken Baby Syndrome is a lifelong treatment. It is an almost impossible task for us to care for our children, to become experts in their care, to advocate for them, to address system changes that will enable them and children like them to get their needs met, and to educate the public about SBS. We need your support, not just for the 'baby' part, but as part of a lifelong process.

7. "Connect us if you can with other parents of SBS victims. If you cannot find any others, make sure we connect with parents of children with severe disabilities, parents of murdered children, or groups like Parents Anonymous as appropriate. Being able to talk with other parents helps to normalize feelings; we do not feel so alone knowing we are not the only ones.

8. "As children's advocates and specialists, don't forget about the siblings who may not understand, but who are also vulnerable to the stressors associated with the lifelong effects of SBS in the family. Like their parents, they may suffer from posttraumatic symptoms and be victims as well. Help us to expect and understand the emotional and behavioral changes that siblings may demonstrate.

9. "Please do not distance yourself from us with your charts, your statistics, your assessments, your professional stance. These are important, but we are real people with real feelings and fears. There is no neutrality with trauma like SBS. Professional distance is not to be used as an illusion or defense. Out of necessity, many of us quickly do become experts too. We ask that you partner with us.

10. "PLEASE take care of yourself. You cannot help us if you are traumatized yourself, burned out, or overwhelmed. Find a group where as a professional, you can talk about and deal with the trauma you have experienced

directly or indirectly, and share your feelings, concerns, and frustrations. As parents, we often feel isolated and alienated and we understand that by doing the kind of work you do, you can feel isolated and alienated at times, too."

NOTES

1. D'Lugoff MI, Baker DJ. Case Study: Shaken Baby Syndrome—One Disorder with Two Victims. *Pub Health Nurs* 1998; 15:243–249.

2. Phillips, MB. Ten Things Parents of Children with SBS Want You to Know. First National Conference on SBS. September 1996.

✧   ✧   ✧

CHAPTER TWENTY

Psychological Aspects

I N THE CONFUSION OF the clinical and legal aspects of SBS, and the intensity of the focus on the well-being of the shaken child, the emotional needs of all members involved, family and professional alike, can be overshadowed. People say, "Here is what the test showed," when they should be asking, "How are you doing?" Emotions run high when an infant has been hurt or killed. Time to cultivate and discuss feelings is what is often most needed to see families and professionals through the rough emotional times typical of SBS. Discussed here are many of the emotions that arise in people affected by such a tragedy.

PARENTS OR CAREGIVERS

Anger

When an infant is shaken, the term anger does not do justice to describe the emotions the child's parents or caregivers feel. Anger can be volatile and misdirected. Statements such as "The doctors aren't doing enough," "I'd like to kill the person responsible for doing this to my baby," "Why did God allow this to happen?" or "I hate myself for choosing that person to watch her while I was out" confirm that one's deepest fears have become reality.

Though difficult for some, anger needs to be expressed appropriately. Physical violence to oneself or others, screaming in public areas, or actively threatening another person are not appropriate ways of dealing with anger. Rather, talking with someone directly, yelling at home when no one is present, hitting a soft pillow, counting to one hundred, or tearing up large sheets of paper into tiny pieces are more effective ways of coping with anger.

Parents and caregivers should always be encouraged to appropriately express their anger so that the stress of their emotions does not intensify. Chronic anger and stress can lead to elevated blood pressure and cholesterol.

Anger can become misdirected at those we love and individuals can isolate themselves in a private, painful world. Yet people *can* work through their anger effectively. Telling the story of the shaking incident is usually emotionally difficult at first. Over time the incident may mobilize a caregiver to deal with the trauma positively by helping others who need to learn about SBS.

Betrayal

Parents often go to great lengths to find people who will adeptly and compassionately care for their infant. When a shaking incident occurs, this element of trust is betrayed. Child care is an immense responsibility, because an infant must rely totally on someone else. Child abuse and shaking are the ultimate acts of throwing away that responsibility, which was given in good faith. Perpetrators of shaking discard this gift of trust.

Spouses or partners of perpetrators will often experience this sense of betrayal more deeply. Spouses or partners believe that the man or woman with whom they are raising a child would be the last person to inflict injury. Shaking usually occurs when the perpetrator is alone with an infant. Their spouse or partner will go shopping or to work, and for the brief time the infant is left alone with the caretaker, tragedy strikes. The spouse or partner is left with a fatally or chronically injured child and a broken sense of trust. Parents whose child was shaken by a person who is nonfamily, such as a daycare worker, nanny, or au pair, will tend to never trust anyone but themselves to do future caregiving.

The final sense of betrayal occurs when there is no justice for the shaking incident. This may be present on many levels of the justice system, including poor police investigation, poor medical documentation, lack of charging for the criminal act, undercharging for the criminal act (such as aggressive assault rather than attempted murder), or poor sentencing (such as house arrest or time served). Many parents of shaken children are left feeling betrayed again and again by a system of persons and policies not always in accordance with the medical, social, and legal facts of SBS.

Denial

Spouses or partners of perpetrators of shaking crimes may very well deny that the person had anything to do with the injury of their child, though all evidence points to this perpetrator. Those who support perpetrators under the guise of denial make statements such as "She didn't mean to do it," "Of course the baby rolled off the bed like my husband said," or "He just shook the baby because he was angered by her crying." Beliefs such as these allow the person to come to terms with a tragic event.

Denial allows the perpetrator's actions to seem reasonable. This is a classic psychological defense mechanism a person develops in order to keep emotionally balanced. Unfortunately, denial does not allow for culpability of those who have done wrong and does not change wrongful behavior.

Even after eight-month-old David McBain's battered, shaken body was taken off life support in Kalamazoo, Michigan, in May 1998, his seventeen-year-old mother clung to the story her twenty-two-year-old boyfriend told: that through a series of accidents, including a fall off a waterbed, the boy was injured. The entire extended family of the baby came to believe that the boy's death was not because of the accidents, but rather a cover-up of medical mismanagement at the hospital. The boyfriend was convicted of second-degree murder. At the sentencing hearing, the victim's and perpetrator's families sat together in unity, asking the judge to be fair. The judge was objective, not entering the family's circle of denial, and imposed a sentence of thirty to seventy-five years in prison.

Depression

Depression is a common emotion after the experience of trauma, especially in the death of a child. Parents and caregivers may have ongoing depressive feelings for weeks, months, or years after a tragic event like shaking.

Even if a child survives, family members may suffer from depression. There may be thoughts of what the child's future might have been like if the shaking had never occurred.[1] Parents and others who care for a shaken child on a daily basis may wonder what it would be like if the child could walk, hear, see, or be free from seizures. Processes such as painful rehabilitation, blood examinations, shunt placements, hip surgery, eye surgery, and so forth affect the entire family and also can promote ongoing feelings of depression.

Some family members may feel suicidal after a shaking incident. These individuals and others who experience feelings of depression need help, especially if the feelings affect sleeping or eating patterns. Medication and therapy are effective treatments for depression. Being reminded of what they can actively do to help others avoid the experience of SBS can also give such individuals hope for a more positive future.

Support groups can be very powerful vehicles for emotional guidance of families dealing with the effects of loss. Different families need different things. Some may need the support of one or two meetings; others need ongoing support over a period of several months. Support groups aid families in working through their grief with the help of others who have had a similar experience.[2,3] Once they have done so, families are emotionally more free to move forward in helping themselves and others who come their way looking for supportive words and guidance.

Disbelief

This emotion is more tempered than the emotion of denial. When a shaking incident occurs, there is often disbelief. One parent from Colorado stated: "I couldn't believe it [the shaking] happened! I trusted this caretaker and she let all of us down. We felt good because she was a parent as well. And she shook our baby!"

Disbelief comes with the initial shock of learning one's child has been shaken. This may occur in a hospital emergency room, at home, at work, or on the phone. Disbelief is not limited to immediate family. Friends, relatives, and community members can all experience a sense of disbelief. It is a sense that a child in their community (or family) has been violated, and their innocence has been taken from them.

Disbelief can also be connected to the perpetrator—"He is a great father. He never could have done this!"—though most times this disbelief is dispelled when medical diagnoses and law enforcement investigations are complete, and the true story of the shaking comes to light. Family members of perpetrators will often feel shame or embarrassment after realizing what this person has done.

There also might be a realization that comes over the family member that the perpetrator is not sorry or does not feel responsible for the crime that has been committed against a child. One mother stated: "It has taken me seventeen months to finally come to terms with what he did and that he feels he did nothing wrong and will never change."

Dreams

Dreams allow emotions to come out in creative, imaginative ways. Sometimes dreams intensify our fears or our passions. People can be very troubled by their dreams and may take them on as truth, instead of subconscious moments of psychological adjustment.

Dreams can be explored by talking about them with supportive others. When dreams are interpreted, they may not give answers, but may provide direction, consolation, or even more questions. Dream interpretation might be easier if individuals put themselves in the places of the different characters in a dream. For example, when running from a "monster," is the person running somehow from his or her emotions? This is often a difficult process for someone who might be quite averse to the idea of being one of the characters, such as an abuser. Even symbolically, the process of dream analysis can bring to light hidden stressors and complexities in a person's life.

When the tragedy of SBS strikes a family, many members will experience deep emotional pain. Dreams may be restless and vivid, playing out fears and other emotions. Dreams and the conscious mind often make one feel that "I could be the victim," a sense that one's internal childhood safety is gone, and what is left is a feeling of vulnerability.

Fear

With the low crime conviction rate in the United States, there comes an element of fear. Perpetrators of shaking crimes have been known to threaten, stalk, and harass families of the children they have shaken.

Custodial parents of shaken children may fear that something similar may happen to other children in the house. If the shaken child survives, they might fear for the child's life—that the perpetrator will have access to the child again and kill him or her.

Fear is a response to our feelings of vulnerability and is often exhibited at night in our dreams. Nightmares can be a constant problem for people dealing with the often-debilitating effects of fear. Yet they can be effectively worked through by sharing them with others and by using effect strategies, such as freezing a monster running after an individual in the nightmare or making it extremely small.

In his remarkable book *The Gift of Fear*, Gavin DeBecker wrote: "Remember, fear says something might happen. If it does happen, we stop fearing it and start to respond to it, manage it, surrender to it; or we start to fear the next outcome we predict might be coming. If a burglar [crashes] into the living room, we no longer fear that possibility; we now fear what he might do next. Whatever that may be, while we fear it, it is not happening."[4]

As no one wants to live in fear, a person can use it to his or her advantage. He or she may become advocates for new child protection laws or stiffer penalties for crimes, may seek social service and law enforcement assistance for protection, or may help others in similar situations by being a support person for them.

Frustration

This is a multifaceted emotion held by many families of shaken children. Frustration can begin in a hospital emergency room. Waiting rooms are aptly named. The frustration and anxiety of waiting for answers, good or bad, can be hard to bear. As SBS can, unfortunately, be misdiagnosed as some other condition, there is an element of frustration when a medical professional says, "We aren't really sure what we are dealing with."

Most frustration occurs during the legal part of the journey that no family asked to be a part of. Slow or inept criminal investigation can be very frustrating, especially when it means the difference in charges being brought against a perpetrator. Even when a proper investigation is done, the case may be poorly prosecuted. Perpetrators may be charged below the enormity of their crime (simple battery), plea bargains can be made (reckless homicide from an initial charge of murder), and cases may be delayed repeatedly.

Frustrations may surface once again in the courtroom, especially if the presiding judge has a propensity to sentence lightly. In a 1997 case from South Bend, Indiana, a man shook his eight-month-old son to death. The prosecuting attorney allowed a $3,000 bond for an initial murder charge. The case was then plea-bargained to reckless homicide, and the accused was ultimately sentenced to two years' house arrest and four years' probation. This was an example of an extremely frustrating outcome for many persons on many levels.

Finally, parents and caregivers may be frustrated in their efforts to seek financial support for surviving children of shaking crimes. Some children may await disability benefits for months and even years. Some children are not eligible for certain durable medical equipment because of their parents or caregivers' insurance. And some social service agencies do not have the experience of working with shaken children. An important step that families can take is to seek out experts. These people might be found as part of an early intervention program, a hospital, or a rehabilitation program. There are professionals in the community who are very willing to guide families newly affected by SBS through the multitude of questions that can lead to feelings of frustration.

Grief

Like depression, grief can be acute or chronic. The difference lies in the intensity and longevity of the emotion. Rabin and Pate identified three aspects to the grieving process: immediate grief, acute grief, and mourning.[5] Immediate grief is the initial reaction of family and others affected by the news or discovery of an injured child. There is a sense of panic and time seems to speed. The feeling of grief can be overwhelming and consuming.

Acute grief occurs after several hours and is accompanied by intense sadness or other painful emotions. This is where the concept of anticipatory grieving develops.[5] Here, a parent, family member, caregiver, or friend will experience a "death watch" for a child who is not expected to live. This grief is very devastating, as the infant or child will be connected to many mechanical devices, and monitors will be sounding, showing the spiked lines of the circulatory, nervous, and respiratory systems. If death does occur, acute grief will be amplified at a wake, funeral, or memorial service. Those making arrangements for services, such as church officials and funeral directors, are greatly affected by the tragic loss of a child as well. Death of an infant or child is an anomaly, because people are not expected to die at a young age. There is a feeling of disbelief.

Mourning follows the acute period and is often a lengthy road. A person experiences a psychological adjustment in his or her life's focus with the loss of a child. Though every year without the child is grief provoking, it is the initial year after a death that is the most hurtful. This is the year for celebrations without the child. It might have been the year of the child's first Thanksgiving, Christmas, or birthday. The anniversary of the shaking is significant as well. Families may remember the day before the event, too, when life was normal. Such days are emotional for families. Sharing memories, pictures, and grief with other loved ones can be helpful.

Other ways that parents and family members can ultimately deal with a SBS loss is through positive coping. This type of coping might mean joining a support group, exercising, listening to music, keeping a personal journal, praying or meditating, going to therapy, or writing in a journal to the child (living or deceased).

As it is never beneficial to grieve alone, parents and other family members should be encouraged to share their feelings with others. Expressing and sharing one's feelings to others can lead to acceptance of the tragedy and an ultimate act of moving forward in life.

Moving forward takes a significant amount of time and every person affected by grief will move at different rates and levels. Sunny Eappen, Matty Eappen's father, has said: "My goal was to get everything back to normal as soon as possible if I could, whatever normal was. I didn't need to be in that sadness. Debbie [his wife] seemed to want to be in this sad place . . . because for her to be sad was to be with Matthew and she didn't want to leave him." This is the experience of many parents and family members of shaken children, where emotional support becomes vital.

The level of stress is so great on couples after the death of a child that relationships have a significantly higher chance of breaking up. Spouses or partners may not want to grieve, but instead bury their emotional pain to avoid dealing with it directly. Tensions can become high, and couples may take their anger out on each other. In actuality, the couple is grieving and does not realize the source of their volatility. They may have both grief for the tragedy of having an infant injured or killed by shaking and past grief that they have not yet resolved.[6]

In the cases of children who survive shaking incidents, families may grieve over the loss of potential. Grief is an emotion that can recur over time, especially when a child is unable to do certain things because of a permanent disability.

Intense feelings of grief can make some people uncomfortable. They prefer that those who are grieving will "get past it," so normalcy can return. Yet normalcy, as was once known, may never return, and this is one of the most damaging results of child abuse.

Each person handles grief differently. Grieving individuals can not be rushed to get beyond their sadness. Instead, they need to be supported with comforting words such as "I'm here for you," "I'm so sorry that this happened," "Let me know when you're ready to talk," and "I will support you any way I can." These words are symbols of true friendship during emotionally difficult times.

Parents of shaken children will never be the same emotionally. Parents hold a responsibility for nurturing and protecting, and when they lose a child, they lose a large part of their work in life. When does a family get over the death or loss of potential of a child? They never totally get over this tragedy. People carry this loss through life, relying on support systems and mechanisms for coping. One grandmother writes: "It's so important to memorialize those we intensely love and have tragically lost as this provides us with a sense of good grief. Bad grief suppresses us, causes depression, separates us from surviving people who love us, and gives us no hope . . . hope that there *is* goodness in this world."

Guilt

Parents or caregivers will typically experience a mental debriefing of thoughts after a shaking incident. Feelings of guilt can play a major role during this time, with thoughts such as "If I only would have listened to myself and not gone to the store, this would not have happened," "Why did I go back to work so soon after he was born? I should have stayed home," or "I should have sought protection from him sooner—now look what happened!" These are statements that are self-blaming. The parent or caregiver may feel responsible for assuming trust in another person. Yet the real blame should instead be placed on the perpetrator of the crime. But this is often a hard concept to incorporate initially.

"I'll always remember the last time I saw [him] alive [he] was crying in her arms. I guess we just have to keep reminding ourselves that there are options for shaking a child and we are not responsible for the option our sitter took." This mother only now understands that it was important not to second-guess her actions on the day her son was shaken to death by a babysitter. Yet these mental images can plague parents and caregivers, which is why emotional support and being allowed to talk through feelings are vital in the recovery process. Counselors, therapists, and social workers can assist individuals who are burdened by feelings of guilt.

People may also feel a sense of shame for being a partner to a perpetrator of a shaking crime. They have a feeling of regret and blame themselves for making a poor choice in this person. Others may feel a sense of guilt for wanting to return to work after their child is born. When Matty Eappen was shaken and impacted to death by au pair Louise Woodward, his mother, Debbie, was persecuted by many for being a working parent, with statements such as "That wouldn't have happened to him if his mother was home" and "She played the part of the rich doctor to go off and leave her son at the hands of a murderer."

People need to work for many reasons, and bad things happen while they are at work. One woman stated: "I do have guilty feelings because I work full time and I'm not able to stay at home with my children and protect them from this awful world we live in. I've been remembering my childhood days and my mother staying at home with us, and thinking about even up through high school years—she was always there."

Guilt is an unfortunate, yet natural, feeling in family members of victims of violence. Thoughts of "If only I had . . ." become recurrent when a person is trying to process the tragedy of SBS. It's vital that people express thoughts and feelings of guilt to others who can be loving and supportive. The more support there is during a time of tragedy, the better the emotional outcome.

Isolation and Loneliness

When attention to SBS cases settles, parents and caregivers of shaken infants can be left with a sense of emptiness. When they return home from the hospital, with or without their child, parents or caregivers often feel very alone. They are left to their own devices to grieve and, if their child survived, to begin the rehabilitation process. Support groups for families of shaken infants are not standard in hospitals, clinics, or social service agencies.

The medical, social and legal aspects of SBS are complex, and parents and caregivers rarely have access to necessary information to help clarify their multitude of questions. They must depend on the knowledge and experience of professionals or do their own research. Yet such professional guidance may not even be available. One mother of a shaken seven-month-old male reported: "I moved to a new area after my son was shaken and met with his new pediatrician. That doctor looked at me surprisingly and stated: 'I have to look that one [SBS] up.' You can imagine how I felt."

Families also need support from other parents and caregivers who have gone through similar recovery experiences. The Internet can bring a wealth of information and support to families of shaken children. Parents and caregivers might also wish to become active SBS prevention advocates in and around their hometown. Reducing the feeling of isolation means the ability to share and glean information that can make one's life and the life of a child more manageable.

Mistrust

Like the feeling of betrayal, mistrust pervades the lives of parents and caregivers of shaken children. After a shaking event, many parents will not leave their children alone with anyone, or they may trust only immediate family members for support. One woman, whose son survived a shaking incident nearly twenty years ago, answered "Never" to the question, "When do you learn to trust your child to the care of others?"

When families experience bureaucratic disappointments by agencies within society, the sense of mistrust becomes elevated. When there are questions that medical professionals just cannot answer, they mistrust the competency of medical decision making.

Parents and caregivers are encouraged to trust cautiously in order that they might regain some semblance of a feeling that there is goodness in the world. Trusting others is usually a very long process for families who have suffered tragedy. For many individuals, there needs to be regular proof of goodness in their lives before they are ready to let down their emotional guard.

Overprotection

As shaken children become older and strive for independence, parents or caregivers may become overprotective in the hope of keeping them from further harm. When a child reaches school age, he or she needs space and time away from adults in their lives. This is vital to their stable emotional growth. A child needs to experience and develop socialization skills. To this end, parents and caregivers are encouraged to allow their children this time of exploration. Even if confined to a wheelchair, a child can and should experience independence. Being overprotective only stifles that independence.

Post-Traumatic Stress Disorder

In children and their families, post-traumatic stress disorder (PTSD) is a real psychiatric phenomenon that can hinder the coping process.[7] Infants and children were once thought to be too young to experience the effects of PTSD. Yet there are symptoms children will exhibit that show the effects of SBS trauma, including emotional blunting, hypervigilance, detachment, loss of interest in activities, irritability, sleep disturbance, and nightmares. These are all examples of the psychological effects of PTSD.[8] These effects can be the same for adults who are also living with the tragedy that SBS has had on their child. Individuals who experience PTSD will feel a sense of foreboding, or that the future is unclear, or that danger is continually present. These feelings are normal reactions after a tragedy has occurred.

The kind of tragedy that families affected by SBS have experienced requires years of emotional healing. It is important for such families to understand and experience their grief fully. Once this is done, individual members will be able to move beyond feelings that may be immobilizing.

Vengeance

Like anger, uncontrolled vengeance can produce devastating results. Many people truly believe that those in society who cause harm to children should not be on this earth. Feelings and thoughts of taking action against the perpetrator of a shaking crime are common. Yet vengeance fulfilled brings its own losses—loss of freedom, loss of family, loss of resources, and possibly loss of life. Those who seek to carry out their vengeful thoughts do so impulsively. It is blind rage that drives individuals into reacting with their own violence.

Thoughts of vengeance can be changed into positive responses, such as efforts toward advocacy, prevention, better legislation, and building support networks. By changing negative thoughts and feelings toward something positive, individuals can become agents for change and avoid the traps of negativity.

✧   ✧   ✧

The information above relates to the emotions of a shaken child's parents and caregivers. What about the child's emotion and others directly affected by SBS? In the section that follows, the reader will see how emotions play a part in the lives of a variety of people.

CHILDREN AND OTHERS DIRECTLY AFFECTED

Child Survivors

As children who have been shaken grow and mature, they may question parents or caregivers about their injuries. Children who are shaken may ultimately ask, "How was I hurt?" "Why was I hurt?" "Why did my father/mother do this to me?"

These questions can be difficult for an adult to answer easily and may need to be addressed in the presence of a therapist or counselor. Some families may never disclose the events surrounding shaking incidents to the children.

Shaken children will have a multitude of issues to work through in order to gain a sense of understanding and stability. They want to know why other children can run, walk, or think normally, when they are unable to. They also want to know how long they will need to see doctors and other specialists for their disabilities. There will be the psychological aspects and physiological pain of medical tests and procedures. And there will be great shifts in mood, deep dependency issues, and anxiety that may not allow the child to fully trust anyone.

Such issues can usually be worked out in a therapeutic setting. One type of therapy that helps children experience trust and openness more fully is play therapy. This type of therapy allows children a chance to play with toys or special items chosen by a therapist and takes the intimidation away from a typical "counseling session." Art therapy, which combines coloring and drawing with conversation to foster communication of feelings, can also be very successful in treating children.

Children who have been shaken have a plethora of psychological needs. Structure within their living environment needs to be based on love. This will be a stabilizing factor in shaken children's lives. Parents or caregivers may try to avoid positive discipline and structure, believing this will somehow be detrimental to the child. On the contrary, most children yearn for a structured environment, especially if structure has been lacking or inconsistent for them growing up. Structure provides a safe environment. In turn, a child has a better chance at giving positive feelings to others.

Grandparents

Loving grandparents can feel isolated after a grandchild has been injured or killed by shaking. They may be privy to limited medical communication and rely on secondhand information about the investigation of the case. Family meetings at the hospital can be arranged by a unit social worker to help clarify information and provide direction for all family members.

Emotionally, grandparents may experience the shame of having either a child or an in-law that was the perpetrator of the shaking. Rumors of the incident may even be told to other family members, friends, and neighbors. Grandparents will then need to face others asking for information.

Denial may be a pervasive emotion for a grandparent throughout the investigation process. They might make statements to those around them such as "My son never could have done such a thing," or "My daughter-in-law is very religious and she would think it a sin to hurt that baby!" Such statements attempt to soothe shameful or guilty feelings. Guilt plays a role if they turned down an opportunity to babysit and the alternative caretaker shook their grandchild.

Grief needs are different with grandparents. They grieve not only for their grandchild who is the victim, but also for their own child who is directly experiencing the tragedy of SBS. Grandparents may not have a support network available in order to debrief about the shaking incident. Powerful feelings of emotion that are stressing can be physically harmful to grandparents without an outlet of support. Grandparents can successfully cope in their own unique ways through counseling, advocacy work, and simple, loving caregiving to a grandchild with any needs.

Ultimately, caregiving responsibilities may fall on the shoulders of grandparents. A shaken infant may be taken away from its parents by protective services and placed with the grandparents. The responsibility of caregiving may also be a voluntary act on the part of the grandparents. This can become complex, especially if it has been a number of years since they were child providers. Giving grandparents options for involvement can increase their self-esteem and help fortify a parent's network of support.

Siblings

Often known as the "forgotten mourners," siblings may be emotionally among the hardest hit in cases of SBS, because violence may be a new concept in their lives. Death and injury are typically uncommon entities as well. One mother expressed the effect that a shaking death had on her family by stating, "What about eight- and nine-year-old brothers who went to the same caregiver and now have lost their baby sister? They loved their sister and loved to make her laugh.

And there is a fifteen-year-old brother who carried her around and held her on his lap while he watched TV, and he has a hard time talking about this."

Siblings affected by SBS have a far more difficult time in knowing how to deal with emotional pain. It often comes out through behavioral responses, such as night terrors, acting out, or withdrawal. Siblings also do not always have the words to express their feelings about the tragedy that has occurred in the family. Allow children to talk when they are ready; they should not feel prematurely pressured to do so.

Safety is a very important issue in the life of a child. For siblings, the after-effects of a tragedy can be handled well by ensuring as much safety as possible. This means that parents or caregivers will readily check under their beds for "monsters," put nightlights on, give secure hugs, and say kind words. Teachers and counselors can provide additional emotional support to children of families working through the stabilization process after SBS.

Siblings may also express the effects of a shaking incident through nightmares, anxiety, abnormal fears, separation anxiety, and poor school behavior and performance. Parents and others need to provide consistent, loving discipline if siblings act out. Siblings may have the feeling of being left out, as much attention is placed on their brother or sister who has been injured or is deceased. Parents are often taken aback by discordant emotions experienced and expressed by their children. Siblings may be angry and express disbelief and denial about the fact that another parent or caretaker could shake their brother or sister. Adults should normalize such powerful emotions in children by encouraging the expression of grief to allow honest feelings to come forth. Kind and supportive words such as "Tell me what you are feeling" or "I'm sorry you are feeling left out; we are all sad about what has happened. How can I help you?" can help guide siblings back to a sense of normalcy. If children need additional help, professional grief therapy should be obtained.

Foster Families

SBS is often a new diagnosis for foster parents, and many are not prepared for the depth of the special needs that accompany survivors of this syndrome.

Like all caregivers in society, there are good and bad foster parents. Some may be involved in caregiving from a benevolent, altruistic incentive, whereas others may be motivated by a financial one. Caring and loving foster parents will provide not only sound caregiving, but also consistent outpatient medical visits for their foster child. Financially motivated, unloving foster parents may delay medical care and are likely to become abusers of the child themselves, frustrated by the multiple needs that take so much of their time.

Individuals who take in SBS survivors as foster children benefit by learning about the characteristics of abusive head trauma and the subsequent needs for medical, social, and legal management. Obtaining a copy of the child's medical record will broaden foster parents' understanding of the child's physical needs and capabilities. Prompt follow-up visits to physician or specialist offices provide good care for the child, as well as answers and direction from the medical providers.

As shaken infants and children grow, there may be emotional crises that foster families experience. Words and behavior of abused children with traumatic brain injury can be extreme. Foster parents need to be prepared for any range of emotions and behavior. Providing loving, concrete guidance will be a key in responding to a child effectively.

Foster parents can help themselves by attending support groups, discussing home needs with their caseworker from protective services, garnering information from medical providers, attending therapy when appropriate, and continuing to provide positive emotional support for all members within the family.

Professionals

Morris Wessel, a pediatrician from the Yale University School of Medicine in New Haven, Connecticut, calls the experience of supporting adults and children in the death of a loved one a "unique opportunity."[9] Unique because the physician is able to fulfill a role that comes with the profession—to enhance the ability of families to "meet stresses in their lives as effectively as possible." The same process is needed for children who have survived an incident of shaking and their families.

Emotional support given, beyond clinical descriptions of what an injured child has suffered, is the greatest gift any medical professional can give to family. For a child who dies from shaking injuries, allowing families time to say good-bye is always in order. These moments might include holding the baby, offering a time of silence, saying a prayer or meditation, or simply talking about the life of the child.[10] Brunnquell and Kohen have stressed the importance of the medical team's response not only to the child, but also to the child's family in pediatric emergencies as this will be key in how families will remember what care the child received.[11]

For spouses or partners of perpetrators of shaking crimes, extra emotional support is needed because the individual is dealing with several losses at once. It is important for medical professionals to acknowledge such losses, for example, "I know everything is emotionally very hard for you at this time. I will do what I can to assure that you have as much information as possible on [child's name] condition and that we as a team will do everything in our power to keep him/her well."

In the presence of an alleged perpetrator of a shaking crime, such professionalism may be difficult to provide. Human emotions can, and often do, get in the way of the nonjudgmental presentations expected of a medical professional. When confronted with a suspected perpetrator, all medical personnel should deliver clinical news directly in an unassuming, nonthreatening way, such as "Based on the findings with your daughter's condition, we find it difficult to understand that her injuries were caused in the way that was described. Can you give us more information?" or "Our first priority as medical professionals is the safety and well-being of our patients. Your son's injuries have prompted the need for investigation by local protective services to assist us in determining what happened."

Emotional attachment to a particular case can be an occupational challenge, often being brought home long after leaving the care facility. A particularly compelling account of such emotions was written by the author of "Remembering

Allison," which describes the range of emotions that can churn in the core of a physician's soul.[12] Medical providers can be seen as aloof by laypersons when dealing with their clinical cases. Yet by providing effective family treatment beyond effective medical treatment, clinicians can keep empathic understanding at the forefront of what they offer to others on a daily basis.

Because occupational burnout can be a challenge to care providers working in emergency departments, pediatric units, and pediatric intensive care units, on-site interdisciplinary support groups can be beneficial. Involvement on hospital child abuse teams or in community child abuse prevention groups can allow clinicians the feeling that they are contributing to the advocacy and prevention work needed daily in any community.

✧   ✧   ✧

Such are the effects of the human psyche. Emotions in the wake of tragedy can bring us down, but we can be built up through our responses. Each person directly and indirectly affected by the challenges of SBS has opportunities for growth. Tragedy does not need to remain catastrophic. Disabling emotions can be renewed into something positive, and that process can be ultimately life-changing and life-enhancing.

NOTES

1. Ravenscroft K. Psychiatric Consultation to the Child with Acute Physical Trauma. *Amer J Orthopsychiat* 1982; 52:298–307.

2. Wheeler SR, Limbo RK. Blueprint for a Perinatal Bereavement Support Group. *Ped Nurs* 1990; 16:341–344.

3. Back KJ. Sudden, Unexpected Pediatric Death: Caring for the Parents. *Ped Nurs* 1991; 17:571–575.

4. DeBecker G. *The Gift of Fear.* New York: Little, Brown; 1997.

5. Rabin PL, Pate JK. Acute Grief. *South Med J* 1981; 74:1468–1470.

6. Smialek Z. Observations on Immediate Reactions of Families to Sudden Infant Death. *Pediatrics* 1978; 62:160–165.

7. Rostain AL, Shumway WE. Acute Psychiatric Manifestations. In: Ludwig S, Kornberg AE, eds. *Child Abuse: A Medical Reference.* 2nd ed. New York: Churchill Livingstone; 1992:357–382.

8. Humphreys J. Children of Battered Women. In: Campbell J, Humphreys J, eds. *Nursing Care of Survivors of Family Violence.* St. Louis: Mosby; 1993.

9. Wessel MA. The Role of the Primary Physician When a Child Dies. *Arch Pediatr Adolesc Med* 1998; 152:837–838.

10. Coleman MF. The Injured Family. In: Eichelberger MR, Pratsch GL, eds. *Pediatric Trauma Care.* Rockville, MD: Aspen Pub.; 1988:199–205.

11. Brunnquell D, Kohen DP. Emotions in Pediatric Emergencies: What We Know, What We Can Do. *Children's Health Care* 1991; 20:240–247.

12. Asta LM. Remembering Allison. *Hippocrates* 1997; 11:24, 25, 29.

CHAPTER TWENTY-ONE

Government Intervention

T HIS CHAPTER DESCRIBES what government programs are in place to assist both families who have experienced SBS and those hoping to avoid it. The issue of infant and child care is addressed as well. In order to work effectively, the agencies of the state and federal government need to be finely tuned with the services that they provide. Unfortunately, this is not yet the case, but efforts in recent years have changed the way the government looks at child abuse and its victims.

Below are various aspects of the federal government that individuals and families affected by SBS and other types of abuse should understand. Many of these agencies have the power to make important changes happen, but a community presence is also necessary to motivate lawmakers to action.

GOVERNMENT AGENCIES AND ASSISTANCE

Child Abuse Prevention and Treatment Act of 1996 (CAPTA)

Known as Public Law (PL) 104-235, CAPTA, under the auspices of the Department of Health and Human Services (DHHS), declares that states will provide certain basic elements in the protection of children, including screening and safety assessment, protecting the safety of children, and placing children in a safe environment. There are certain eligibility requirements for CAPTA that need to be met by all states. PL 104-235 was signed into law on October 3, 1996, was authorized through the year 2001 providing $21 million for state grants and $14 million for discretionary grants.

There have been specific changes to child protection laws under this act; for example, unrestricted immunity had formerly been given to all reporters of child abuse and neglect, but wording has now been changed to provide immunity for reports made in "good faith."

CAPTA also lists persons who may access confidential Child Protective Service (CPS) records, including those persons who are the subject of reports, law enforcement officials and anyone else authorized by law for a legitimate purpose (attorneys, citizen review panels, child fatality review panels, grand juries or courts). States are also now required to allow people who disagree with CPS findings of abuse or neglect to appeal these findings.

CAPTA set into motion a requirement for states to create citizen review panels, similar to child fatality review panels. Such groups would review active cases of CPS, along with policies and procedures.

Finally, under recent changes to CAPTA, states are required to certify that reunification of surviving children with an offending parent should not occur when a court has found that a parent committed murder or voluntary manslaughter of one of their children; aided or abetted, conspired, or solicited to commit one of these two acts; or committed a felony assault resulting in serious injury to their child. Convictions for the offenses are grounds under state law for termination of parental rights, though within the sole discretion of the state.

CAPTA reauthorization was approved by the House education subcommittee in August 2001. Advocates of the bill called for an increase of funds by several hundred million dollars, primarily targeting child abuse prevention efforts.

Children's Bureau

The Children's Bureau is the agency within the federal government that is responsible for assisting state child welfare systems to promote continuous improvement in child welfare services. Under the guidance of DHHS, the Children's Bureau helps state officials, advocates, and others in the field of child welfare work together to identify problem areas and develop measures to accomplish specific goals.

A report presented annually by the Children's Bureau to Congress details certain aspects of the U.S. child welfare system. It includes the number of children reported for abuse or neglect, the number found to be victims of maltreatment, the number in out-of-home care, and the number of adoptions. These reports help Congress assess state performance by recording changes in each state's performance on certain measures.

One ultimate objective is to document either a pattern of continuous improvement or performance problems. This helps legislative bodies hone in on areas of child welfare in need of further attention. The Children's Bureau does not, per se, target SBS prevention initiatives, but does report on injury and death by abuse and can make recommendations.

Financial Assistance

Medicaid is a federal medical insurance that covers children and adults who are uninsured and have a financial need. This program has strict income requirements, but children who are disabled, in this case due to SBS, may qualify. Medicaid thus becomes a medically necessary source of coverage.

Social Security Disability (SSD) and Supplemental Security Income (SSI) allow children to receive regular monthly payments for their care by the federal government. To qualify, children need to be identified as disabled. The distinction between the two is based on income of the parents or guardians. If, over time, there is significant rehabilitation and recovery, financial assistance from SSD or SSI may be eliminated.

Children's Health Insurance is another federal program designed to cover children who have no medical insurance but are not eligible for Medicaid due to higher family income. Information about applying for such insurance can be acquired at a county health department or through a hospital's patient financial services department.

Protective Services

Child Protective Service (CPS) caseworkers in the United States are part of a larger system of child welfare programming that has been in place since the early part of the twentieth century. They investigate allegations of child abuse and neglect based on reports given to them by families, social workers, law enforcement officials, medical personnel, and teachers.

CPS caseworkers typically do not have social work degrees. Some start out with human service backgrounds, but most are new to the field of children and family services. Each worker typically has a large caseload and frequently appears in court to appeal for judicial protection. Because of the intensity of the work, low government pay, and the nature of some cases, a high rate of turnover is typical. When caseworkers come and go within an agency, families are left without a continuity of care, and this becomes a problem when dealing with at-risk families.

While a CPS caseworker is investigating a report of abuse or neglect, a child may be taken from his or her living environment to keep him or her safe. Because cases of SBS are sometimes difficult to investigate, a child may be taken away even if an out-of-home caretaker is the suspected perpetrator, and placed in short-term foster care or with relatives. Relatives can appeal to the CPS worker to assume temporary custody while an investigation proceeds.

A large majority of citizens and legislators believe that many changes are in need within the child protection system. Several years ago, the National Commission on Children, chaired by Sen. John Rockefeller, found that only 25 percent of child welfare workers were professionally trained social workers, and only 50 percent of child welfare staff had any experience in working with families. CPS staff who are adequately trained and experienced can make more competent decisions that will ensure proper casework.

In 1996, New York City developed a new program of child protection whereby a child would be taken from his or her home if it represented a risk to the child's safety. This decision has been supported highly by child abuse prevention advocates, as too often children at risk who are left in homes suffer repeat abuse and even death. In determining whether there is imminent danger, CPS workers often proceed with the mindset "When in doubt, take them out." A follow-up program was started in New York that arranges for a meeting between relatives, social workers, and teachers within seventy-two hours of a child being removed from home to determine when and if the child can safely return. However, a group of New York parents filed a class-action lawsuit against the city's child welfare agency, with claims that protective service workers routinely take children from their families when they are not in danger. Most state laws allow workers to remove children from their homes only when children face "imminent danger" to their health or life. This particular group charged that their city's CPS workers often violate the "imminent danger" law and needlessly place children in foster care without follow-up means for family reunification.

Congress has asked state child welfare agencies to report on the status of protective service cases. These reports need to include the number of children who receive services, who are removed from home, who are returned home, who receive prevention services, and who die because of repeat abuse. States also need to report on the methods of response to case reports, the size of caseloads, disposition of children, and follow-up services.

✦ ✦ ✦

All the key elements are in place for an efficient and workable child welfare system. There now needs to be training, research, and persons in power committed to the welfare of children. Government control can become government guidance, but only when the right people are doing the right intervention for the prevention of child abuse.

INFANT- AND CHILD-CARE ISSUES

Many citizens believe that the government should avoid involvement in certain activities performed by privately owned businesses. Privacy in this instance is often seen as a basic right for individuals. Yet when it comes to the safety of children, government involvement and regulations are vital.

Too many children are injured or killed while being watched by caretakers who are not the children's parents. Both accidental and nonaccidental injuries occur in licensed and unlicensed facilities, and in children's homes. State regulations for child-care facilities and homes are difficult to enforce, at best. The majority of child-care providers do follow state regulations, simply because it is the right way to provide care. But others, such as unlicensed in-home care, have no system of review and may have no established rules of safety.

Few states check the backgrounds of professional child-care workers. Even fewer states require basic child-care training, including topics such as recognizing signs of physical abuse and warnings that shaking children is dangerous. This is a dangerous and faulty system. Listed below are key issues that relate to child-care and some possible ways of improving what is typically an unregulated system at present.

Advocacy

Injuries or deaths that occur within child-care facilities or homes are typically ruled as accidental, and charges may not be filed. Providers often then continue caring for children as if nothing has happened. Because parents may have limited choices in finding new care, they frequently continue to have their children attend programs where tragedy has occurred, not realizing that changing providers can be life-saving.

Cases of abuse are usually only recognized in hindsight. A parent may have seen a bruise on his or her child or have been informed about an injury that was described as accidental, and passed it over as an isolated incident. Several weeks later, a child ends up dead or seriously injured. Only then will a group of parents talk with each other and compare the frequency of injuries among a large number of children.

Parents, former and present, may support child-care providers when child abuse allegations are made. They may even testify that they believe the provider is incapable of inflicting injuries on any of their children, despite physical evidence of child abuse. Other parents may refuse to have doctors examine their children for abusive injuries, as they are blind to even considering that the provider in question would hurt their child.

For parents who are vocal about child abuse allegations, this often leaves them feeling alone in their cause. Yet it is by embracing a cause that individuals force change to occur. Advocacy groups who are influential can make legislative change happen. It is vital for groups of parents to get involved in seeing that laws are passed mandating safety for children in child care, and training, including child abuse prevention, for their providers.

Daycare Centers

Daycare centers throughout the United States have a record for care that is poor to fair. Improved care is not only the responsibility of the individual care center, but also the responsibility of the government. Problems that are identified include poor child–staff ratios, inadequate pay and supervision, and inconsistent inspection. Parents place their children in daycare centers trusting that personnel will provide more-than-adequate care. But such care is often less than adequate.

Working Mother magazine puts together an annual state-by-state rating of child care.[1] The magazine assesses child-care centers, as well as in-home care. The outcome is usually not favorable. Various states were identified as needing to increase funding for child care and to sponsor educational programs. Few states targeted funds for training, and even fewer set legislation to monitor child-care providers.

The National Association for the Education of Young Children (NAEYC) is the preeminent organization for standardized quality child-care programming in the United States. Child-care centers can become accredited by this organization by meeting several key standards, which include training and supervision. Many states have even begun to pay higher rates to centers that are accredited through NAEYC. Parents rightly feel more emotionally secure in placing their child in such an accredited facility.

For the prevention of SBS, and other types of physical child abuse, the following areas within the arena of child-care need to be improved: background checks for child-care providers, decrease in child–staff ratios, better pay, increased training, frequent inspection of facilities, and accreditation of facilities. If all these issues could be formally addressed and served by state legislation, then child abuse tragedies would occur at a far lower rate.

Family Child Care

The National Association for Family Child Care (NAFCC) is an organization that supports and accredits caregivers who operate out of their own homes. This organization is important because the vast majority of family child-care homes are unlicensed and fail to provide standardized health and safety measures, so that they offer a greater risk for physical child abuse.

A family child-care provider who applies for licensing or registration in his or her county must meet certain criteria. One state guideline is a limit on the number of children that can be resident in the home before such licensing or registration is given. Most states allow a limit of one to six children in a home.[1]

Parents often use family child care, as family homes are typically less expensive than formal facilities. Parents will also use certain homes based on reputation of care. Yet one parent's positive experience may also become another parent's tragedy.

In-Home Care

Nannies, au pairs, and other in-home providers often fail to understand the true demands of their assignments. Parents will assume that these women are qualified, trained, and ready to take on the role of caregiver. Younger nannies and au pairs come overseas excited to be in an American home. Yet actually, living out the day-to-day tasks of caretaking infants and children can be disappointing. Such was the case with au pair Louise Woodward.

Great Britain put into place a tighter control over nannies with the introduction of voluntary standards for supervising agencies. One measure used is to conduct background checks on potential nannies. Agencies that carry out such important quality measures are recognized publicly by the government. The British government has also sought greater regulatory and enforcement powers over child care and is providing guidance to parents on how to choose a nanny. Regulation in the United States of nanny and au pair services to ensure a minimum standard of child development education should be in place for every employee.

Other in-home providers are more difficult to regulate. Many women have their own in-home child-care businesses, not subject to any type of outside regulation. They are allowed in parents' homes on the basis of references and work history. At a minimum, parents should sit down with individuals they employ and review their expectations for proper child care. Included in this discussion should be a statement such as "We will not allow any physical discipline of our daughter, and never, ever shake her. If you need us to assist you, we expect that you will call us." All parties can then sign a formal agreement. This is a clear, up-front way to take preventive measures when using in-home providers. Such a statement may not stop a shaking incident, but it will provide a basis for the care-taker to understand what the parents expect.

Information for Parents

Parents who place their children in child-care programs should have specific information available that details their state's child-care regulations. Keeping parents more informed and updated on resources will make them better consumers. Child-care programs should also provide written information on their internal policies for safety and for the training and hiring of workers.

If a child is abused at a care facility or if there is a question of abuse, all parents should be informed that an investigation is in progress. Facility directors should openly share this information. On the other hand, parents of the injured child should never discuss an investigation with other parents, due to issues of liability if abuse allegations are not found to be substantiated by investigators and protection workers.[2]

Inspections

Most states require regular, unannounced visits by state officials for both day-care and family child-care centers. This allows for proper oversight to ensure quality programming. Unfortunately, many states do not have a requirement for annual child-care facility inspections. Family child-care centers are even more rarely inspected. These facts fail to meet child-care legislation. Even when legislation requires a minimum number of visits, state employees often claim a lack of personnel as an excuse for irregular inspections.

Legislation

In 1998, the Clinton administration proposed a child-care act that would funnel millions of federal dollars to states for the purpose of keeping America's children safer. The act set in place specific requirements for all child-care providers that would mandate better safety, education, training, and care. This was just one step in the direction of more competent child care on a national level.

Pamela Rowse, grandmother of Kierra Harrison, who died from abusive head trauma at the hands of a daycare worker, has a more aggressive strategy and developed a vision for a Child Welfare Committee within the U.S. government. This committee's charge would be to develop a program that sets minimum guidelines and standards for daycare operation. She proposed that there be mandatory regulation regarding child–staff ratios; environmental and equipment standards; curriculum and educational standards; licensure application and review standards; monitoring; reporting processes; 911 response guidelines; emergency first-aid and CPR training requirements; education requirements for directors, owners, aides; and ongoing in-servicing before a license is granted. Accreditation would be granted only to centers or providers adhering to all requirements. While these recommendations are strict, they are a necessary part of what is needed for today's children.

Many advocates believe that when there are claims of child abuse against child-care providers, there should be a process for automatic suspension of a provider's license until an investigation of the charges has been completed. This is a basic issue of safety for other children in the care of the individual in question. In any other profession, if there is a question of wrongdoing, a person is temporarily suspended. Why is this not a standard in the field of child care?

Criminal background checks of child-care workers is another topic that has been debated in recent years. Currently, the only standard for this type of investigation is in California. Known as TrustLine, this system fingerprints potential child-care workers and performs background checks through the Department of Justice for any criminal history or listing on child abuse registries. Law enforcement personnel in every state can be more actively involved in education on child-care abuse investigation.

Finally, education regarding SBS and other forms of physical child abuse should be mandatory for all child-care providers. Personnel would learn about the dangers of shaking infants, positive alternatives for soothing children who are crying, and when to suspect and report child abuse on the part of the parents.

Liability Insurance

Most states require daycare centers to carry liability insurance in the event of accident, injury, or death of a child or worker, but for family child-care centers, only *four* states require some form of liability insurance. Carrying such insurance is important for two reasons. It helps validate a child-care worker's responsibility for the provision of good care, and it helps cover any medical costs that families of injured or abused children may face in their future. All states should require such insurance for daycare and family child-care centers. In civil cases against perpetrators of shaking crimes, it is typically a person's liability insurance that will cover the cost of a trial and any subsequent penalties.

❖   ❖   ❖

The government assumes a large part of the responsibility for safe child care, and many legislators fight an annual battle to bring about positive regulatory change. But much more can and should be done in order that crimes against those most innocent are not allowed to occur. If state and federal governments consider recommendations that have been put forth by advocacy groups, then welcome change will occur.

NOTES

1. Fragin S. Who Cares for Kids? *Working Mother* November 2000; 57–75, 122–125.

2. Barasch DS. Would You Hurt This Baby?: How a New Wave of Apathy Puts All Children at Risk." *Redbook* December 1998; 124–144.

CHAPTER TWENTY-TWO

Prevention

IN 1974, JOHN CAFFEY'S SECOND DISCOURSE on "Whiplash-Shaken Infant Syndrome" called for a nationwide educational campaign against shaking.[1] This would not occur until 1989, fifteen years after the clarion call.[2] The number of infants killed and disabled as a result of SBS during that span of time can only be presumed. This syndrome carries with it high morbidity and mortality rates. For years it was ignored and poorly serviced by the medical and legislative communities. Prior to 1990, there were less than twenty articles and books that referred directly to SBS. It appeared as though abuse of children continued to hold a low priority.

Prevention of a syndrome, especially SBS, can be a relatively easy process. The concept that shaking infants is potentially fatal should be an ingrained part of society, similar to the prevention message of "Don't Drive Drunk." Carol Kandall, a physician in New Haven, Connecticut, wrote a simple letter in 1990 to the editors of the *American Journal of Diseases in Children*, imploring pediatricians and other medical personnel to listen to parents and other caregivers frustrated by the cries of their children.[3] She felt that in some way, prevention efforts could reduce the wider incidence of SBS.

There are three types of prevention: primary, secondary, and tertiary. *Primary prevention*, being the most direct, targets an entire community to prevent abuse before it starts. It sets in place community policies and programs to have a concrete effect on parents and caregivers so abuse will be less likely to occur. General public awareness campaigns are an example of primary prevention.

Secondary prevention comes in the form of intervention after there are early signs of abuse. Any "at-risk" parents or caregivers are the focus for intervention services to provide positive options and support. Problems are treated and efforts are strengthened. Regular clinic or home visits are examples of secondary prevention.

Tertiary prevention is treatment given after abuse has occurred. This type of prevention is aimed toward eradication of further abuse. If successful, these efforts will halt the cycle of abuse from generation to generation. Group therapy, home visitation, crisis drop-off centers, and foster care are examples of tertiary prevention.

Public education along with sound intervention programs appears to be the best type of prevention.[4] Such programming is very inexpensive compared with the cost of even one case of abusive head trauma (with 92 percent of the care costs being nonmedical).[5]

Community-wide child abuse prevention programs work in theory but their overall effectiveness has not been measured. As a result, prevention programs may be infrequently accepted or supported in some communities. Suppose that in one county, the number of infants shaken drops dramatically from the previous year. Such a result could be attributed to an SBS prevention program. It might also mean that more shaken infants were missed or not reported. Or it might mean that more perpetrators did not seek medical attention for these children. Regardless of the statistics, prevention programs are a vital part in protecting our children.

Successful prevention programs provide parents and other caregivers with positive options for dealing with the multitude of stressors associated with caring for an infant. These programs also save lives. It would be ideal for SBS prevention programs to be a part of every segment of the community, but this is typically not financially or logistically feasible. Instead, those most at risk would need to be the focus of direct SBS prevention and education.

SETTINGS FOR PREVENTION PROGRAMS

Babysitting and Parenting Classes

Caring for an infant brings a multitude of emotions and challenges. Many experiences can be frustrating and, in turn, cause feelings of anger. Individuals may even be left with the responsibility of having to care for a child when they want to be doing other activities. New parents and other caregivers need to be educated on properly caring for an infant to prevent shaking and abuse from ever happening.

Part of that education should cover the dangers of shaking infants. This can occur through a "ground-zero" approach for prevention. Such an approach capitalizes on an audience of students, as in a babysitting, Lamaze, or new parents class, and includes SBS prevention within a curriculum. Childbirth education classes typically include a section on newborn care and even a discussion on how to soothe a crying baby. This lends a perfect opportunity to bring up the topic of SBS. It is also a good opportunity to briefly discuss the importance of knowing and trusting others who may care for a couple's baby. The couple can then be the ones instructing babysitters, relatives, and other caregivers never to shake their child and how to contact them for help.

There are national programs that target at-risk parents that use specific interventions to enhance basic child care and assist in stress management, such as Parent Effectiveness Training (PET) and Systematic Training for Effective Parenting (STEP). Such programs have been proven to reduce the risk factors associated with physical child abuse. Parents Anonymous is one type of mutual support group that allows members to increase social contacts at the same time as assisting each other with child-development strategies. There are other types of programs that focus on mutual support of parents who find themselves in similar circumstances that produce a tense living environment.

Children in babysitting instruction classes can be successfully involved in SBS education through the use of demonstrations and open discussion. There is a significant impact on students in babysitting classes who observe a demonstration with an egg broken into a small plastic container. If the container is dropped three feet, the yolk usually remains intact. If the container is shaken, the yolk scrambles.

Unfortunately, not all new parents and caregivers will be reached. Many will not want to participate in SBS prevention instruction. It is the duty for all members of the community, professional and layperson alike, to set in place avenues for prevention and education. There are untapped areas where a great deal of abuse happens. Anyone can become a community advocate for how SBS information is provided. This process may start by simply hearing about this information in a classroom setting. The word can then be spread to reach those who need it most.

Child-Care Facilities and In-Home Care Services

SBS prevention efforts need to be on the same front line as other types of prevention that are emphasized at child-care facilities, such as injury prevention. Child abuse is one of those life issues that is not discussed within wide circles. Because of this, licensing requirements established to prevent child abuse injuries might be minimal at best in many states.

Directors of child-care facilities may have the mindset of "not in my backyard" when it comes to abuse happening in their facility. Adjusting this thinking can lead to the implementation of a plan that epitomizes safe child care. Such a plan would require education about SBS and other acts of physical abuse for all providers. This plan would also have a requirement for a minimum number of hours of care experience for all employees. Directors would be charged to keep in the forefront of their programming ways to keep employees regularly trained on proper child-care techniques.

Parents and caregivers have a role in the prevention of potential abuse that may occur to their child by a child-care provider. Examining materials about potential child-care providers could be an initial step in developing educated and informed child-care choices. Many communities have agency licensing files that may be perused. Child-care resource and referral agencies are also in place to provide guidance in the selection process of reputable child-care facilities. Parents and caregivers should also interview directors of potential facilities to learn the training background requirements of workers. Directors of facilities should be asked about ongoing child abuse training offered to the staff. Finally, unannounced visits by parents and caregivers, after a child begins attending a facility, are reasonable and should be welcomed.[6]

SBS and other acts of abuse can never be completely prevented within any type of child-care system. There are always people who intentionally misuse their positions to hurt and control those under their watch. Parents and caregivers need to avoid blaming themselves if abuse does occur. These incidents are never expected and breach all aspects of trust.

A strong message was sent to au pair and nanny agencies throughout the world when Louise Woodward was convicted in 1998 of the manslaughter death of Matthew Eappen. The message called for greater safety and care of infants and children under the care of these specialized employees. Agency directors did not want the stigma or liability of the maltreatment of children, so screening criteria were improved in many companies, and educational programs on proper care were increased.

Many parents with in-home services made changes in light of the Eappen case as well, whereby the sales of video surveillance units in homes skyrocketed. Such provisions are a state of what our society has become. Sad though they may be, this is an example of actively securing prevention of child abuse injuries in the home.

Training programs for au pairs and nannies that emphasize safety and choice need to be the foundation of any in-home service agency. SBS prevention information should be a basic part of this training. Other things can also lessen the risk of hiring a potentially abusing caretaker, including complete criminal background checks, quality references, and a required minimum number of hours of caregiving experience.

Parents should also be active in their measures to secure safety at home by researching an agency they may use for au pair or nanny services. Hiring caregivers from licensed and insured agencies with good references should only be a starting point. Parents should also interview prospective au pairs or nannies as to the types of care they provide, their knowledge of SBS, how they soothe crying babies, and so on. These steps are active ways parents can help protect their children.

Community Agencies

Professionals who are a part of the front line in working with children and families can provide methods for SBS prevention. Basic childhood injury prevention has been studied in depth for years. The tenets of such programs include defining the injury, targeting resources and persons to carry out the program, and determining which strategies and interventions will be used in the program.[7] Tools of these prevention programs include posters, brochures, billboards, television public-service announcements, giveaways, radio programs, and newspaper articles. The same structure can be used in SBS prevention (see figure 22.1).

Community agencies have a duty in providing crisis management for all families who have children at risk for being shaken and abused. One of the main reasons why a child is shaken is that the caretaker feels no support is available. Community agencies can solve this easily by putting services in place. Free crisis

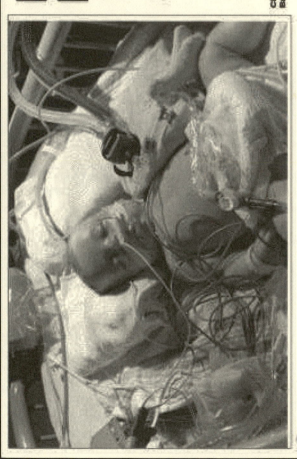

NEVER, NEVER, NEVER SHAKE YOUR BABY!

Christian, Age: 4 Months
Brevard County, Florida

Shaken Baby Syndrome is the medical term used to describe the violent shaking and result sustained from shaking. Those injuries can include: Brain swelling and damage, subdural hemorrhage, mental retardation, and death. Shaken baby syndrome can occur when children are violently shaken as part of a pattern of abuse or simply because an adult has momentarily succumbed to the frustration of responding to a crying baby. Because babies have large heads and underdeveloped necks, the whiplash action created by shaking causes the brain to bounce around in the skull, often tearing blood vessels that connect the brain to the skull. This can result in brain seizures, paralysis, blindness or death. If you feel like you are losing control and have the urge to shake your baby, STOP, place your baby in a safe position, and walk away. Call someone, walk outside and take a few deep breaths, do anything to calm yourself down. Do this for your baby's sake.

Special care must be taken when handling children in the infant to 2 year age range and remember, children must never be shaken for any reason.

FIGURE 22.1   *Christian Knight Shaken Baby Syndrome Prevention Poster—Yellow Umbrella Project, Florida.*

hotlines, low-cost crisis drop-off centers, experienced crisis sitter service, and crisis counseling should be available for families with such needs. Immediate support can save lives either over the phone or through in-person counseling and assistance.

Community agencies can obtain grants to defray the cost of such programming. Hundreds of national organizations give away millions of dollars annually. Most grants need to be very specific, detailing both target audience and method of implementation. Upon completion of the grant, feedback on the program's outcome is typically required in order to receive funding for future initiatives.

Many communities have developed neighborhood-based programs that provide counseling and support. Neighborhood centers can focus on heightening the involvement of parents and caregivers with their children on a more positive and consistent basis. These programs could also support efforts to improve community services, from housing to transportation. When individuals are given options, their sense of esteem increases, as does their sense of control. These positive efforts can influence families and make them less likely to abuse their children.[8]

Finally, representatives from community agencies can come together on a regular basis to share ideas regarding SBS prevention. Simply discussing what is available and what is lacking in a community can create opportunities. Developing an SBS prevention task force requires both telephone calls and follow-up. Community agencies typically come together after a tragedy has already occurred. Enlisting help for primary, rather than tertiary, SBS prevention is the path that makes most sense.

Home Visiting

Home visiting is a concept that was originated by C. Henry Kempe, the lead author of the trailblazing article "The Battered Child Syndrome."[9] The home visiting programs of social service agencies and hospitals over time have established a great rate of success in preventing abuse and neglect in families at risk. Home visiting provides one-on-one guidance and care by a professional. Agencies use nurses, social workers, and volunteers to provide these services. The visitors need to be adequately trained in order to provide thorough education and be positive role models.

The effectiveness of home visiting programs depends on several factors. The parents or caregivers that are the focus of the visits need to be accepting of the services that are presented to them. They also need to be consistently present in the lives of their children in order to learn appropriate caregiving from the home visitors. And finally, they need to have their basic emotional and physical needs met. Otherwise the services that are presented will not be effective.

Several communities have adopted a program for new parents whereby a physician recommends visits to a newborn's home by a perinatal coach for several weeks. The coach keys into many important issues with the new parents, especially coping mechanisms for frustrating situations, developing a support system, and the importance of teamwork to maximize success in their parenting roles. The program is offered while the mother and newborn are still in the hospital and is free of charge. This program is usually sponsored by a hospital or community social-service agency.

Hospitals

Medical providers have the chance to heavily influence parents and caregivers they feel are at risk for child abuse. As Kanev suggests, "At the very minimum . . . each of us in medicine and related health care professions must maintain the highest index of suspicion of child abuse."[10]

Health-care providers, by the nature of their work, are on the front line of child abuse prevention. They can assess whether a parent or caregiver is in need of support during an emergency room visit. They can involve Child Protective Services if abuse is suspected. They can evaluate siblings of injured children for abuse. And they can openly discuss findings with parents and caregivers to foster communication. These are all avenues to use to protect a child from further harm.[11,12]

It is imperative that health-care providers maintain some semblance of suspicion in *all* cases of injuries to infants and children. Such vigilance can be one's greatest prevention tool. This requires both training and experience on the part of providers. Looking at issues such as injuries without relevant explanation, or caretakers seeking medical care at odd hours, as true red flags are important in determining the cause of a child's injuries.[13]

All medical institutions can benefit from a child abuse team. A cross-discipline team will have the advantage of different perspectives about certain cases.[14] Once a team is in place, there can be ongoing discussion about prevention services within the hospital. If medical providers in the hospital setting can stay abreast of the latest information on SBS, they will be better equipped to identify and treat associated injuries more thoroughly.

Hospital administration can do their part in the prevention of SBS by the sponsorship of prevention-education programs. Showers's program "Don't Shake the Baby" was the first nationwide SBS prevention program and has been successful in raising parental awareness about the dangers of shaking.[15] Two other hospital-based prevention-education programs have also developed in recent years. One, from Peinkofer Associates, has a hospital-based prevention and education program that provides the latest educational training for all medical personnel, specific to their areas of care, in addition to brochures, medical placards, and more. This program also incorporates the use of a statement for new parents to sign in obstetric units that asserts their acknowledgment of the dangers of shaking an infant. Such a statement has been found to be successful in reducing the number of SBS cases in certain areas of the country. The other program, from the National Center on Shaken Baby Syndrome, uses posters, brochures, and in-service training, among other things, as the basis for their curriculum.

Obstetric Offices

Obstetric (OB) offices can easily provide basic information on SBS prevention and are important places for early intervention processes to begin. For example, Peinkofer Associates uses its brochure "Preventing Shaken Baby Syndrome" in OB offices to give expectant parents positive options and information in their new roles as primary caregivers. Posters and other types of prevention materials are also beneficial ways of communicating early the dangers of shaking to expectant parents.

Medical providers can encourage the psychological bonding between parents and the unborn child through methods that draw the couple closer together. The expectant parents can develop a birth plan that lists their criteria for an optimum birth. They can be encouraged to attend prenatal visits together. They can attend a childbirth education class together. The expectant father can attend a parenting workshop designed specifically for men, such as the nationally recognized Boot Camp for New Dads. And if the medical provider observes any signs that the parents may be at greater risk for abuse, they can be guided toward more extensive help, such as through a hospital or community social worker.

Physician Offices

Family practice and pediatrician offices are good examples of places where there is an opportunity to educate parents and caregivers about SBS and how to identify symptoms after a shaking incident has occurred. Medical providers typically see a high volume of patients throughout the day. They often do not take the time to assess parenting skills or hear concerns about other caregivers.

Providing education about SBS should be a standard medical practice. This can be done in person by the medical provider or through prevention materials. At an initial visit, providers can talk with parents and caregivers about the physiology of an infant's head in relation to its neck and explain that it must be adequately supported. Warnings about shaking and symptoms that might be evident are basic topics that require minimal time but can save hundreds of lives annually. Some pediatrician offices nationally have been providing or endorsing Peinkofer's book *101 Ways to Soothe a Crying Baby*[16] to promote safe, effective caregiving during potentially stressful times in parents' lives.

Many believe that physicians should treat the parents of potentially abused children *first* to prevent the abuse from occurring.[17] Such basic, primary prevention includes assessing parental stressors, identifying family social problems, offering social work services, home visitation or parenting classes, and providing options that discourage negativity in the home environment.

Schools

Many schools around the country are including SBS as an educational topic each April, which is Child Abuse Prevention Month. By considering SBS as not merely a problem of parents or child-care providers, school systems take a proactive approach.

Many prevention programs, such as the "Don't Shake the Baby" campaign, have age-appropriate presentations for children as young as preschool-age, which educate them on the dangers of shaking an infant. Programs for older children, who may have the responsibility in their homes of caring for infants or children, are provided with options that can be used for an inconsolable child under the student's care.

Some schools even go so far as developing their own SBS prevention campaigns. The La Vega football team, of Waco, Texas, began a campaign in the autumn of 1998 with the inclusion of "Never Shake a Baby" banners at their games and similar messages on their helmets. Such innovative programs receive good media coverage and send out important motivational messages to other students, parents, and teachers.

As in any prevention program, the younger the child when he or she first hears the message, and having it repeated over time, the more successful the outcome. Students learn that shaking and other types of abuse toward infants and children should not be tolerated.

Training Programs

All professionals from the realms of medicine, law, and law enforcement may personally experience a case of SBS at some time in their career. Because of this, there needs to be preparedness training. A standard curriculum can be developed, similar to CPR training classes, whereby professionals learn about the unique physiological and social aspects of SBS to help with aspects of investigation.

Annually, medical, legal, and law enforcement personnel should receive information and updates on the physiology of abusive head trauma, a study of local SBS cases, and ways of improving prevention efforts. These steps will allow for more thorough evaluation of children who are suspected of being shaken and for a more complete investigation leading to more consistency in prosecution.

One organization has already incorporated SBS prevention in its training programs. The American Red Cross has developed an activity on SBS that is included in its *Babysitter's Training Instructor's Manual*. The course instructor leads students through an activity that describes a scenario of an infant who will not stop crying. Students brainstorm as to how they would correctly handle the situation, and then act out the scenario. Follow-up discussion educates participants about the dangers of shaking an infant. Students also learn positive ways to soothe infants in their care. Similar training programs for people in a variety of disciplines can make SBS prevention a standard topic in areas where it is most needed.

Whenever an infant is shaken, anyone who potentially has an influence on prevention should pause and ask two questions: "Why did this happen?" and "What can I do to prevent further cases like this from happening?" Prevention programs need to work to stop SBS tragedies. Anyone may be a unique position to help save lives and families.

NOTES

1. Caffey J. The Whiplash-Shaken Infant Syndrome: Manual Shaking by the Extremities with Whiplash-Induced Intracranial and Intraocular Bleedings, Linked with Residual Permanent Brain Damage and Mental Retardation. *Pediatrics* 1974; 54:396–403.

2. Showers J. Shaken Baby Syndrome: The Problem and a Model for Prevention. *Children Today* 1992; 21:34–37.

3. Kandall CL. Education Concerning Whiplash Shaken Infant Syndrome: An Unmet Need (letter). *Amer J Dis Child* 1990; 144:1180.

4. Thomas N. Shaking Infants: A Case for Public Education? *Prof Care Mother & Child* 1994; 4:59–60.

5. Grabow JD, Offord KP, Rieder ME. The Cost of Head Trauma in Olmsted County, Minnesota, 1970–74. *Am J Pub Health* 1984; 74:710–712.

6. Wissow LS. Causes and Prevention of Maltreatment. In: Wissow LS, ed. *Child Advocacy for the Clinician: An Approach to Child Abuse and Neglect*. Baltimore: Williams & Wilkins; 1989:225–232.

7. Micik S, Miclette M. Injury Prevention in the Community: A Systems Approach. *Ped Clin N Amer* 1985; 32:251–265.

8. Kruger N. Shaken Baby Syndrome: Identification and Prevention by Early Childhood Educators. *S Afr J Educ* 1997; 17:107–112.

9. Kempe CH, Silverman FN, Steele BF, et al. The Battered Child Syndrome. *JAMA* 1962; 181:105–112.

10. Kanev P. Taking Responsibility for Child Abuse. *Headlines* September–October 1993; 36.

11. Wissow LS. Treatment Decisions. In: Wissow LS, ed. *Child Advocacy for the Clinician: An Approach to Child Abuse and Neglect*. Baltimore: Williams & Wilkins; 1989:218–224.

12. Pollack CB. Early Case Finding as a Means of Prevention of Child Abuse. In: Ellerstein NS, ed. *Child Abuse and Neglect: A Medical Reference*. New York: Wiley; 1981:149–152.

13. Rivara FP, Kamitsuka MD, Quan L. Injuries to Children Younger than 1 Year of Age. *Pediatrics* 1988; 81:93–97.

14. Deden S. Why Your Hospital Needs a Child Abuse Team. *Headlines* September–October 1993.

15. Showers J. Don't Shake The Baby: The Effectiveness of a Prevention Program. *Child Abuse & Neglect* 1992; 16:11–18.

16. Peinkofer J. *101 Ways to Soothe a Crying Baby*. Chicago: Contemporary Books; 2000.

17. Betha L. Primary Prevention of Child Abuse. *Amer Fam Phys* 1999; 59:1577–1585.

Conclusion and
Recommendations

✧   ✧   ✧

In the wake of the Matthew Eappen case and a progression of studies and reports made in the medical literature, society understands SBS more completely. But even in light of this understanding, hundreds to thousands of infants are still being shaken each year. Prevention initiatives are springing up in every section of our nation, but so far they have had only a limited effect. There are still parents and caretakers who believe that shaking is an acceptable way to calm or manage a crying child, even though prevention efforts against shaking have been in place for years. Medical schools are only beginning to incorporate into their curricula the process of identifying signs and symptoms of physical child abuse. Yet cases are consistently being misdiagnosed.

Even when perpetrators of shaking crimes are established, their prosecution becomes difficult, largely due to the ignorance of juries and judges. Scene investigation and autopsy protocol are not standard and up to par in many jurisdictions of the country. Training and other educational efforts seem to be important vehicles to heighten the understanding of SBS among a variety of professionals.

Families of shaken children are typically left to fend for themselves. There are no nationally recognized support groups specific to SBS. So the process of the long-term effects of the syndrome becomes emotionally oppressive. It is as if families are going through uncharted territory without a guide. They are unsure of the medical, legal, and social questions to ask. Often the experience of SBS is new to the professionals who handle their cases.

Some recent provisions of support have been set up for both families and professionals. Until 1997, there had been no national front to collectively explore the various aspects of SBS. In the autumn of 1997, Kim Kang, a mother of a SBS survivor, began an Internet mailing list devoted to the families of shaken children and the professionals that worked with them. It quickly became an oasis for many people who had directly experienced the tragedy of such violence. On the computer screen, they could share stories, advice, and care. In 1998, the first national group made up of families of shaken children was established. The Shaken Baby Alliance assists families who have experienced shaking incidents on all levels, from treatment issues to courtroom support. Chapters of the alliance quickly formed around the United States to offer support and information to anyone in need, family and professional alike.

Every two years, Primary Children's Medical Center, National Center on Shaken Baby Syndrome, and SBS Prevention Plus host the National Conference on Shaken Baby Syndrome. In 2000, over 650 individuals attended the conference to hear about the latest research, prevention programs, and family stories. The more individuals learn and talk about this tragic syndrome, the better treatment of children and families will be.

In an effort to encourage others to develop strategies to keep children safer, to help treat victims, and to ultimately prevent this terrible form of child abuse, the following are recommended:

- Long-term studies of the developmental processes of shaken infants and children
- Various types of treatment that focus on better quality of life for shaken infants and children
- Continued studies on diagnosing SBS through imaging evaluation and blood chemistry evaluation
- Mandated education on child abuse injuries, diagnosis, and treatment in medical schools
- Studies on timing and forces involved in SBS
- National tracking of cases identified as SBS
- Improved child-care and monitoring statutes
- Changing of criminal statutes for physical child abuse injuries and death within states
- Mandated SBS-prevention education in hospitals and schools
- Standardizing a system within hospitals for identifying, reporting, and discussing cases of suspected child abuse
- Federal financial support for families of shaken infants and children
- Mandated education on SBS for law enforcement personnel
- Mandated education on SBS for prosecuting attorneys and judges
- National support group network for families of shaken infants and children
- Coordinated multicenter hospital studies of SBS processes, including symptoms at presentation, laboratory findings, and treatment
- Development of a computerized tool for hospitals to use to help identify likely perpetrators of SBS at presentation to the hospital

- Screening to reduce irresponsible testimony by expert witnesses at SBS trials
- County reviews of closed cases of infant deaths of the past to determine whether the cause might now be changed to nonaccidental and their perpetrators brought to justice.

"Little Boy Blue"

The little toy dog is covered with dust
    but sturdy and staunch he stands
The little toy soldier is red with rust
    and his musket molds in his hands.

Time was when the little toy dog was new
    and the soldier was passing fair
And that was the time when our little boy blue
    kissed them and put them there.

"Now don't you go till I come," he said,
    "and don't you make any noise."
So toddling off to his trundle bed
    He dreamt of his pretty toys.

And, while he was dreaming an angel's song
    awakened our little boy blue.
Oh, the years are many, the years are long
    but our little toy friends are true.

Aye, faithful to little boy blue they stand,
    each in their same old place.
Awaiting the touch of the little hand,
    the smile of the little face.

And they wonder as waiting these long years through
    in the dust of that little chair,
what has become of our little boy blue
    since he kissed them and put them there.

—EUGENE FIELD, 1872*

*From *Poems of Childhood* (New York: Charles Scribner's Sons, 1904).

Appendix:
Developmental Milestones

✦   ✦   ✦

At 3 to 6 months, a baby will:

• coo, babble, and laugh
• follow with eyes
• smile in response to another smile
• raise head and shoulders when lying on stomach
• turn head in direction of a sound
• cease crying when caregiver enters room
• recognize familiar faces and objects
• kick out legs vigorously
• actively hold rattle
• pull at blanket or clothes
• sit with support.

At 6 to 9 months, a baby will:

• play with toys and own hands
• imitate sounds
• babble using simple sounds ("ma," "mu," "da")
• bite and chew objects and some solid food
• grasp small objects
• roll from back to stomach
• sit unsupported with back straight and head steady

- transfer objects between hands
- have strong head control
- drink from a cup held to the lips
- lift chest and upper abdomen when lying on stomach
- stand while caregiver holds hands
- adjust position to see a toy
- hold a bottle
- possibly begin crawling.

At 9 to 12 months, a baby will:
- say simple words ("mama," "dada")
- sit steadily for several minutes
- crawl well
- pull self to standing position
- stand holding on to furniture
- grasp small objects between thumb and index finger
- look for a toy seen hidden
- play peekaboo
- roll a ball.

At 12 to 18 months, a baby will:
- first walk with both hands held, then walk without help
- follow rapidly moving objects with eyes
- first say two words, then several more, including names
- understand simple verbal commands
- show emotions such as anger, fear, affection, jealousy
- stand up without support
- drink from a cup without help
- show intense interest in pictures
- ask for objects by pointing
- understand "no"
- tolerate some separation from caregiver.

At 18 to 24 months, a baby will:

- walk up stairs at first with one hand held, then alone holding on to a rail
- throw ball overhand without falling
- jump in place with both feet
- pull and push toys
- eat with spoon well
- turn pages in book, two or three at a time
- say ten or more words
- pick up toy without falling
- run fairly well.

Glossary

✧   ✧   ✧

abrasion   a scrape of the skin as a result of injury

activated coagulation   coagulation occurs when the blood clotting mechanisms are activated throughout the body

acute bleeding   fresh blood

anoxia   a deficiency of oxygen within the blood

anterior   relating to the front section of an area

apnea   temporary cessation of breathing

arachnoid membrane   a delicate membrane attached to the innermost layer around the brain and spinal cord by weblike fibers that allow for movement of cerebrospinal fluid

atrophy   a decrease in size of an organ or tissue

avulsion   a forcible separation from a connecting structure

Babinski's reflex   a reflex that occurs where the big toe flexes toward the top of the foot and the other toes fan out when the sole of the foot is firmly stroked; normal in infants, but abnormal after two years of age. The presence of a Babinski's reflex indicates damage to the central nervous system

burr hole   a surgical procedure whereby small holes are drilled into the skull to relieve blood and pressure.

calcification   new bone formation during the healing process of a fracture

callus   a woven network of new bone that develops over time following a fracture

cerebral edema   swelling of the brain

cerebral ischemia   localized deficiency of blood supply to an area of the brain

cerebrospinal fluid (CSF)   a clear liquid produced in the ventricles of the brain. Also known as spinal fluid

cervical   related to the neck

chorioretinal   pertaining to the choroid and retina

choroid   a thin vascular coat of the eye that supplies blood to the retina, extending from the ora serrata to the optic nerve

coagulation   the process of clotting blood

coagulopathy   abnormality in clotting of blood

concussion   a state of unconsciousness after an impact to the head

conjugate deviation of gaze   both eyes deviating from center; a sign of brain trauma

contusion   a bruise

cortex   the surface area of an organ in the body

coup/contra-coup   specific area of brain injury underneath a site of impact to the head; specific area of brain injury located directly opposite to the site of impact to the head

craniotomy   a surgical procedure, whereby a section of the skull is removed temporarily for the purposes of neurosurgery

cranium   the skull

CT/CAT scan   computerized tomography, a diagnostic procedure combining an X-ray with a computer to produce detailed cross-sectional pictures of the body

cutaneous   related to the skin

cyanotic   the skin bluish in color, signifying poor oxygenation

diaphysis   the shaft of a long bone

differential diagnosis   the determination of at condition or disease a person may have by comparing and contrasting the clinical findings

diffuse axonal injury (DAI)   injury to the delicate axonal nerves of the brain, whereby they are stretched and/or torn

distal   a point farthest from the center or trunk of the body

dura mater   the outer membrane covering the brain and spinal cord

ecchymosis   large hemorrhagic areas beneath the skin due to injury

embolus   a foreign article or clot that moves through the bloodstream and becomes lodged in a blood vessel

enuclation   removal of an eye

epidural hematoma   a collection of blood between the skull and the dura membrane *epiphysis*   the end of a long bone

focal   in a specific, defined area

fontanelle   soft areas of an infant's cranium that allow the skull to mold during the birth process

fovea   a tiny pit in the center of the macula for seeing sharp visual images

frenula   small folds of skin connecting the tongue to the floor of the mouth and the lips to the gums

frontal   pertaining to the front area of the brain or skull

fundus   the retinal area at the back of the eye

funduscope   a device used to view the inner area of the entire eye

ganglion   a group of nerve tissue cells

gastroenteritis   inflammation of the stomach and intestinal tract

gray matter   areas of the brain that appear gray, such as the surface (cortex) of the brain, basal ganglia, and thalamus

hematoma   a mass or collection of blood caused by a break in a vein

hemiparesis   muscle weakness or partial paralysis on one side of the body

hemorrhage   continuous flow of blood from a break in a vein

hydrocephalus   constant accumulation of cerebrospinal fluid within the ventricles of the brain, leading to disproportionately sized heads in infants

hyperemia   increased blood flow to an area of the body

hyperflexion   increased flexibility of the joints, usually as a result of trauma

hyphema   bleeding within the front area of the eye

hypothermia   below-normal body temperature

hypoxia   deficiency of oxygen

infarction   an area of dead tissue as a result of stopped or blocked blood flow

intracranial   within the cranium

intraocular   within the eye

ischemia   a deficiency of blood supply to an area of the body due to trauma or disease

laceration   tearing of the skin from blunt trauma

lateral   relating to the side section of an area

lesion   an injury or wound

long bones   arm and leg bones

lumbar puncture   spinal tap

macula   a yellow circular area at the center of the retina that is responsible for acute vision *medial*   related to the middle section of an area

meninges   all three membranes that cover the brain

metaphysis   area between the shaft and end of the growing bones of infants

MRI   magnetic resonance imaging, a diagnostic procedure combining electromagnets, radio frequency waves, and a computer to produce highly detailed pictures of the body

myelinated   having a formed sheath around an axonal nerve, strengthening and protecting it

neurological   related to the system of nerves and their functioning within the body

nuchal rigidity   the nape or the back of the neck being tense; a sign of neurological impairment

nystagmus   involuntary eye movement; in SBS, this is a result of brain trauma

occipital   related to the back part of the head

optic nerve   a nerve that originates in the brain and carries sensory impulses for sight to the retina

optic sheath   the covering of the optic nerve

ora serrata   the irregular ridge on the anterior part of the retina

orbit   the outside of the eye

parenchyma   the actual substance of the brain

parietal   related to the bones on the back and side of the skull

pathognomonic   having characteristic signs or symptoms indicative of a certain disease or condition

pathology   the study of the cause of trauma and disease; typically done after death

periosteum   a membrane that serves as a covering for the bones

petechiae   tiny spots of hemorrhagic blood found on the skin or within the organs of the body; related to trauma in infants

pia mater   the innermost membrane covering the brain and spinal cord

posterior   relating to the back section of an area

posturing   stiffening and tensing of the body, as seen during seizures

prothrombin time (PT)   a measure of how quickly the blood coagulates (or clots)

proximal   a point closest to the center or trunk of the body

reflux   abnormal backflow of fluid, as occurs in the esophagus

retinal   related to the retina, the main area for vision in the eye

retinoschisis   splitting of the retina from trauma

roentgenogram　an X-ray

sclera　the white outside part of the eye

seizure　sudden, uncontrolled contracting and relaxing of the muscles, often accompanied by unconsciousness

sepsis　blood infection

shunt　a device to divert the buildup of fluids within the brain to another area of the body

skeletal survey　a series of X-rays studying all the bones within the body

subarachnoid　an area below the arachnoid membrane, within which cerebrospinal fluid flows

subdural　an area below the dura mater, within which bridging veins of the brain may stretch, tear, and bleed during and after an incidence of shaking

subgaleal　related to the area just under the scalp

subhyaloid bleeding　bleeding in front of the retina; also called preretinal bleeding

subperichondrial　area below soft cartilage

superior sagittal sinus vein　a major vein within the brain that drains blood away from the brain

temporal bone　the bone on each side of the base of the skull

tentorial　tent-like area of the brain that supports the occipital lobes and covers the cerebellum

tetraplegia　muscle weakness affecting all four limbs

thorax　the area of the body that includes the chest and upper back

ventricles　the inner cavities of the brain where cerebrospinal fluid is made

vitreous body　a transparent, gelatinous fluid that fills the globe of the eye

white matter　connecting nerve fibers of the brain that appear white

xanthochromia　brownish yellow discoloration of the cerebrospinal fluid signifying older intracranial blood

Resources

✧ ✧ ✧

BOOKS RELATED TO CHILD ABUSE, REHABILITATION, AND ADVOCACY

The Battered Child. R. Kempe, ed. 4th ed. Chicago: University of Chicago Press, 1997.

Child Abuse: Medical Diagnosis and Management. R. Reece, ed. Philadelphia: Lea & Febiger, 1994.

Child Maltreatment:: A Clinical Guide and Reference. J. Monteleone and A.E. Brodeur. 2nd ed. St. Louis: G.W. Medical Publishing, 1998.

Children's Head Injury: Who Cares? D.A. Johnson, D. Uttley, M.A. Wyke. Bristol, PA: Taylor & Francis, 1989.

Children with Epilepsy: A Parent's Guide. H. Reisner, ed. Washington, DC: Woodbine House, 1988.

Death in White Bear Lake. R. Siegel. New York: Bantam Books, 1990.

Death of Innocents. R. Firstman and J. Talan. New York: Bantam Books, 1997.

Diagnostic Imaging of Child Abuse. 2nd ed. P.K. Kleinman. St. Louis: Mosby, 1998.

Occupational Therapy for Children with Disabilities. D. Penso. Rockville, MD: Aspen Publishers, 1987.

Pediatric Brain Injury: A Practical Resource. C.W. Sellars and C.H. Vegter. Tucson: Communication Skill Builders, 1993.

Rehabilitation of the Adult and Child with Traumatic Brain Injury. 2nd ed. M. Rosenthal, E.R. Griffith, M.R. Bond, and J.D. Miller. Philadelphia: F.A. Davis Company, 1990.

Representing Children in Child Protective Proceedings. J.K. Peters. Charlottesville, VA: Lexis Law Publishing, 1997.

Seizures and Epilepsy in Childhood: A Guide for Parents. J.M. Freeman, E.P.G. Vining, and D.J. Pillas. Baltimore: Johns Hopkins University Press, 1990.

Signs and Strategies for Educating Students with Brain Injuries: A Practical Guide for Teachers and Schools. G. Wolcott, M. Lash, and S. Pearson. Houston: HDI Publishers, 1995.

Tears of Rage. J. Walsh. New York: Pocket Books, 1997.

Therapeutic Education for the Child with Traumatic Brain Injury: From Coma to Kindergarten. D. McKerns and L.M. Motchkavitz. Tucson: Therapy Skill Builders, 1993.

What Happened to Christopher: An American Family's Story of Shaken Baby Syndrome. A.J. Morey. Carbondale: Southern Illinois University Press, 1998.

ORGANIZATIONS RELATED TO CHILD ABUSE, REHABILITATION, AND ADVOCACY

ABA Center on Children and the Law, 740 15th Street, NW, Washington, DC 20005 (202-662-1720; fax: 202-662-1755) <www.abanet.org/child>.

American Academy of Neurology, 1080 Montreal Avenue, St. Paul, Minnesota 55116 (651-695-1940) <www.aan.com>.

American Foundation for the Blind, 11 Penn Plaza, Suite 300 New York, NY 10001 (800-232-5463; 212-502-7600) <www.afb.org>.

American Occupational Therapy Association, Inc., 4720 Montgomery Lane, Bethesda, MD 20814-3425 (301-652-2682; fax 301-652-7711) <www.aota. org>.

American Physical Therapy Association, 1111 North Fairfax Street, Alexandria, VA 22314 (703-684- APTA; fax 703-684-7343) <www.apta.org>.

American Prosecutors Research Institute (APRI), 99 Canal Center Place, #510, Alexandria, VA 22314 (703-549-4253; fax 703-549-6259) <www.ndaa.org/ apri/index.html>.

American Society for Deaf Children, P.O. Box 3355, Gettysburg, PA 17325 (parent hotline 800-942-2732; 717-334-7922; fax 717-334-8808) <www.deafchildren.org>.

American Speech-Language-Hearing Association (ASHA), 10801 Rockville Pike, Rockville, MD 20852 (action center 800-638-8255; 301-897-5700; fax 301-571-0457) <www.asha.org>.

The Arc of the United States, 1010 Wayne Avenue, Suite 650, Silver Spring, MD 20910 (301-565-3842; fax 301-565-3843) <www.thearc.org>.

Blind Children's Center, 4120 Marathon Street, Los Angeles, CA 90029-3584 (800-222-3566; fax 323-665-3828) <www.blindcntr.org/bcc>.

Brain Injury Association, Inc., 105 North Alfred Street, Alexandria, VA 22314 (703-236-6000; fax 703-236-6001) <www.biausa.org>.

Council for Exceptional Children, 1110 N. Glebe Road, Suite 300, Arlington, VA 22201-5704 (888-CEC-SPED; 703-264-9446; fax 703-264-9494) <www.cec. sped.org>.

Disability Rights Education and Defense Fund, Inc., 2212 Sixth Street, Berkeley, CA 94710 (ADA hotline 800-466-4232; 510-644-2555; fax 510-841-8645) <www.dredf.org>.

Family Resource Center on Disabilities, 20 East Jackson Boulevard, Room 900, Chicago, IL 60604 (800-952-4199; Illinois only 312-939-3513; fax 312-939-7297) <www.ameritech.net/users/frcdptiil/index.html>.

The Kierra Harrison Foundation for Child Care Safety, 1982 N. Rainbow Boulevard, Suite 258, Las Vegas, NV 89108 (702-656-4866) <www.kierraharrison.com>.

Laurent Clerc National Deaf Education Center. Gallaudet University, 800 Florida Avenue, NE, Washington, DC 20002-3695 (202-651-5051; TDD 202-651-5052; fax 202-651-5054) <clerccenter.gallaudet.edu/index.html>.

Low Vision Information Center, 7701 Woodmont Avenue, Suite 302, Bethesda, MD 20814 (301-951-4444; fax 301-951-0078) <members.tripod.com/~Low_Vision_Info/index.html>.

The Matty Eappen Foundation, P.O. Box 14597, Chicago, IL 60614-0597 (312-409-5645) <www.mattyeappen.org>.

National Association for Parents of the Visually Impaired (NAPVI), P.O. Box 317, Watertown, MA 02272 (800-562-6265; 617-972-7441; fax 617-972-7444) <www.spedex.com/NAPVI>.

National Association of Social Workers (NASW), 750 First Street, NE, Suite 700, Washington DC 20002-4241 (202-408-8600; fax 202-336-8311; TDD 202-408-8396) <www.socialworkers.org>.

National Center for Prosecution of Child Abuse, 99 Canal Center Plaza, Suite 510, Alexandria, VA 22314 (703-739-0321; fax 703-549-6259).

National Center for the Victims of Crimes (NCVC), 2000 M Street, NW, Suite 480, Washington, DC 20036 (800-394-2255; 202-467-8700; fax 202-467-8701) <www.ncvc.org>.

National Center on Shaken Baby Syndrome, 2955 Harrison Boulevard, #102, Ogden, UT 84403 (888-273-0071; 801-627-3399; fax 801-627-3321) <www.dontshake.com>.

National Clearinghouse on Child Abuse and Neglect Information, 330 C Street, SW, Washington, DC 20447 (800-394-3366; 703-385-7565; fax 703-385-3206) <www.calib.com/nccanch>.

National Easter Seals Society, 230 West Monroe Street, Suite 1800, Chicago, IL 60606 (800-221-6827; 312-726-6200; fax 312-726-1494) <www.easter-seals.org>.

National Exchange Club for the Prevention of Child Abuse, 3050 Central Avenue, Toledo, OH 43606 (800-924-2643; 419-535-3232; fax 419-535-1989) <www.preventchildabuse.com>.

National Institute on Deafness and Other Communication Disorders (NIDCD), National Institutes of Health, 31 Center Drive, MSC 2320, Bethesda, MD 20892 (301-496-7243; TDD 301-402-0252; fax 301-402-0018) <www.nidcd.nih.gov>.

National Organization for Victim Assistance (NOVA), 1730 Park Road, NW, Washington, DC 20010 (800-879-6682; 202-232-6682; fax 202-462-2255) <www.try-nova.org>.

The National Organization of Parents of Murdered Children, Inc., 100 East Eight Street, Suite B-41, Cincinnati, OH 45202 (888-818-POMC; 513-721-5683; fax 513-345-4489) <www.pomc.com>.

National Respite Locator Service, 800 Eastowne Drive, Suite 105, Chapel Hill, NC 27514 (800-773-5433) <www.chtop.com/locator.htm>.

Office for Victims of Crimes (OVC) Resource Center, Box 6000, Rockville, MD 20849-6000 (800-627-6872) <www.ojp.usdoj.gov/ovc/ovcres>.

Parents Anonymous, 675 W. Foothill Boulevard, Suite 220, Claremont, CA 91711-3475 (909-621-6184; fax 909-625-6304) <www.parentsanonymous-natl.org>.

Peinkofer Associates, P.O. Box 1376, Mishawaka, IN 46546 (888-823-4122; 574-256-6825) <members.aol.com/piney94; www.silencedangels.com; www.sootheababy.com>.

Prevent Child Abuse America, 332 South Michigan Avenue, Suite 1600, Chicago, IL 60604 (312-663-3520; fax 312-939-8962) <www.preventchildabuse.org>.

SBS Prevention Plus, 649 Main Street, Suite B, Groveport, OH 43125 (800-858-5222; 614-836-8360; fax 614-836-8359) <www.sbsplus.com>.

The Shaken Baby Alliance, P.O. Box 150734, Fort Worth, TX 76108 (877-636-3727) <www.shakenbaby.com>.

United Cerebral Palsy Association, 1660 L Street, NW, Suite 700, Washington, DC 20036 (800-872-5827; fax 202-776-0414) <www.ucpa.org>.

Yellow Umbrella, 1333 Gateway Drive, Suite 1024, Melbourne, FL 32901 (321-951-7179; fax 321-722-5942).

WEB SITES RELATED TO CHILD ABUSE, REHABILITATION, AND ADVOCACY

American Academy of Ophthalmology <www.aao.org>.

American Association for Pediatric Ophthalmology and Strabismus <med-aapos.bu.edu>.

American Professional Society on the Abuse of Children <www.apsac.org>.

Children's Health Insurance Program <www.hcfa.gov/init/children.htm>.

Disabilities Resources, Inc. <www.disabilityresources.org>.

Epilepsy Foundation of America <www.efa.org>.

Find Law—Internet Legal Services <in-137.infospace.com/info.law/blue/my-state.html>.

Government Directory <www.findlaw.com/directories/government.html>.

House of Representatives <www.house.gov/writerep>.

Legal Cases/Codes <www.findlaw.com/casecode>.

National Library of Medicine Medline <www.nlm.nih.gov>.

Parent Advocacy Coalition for Educational Rights (PACER) <www.pacer.org>.

President of the United States <www.whitehouse.gov>.

Senators <www.senate.gov>.

Shaken Baby Syndrome Resource Centre <www.geocities.com/HotSprings/Spa/4069>.

State Court Directory <www.findlaw.com/11stategov/directories/courts.html>.

State Legislatures Guide <www.congress.org>.

State and Local Governments <www.piperinfo.com/state/states.html>.

Index

✧ ✧ ✧

About the Author

JAMES R. PEINKOFER is a licensed clinical social worker on the pediatric unit at a midwestern hospital. He has trained hundreds of professionals across the country about all aspects of Shaken Baby Syndrome (SBS) and has consulted on SBS-related cases with law enforcement professionals and prosecuting attorneys in a variety of states. He has his own health care consultation agency specializing in SBS prevention and education.